Cancer Drug Discovery and Development

Series Editor
Beverly A. Teicher
National Cancer Institute, Rockville, MD, USA

For further volumes:
http://www.springer.com/series/7625

Peter J. Quesenberry • Jorge J. Castillo
Editors

Non-Hodgkin Lymphoma

Prognostic Factors and Targets

Humana Press

Editors
Peter J. Quesenberry
Division of Hematology & Oncology
Rhode Island Hospital
Providence, RI, USA

Jorge J. Castillo
The Miriam Hospital Division of Hematology and Oncology
The Warren Alpert Medical School of Brown University
Providence, RI, USA

ISBN 978-1-4614-5850-0 ISBN 978-1-4614-5851-7 (eBook)
DOI 10.1007/978-1-4614-5851-7
Springer New York Heidelberg Dordrecht London

Library of Congress Control Number: 2012954773

Printed on acid-free paper

Humana Press is a brand of Springer
Springer is part of Springer Science+Business Media (www.springer.com)

Contents

Part I Biology

Part II Prognostic Factors

Part III Therapy

Part I
Biology

Cancer Stem Cells: A Matter of Perspective

Peter J. Quesenberry, J. Reagan, B. Ramratnam, and L. Goldberg

Abstract Chronic myelogenous leukemia (CML) is a disease in which a small number of primitive renewing stem cells give rise to more differentiated hematopoietic cells. The stem cells are the basis for continuation and recurrence of the disease. Recent reports have suggested that most cancers are driven by rare stem cells which may have a different sensitivity to therapeutic agents and must be eliminated in order to obtain a cure of the disease. It would appear most likely that there is a spectrum of "stemness" in cancers with some cancers such as acute myeloid leukemia (AML) consisting almost totally of stem cells, with many carcinomas being a mixture of stem and differentiated cells and a disease such as CML being generated by rare stem cells. Therapeutic relevance lies in tumors of the latter class.

Introduction

The existence of cancer stem cells has been a given for hematologists due to CML, a disease in which primitive cells differentiate into mature classes of myeloid cells. The observations that therapy with imatinib (Gleevec®) could induce a complete hematologic remission and then that the disease could recur when imatinib was discontinued indicated the existence of a rare primitive cell with the capacity to create the disease—a stem cell. However, the major question is the rarity of such a cell in different cancers. The "differentiating" tumors, i.e., CML, are clearly a different class of cancer, separate from the undifferentiated cancers, i.e., CML, in blast crisis or perhaps glioblastoma multiforme or the differentiated frozen cancers,

P.J. Quesenberry, M.D. (✉) • J. Reagan • B. Ramratnam • L. Goldberg
Department of Medicine, Division of Hematology/Oncology, Rhode Island Hospital and Brown University, Providence, RI 02903, USA
e-mail: pquesenberry@lifespan.org

P.J. Quesenberry and J.J. Castillo (eds.), *Non-Hodgkin Lymphoma: Prognostic Factors and Targets*, Cancer Drug Discovery and Development,
DOI 10.1007/978-1-4614-5851-7_1,

Table 1 Cancer stem cell concepts

Concept	Examples
Rare cells differentiating into cells that form the bulk of the cancer	CML, Multiple myeloma
Cancers in which all the cells have cancer renewal potential—the primitive cell neoplasms	AML, Glioblastoma multiforme
Fixed phenotype cancers in which variable percentages of the cancer population may have stem cell potential	Adenocarcinoma breast, colon carcinoma
Evolving cancers in which initially there are rare cancer stem cells (CML) which then evolve into a cancer in which virtually all the cells are cancer stem cells	CML in blast crisis

i.e., adenocarcinoma of breast or colon. In a similar vein, cell populations at different stages of cancer development may progress from a tumor with only rare stem cells to a tumor consisting totally of stem cells. A major question as to the importance of the cancer stem cell concept is whether they are rare cells, separate from the majority of the cancer cells in a neoplasm and giving rise to those cells, or whether virtually all cells in a cancer have cancer-initiating potential and are thus cancer stem cells. As noted above, this may vary with type of tumor and stage of tumor development. If most cells in a cancer have cancer-initiating capacity, then the cancer stem cell concept does not advance our knowledge of cancer and is of little benefit therapeutically. However, if certain cancers have rare stem cells which drives the cancer, then this would be the target for therapy and would forward our understanding of cancer (Table 1).

It is apparent that only those cancers in which the stem cells are rare and in which their sensitivity to different therapeutic interventions is different from the bulk of the cancer population would be of significant interest as to different therapeutic strategies for cancer.

The concept that there are stem cells for cancer is not new. Early studies established that single cells could cause a cancer [1]. These assumed that most cells in a cancer were cancer-initiating cells. The concept of rare clonal units driving cancers recurred and, in the early 1970s, it appeared that Hamburger and Salmon had developed an in vitro soft agar clonal assay for tumor stem cells [2]. Tumor stem cell colonies in soft agar were described from different cancers and showing varied colony growth characteristics and morphology. In a small number of studies on 9 patients with multiple myeloma and 9 patients with ovarian cancer treated with standard chemotherapy, unique in vitro patterns of chemosensitivity and resistance to the 6 agents tested were demonstrated, and it was felt that the assay "showed promise" for further study [3]. In continuing studies, tissue from 100 patients with ovarian cancer was evalvated, and a maximum plating efficiency of 1% was observed [4]. Tissue from 65 patients with non-Hodgkin's lymphoma was grown in soft agar, and growth was found for 61% with a bone marrow source and 50% with a lymph node source. Plating efficiency ranged from 0.001% to 0.1% [5]. Myeloma colonies when studied showed a plating efficiency of 0.1%. In general, it appeared that these clonal units were actively proliferating cells.

There was a good deal of work done in this area of research with a clear emphasis on utilizing the assay to predict for chemotherapy responsiveness. Commercialization followed and eventually it became clear that the assays were no more predictive than standard clinical and pathological information on the patients. The negative evolution of this work is summarized by Weisenthal and Lippman in 1985. "Neither theoretical concepts nor direct experimental data or clinical correlations support the alleged superiority of clonogenic assays. Clonogenic assays may not be advantageous compared to other more practical methods of estimating the general chemosensitivity of proliferating cells. In contrast, there is a growing body of literature which indicates that early evidence of cell damage in the entire tumor cell population may accurately predict for a multiple-log stem cell kill and meaningful clinical response" [6].

Interest in these approaches receded and essentially disappeared until the current flurry of activity on cancer stem cells was initiated by reports in 1994 on the existence of a cell initiating human acute myeloid leukemia (AML) after transplantation into SCID mice. In this report, Lapidot and colleagues [7] reported that CD34+CD38- was a leukemic stem cell. They showed by limiting dilution analysis that the frequency of leukemia-initiating cells in the peripheral blood of AML patients was one engraftment unit in 250,000 cells. Previous studies of hematopoietic stem cells and surface markers which characterize these stem cells formed a basis for these studies. The basic assumption was that there was a hierarchy of cancer cells; only a few of which could actually propagate tumors. The antibodies, CD34 and CD38, had been characterized on various hematopoietic cell populations and could be used with fluorescent-activated cell sorting to purify and separate classes of leukemic cells, just as they are used to separate classes of normal hematopoietic cells. There followed work indicating the presence of cancer stem cells in a variety of solid tumors.

Al-Hajj et al. [8] reported that breast cancer cells were heterogeneous and that down to 100 CD44+CD24-/low cells could form tumors in immunodeficient mice. Tens of thousands of breast cancer cells with alternate phenotypes did not form tumors. There followed reports of cancer stem cells in many other cancers (Table 2) using surface epitope labeling, separation by FACS, and growth in immunodeficient mice.

The general theme here was that using markers that are common to a number of cell types, a subset of cancer cells could be isolated from different cancers which could differentially grow in immunodeficient mice. It appeared to some to represent a breakthrough in the biology of cancer, offering new targets for chemotherapy. Many inconclusive studies followed on whether the so-called cancer stem cells would show a differential sensitivity to radiation or chemotherapy. Studies on the regulation of these cells proceeded. A continuing observation was that the transplanted tumor stem cells recapitulated at least some of the heterogeneity in the parent tumor [32]. Many analogies were drawn to the hierarchical system of hematopoietic stem cells in which a single stem cell which could be purified, gave rise to a series of cells which progressively gained differentiated characteristics and lost proliferative and renewal potential.

Table 2 Cancers and their stem cell markers

Primary tumor	Stem cell markers	References
Acute myelocytic leukemia	CD34+CD38-CD0−IL-3R+CD71-HLA-DR-CD117-	[9–13]
Breast	CD44+CD24-Lin-ALDH1+	[8, 14]
Brain	CD133+	[15, 16]
Melanoma	CD20+ ABCB5+	[17, 18]
Colorectal	CD133+, epCAm+CD44+ALDH1+	[19–22]
Lung	CD24+CD44+CD133+	[23, 24]
Sarcoma	CD105+, CD44+Strol+	[25]
Head and Neck	CD44+	[26]
Liver	CD133+CD90+CD44+	[27, 28]
Pancreatic	CD44+CD24+ESA+CD133+	[29, 30]

Adapted from Table 1 in, "The cancer stem cell paradigm: a new understanding of tumor development and treatment" Ebben JD, Treisman DM, Zorniak M, et al. (2010). Exper Opin Ther Targets 14:621–632 [31]

Two critical questions were not rigorously addressed by the cancer stem cell investigators: (1) Is the xenogeneic model an adequate model for these studies? and (2) Is the system stable or could it be on a continuum of reversible change as some claim the hematopoietic stem cells system to be? These two questions are critical to determining the validity of the cancer stem cell system as recently put forward.

The question of the validity of the assay is of course paramount. This was addressed by Kelley and colleagues [33] in studies that suggested that observations on leukemic stem cells were artifacts of the transplant model. They demonstrated that when murine lymphoma or leukemia cells were carried out in a syngeneic system, a very high frequency of stem cells (1 in 10) was able to induce malignant disease. They studied cells from Eu-myc pre B/B lymphoma, Eu-N RAS thymic lymphoma, and acute myeloid leukemia in Pu.1-/- mice injected into C57BL/6 nonirradiated hosts. They found that single cell transfer in 3 of 8 recipients gave lymphoma in 33–76 days. They suggested that the low frequency of leukemia-initiating cells in xenogeneic transplant models might represent the effect of a hostile xenogeneic environment. Similar results showing a relative high frequency of leukemia-initiating cells in MLL-AF9 AML model were reported [34], and using the same model, Krivtsov et al. [35] showed transfer of leukemia with injection of 4 cells. In many of the other cancer stem cell models, a relatively high percentage (<up to 20%) of the cells were marked as stem cells. Studies on melanoma cancer stem cells are informative and probably applicable to many of the other solid tumor stem cells. Initial studies indicate that there was a frequency of 1 in a million for cancer induction [18]. Quintana et al. [36] studied melanoma cells from 12 different patients in a modified immunodeficient model of Nod/Scid IL-2 receptor gamma chain null mice and showed that leukemia induction was increased by orders of magnitude. In single cell transplants, an average of 27% of unselected melanoma cells from 4 different patients formed tumors. Boiko et al. [37] used CD271 as a marker and showed a melanoma cancer stem cell frequency of between 2.5% and 41%, but Quintana et al. [36] subsequently showed that single primary

melanoma cells could initiate tumors at frequencies of at least one in four. These studies indicate that details of the transplant model may totally alter outcomes and that at least some of the reported characterizations of cancer stem cells, especially leukemic cancer stem cells, are flawed. The reasons for relatively poor growth in xenogeneic models could be a failure of cytokine or accessory cell support, or other less well-defined toxic influences.

The interpretation of the cancer stem cell results also depends upon the assumption that the phenotype of the cancer stem cell is stable; it probably is not. The original model for the stem cell in AML was the murine hematopoietic stem cell hierarchical model in which a stable dormant long-term repopulating stem cell (LT-HSC) gave rise to a hierarchical system of progressive differentiation and loss of renewal and proliferative potential. Although controversial to some, the extant data now indicates that this model is incorrect. The system is rather a continuum of potential linked to cell cycle passage, and when whole marrow is interrogated, the long-term multilineage repopulating marrow stem cells in the mouse are in active cell cycle [38]. The hematopoietic stem cell phenotype is continually changing, and while the population maybe relatively stable, the individual cells are not. That this probably holds for AML stem cells is supported by recent studies on the heterogeneity of AML stem cell and AML at large. Thus, the concept that a single isolated phenotype will represent a cancer stem cell is also probably wrong.

Is there validity to the concept of a cancer stem cell? There probably is, but whether xenogeneic systems are valid is a major concern. The disease CML is a clear example of a cancer stem cell disease. It is a differentiating cancer, and any cancer with these characteristics probably is fed by rare primitive stem cells. This is evidenced in CML by relapses seen after withdrawal of imatinib therapy; these had to derive from a stem cell population. It is of interest here that therapy with imatinib seems to eliminate the bulk of CML cells and not the stem cells. This, of course, is not "stem cell therapy" although efforts to eliminate the resistant stem cells continue.

Recent work has described cancer stem cells in Hodgkin's disease, mantle cell lymphoma, and multiple myeloma with interesting differential sensitivities to possible therapeutic agents. The identity of the stem cell for multiple myeloma has been controversial with some claiming CD138+ cells engrafting in SCID-hu mice as the key cell [39], while others have defined a CD138-CD19 + CD20 + CD27 + aldehyde dehydrogenase-positive cell growing in Nod/Scid mice as the relevant stem cell [40]. Studies from the Johns Hopkins group have indicated that these cells are sensitive to anti-CD20 antibodies and also may be differentially sensitive to hedgehog inhibitors (GDC-04449) and to telomerase inhibitors (imetelstat). These cells were relatively resistant to dexamethasone, cyclophosphamide, lenalidomide, and bortezomib, agents that are quite active against the bulk of myeloma cells. Matsui and colleagues felt that clonotypic B cells constituted the stem cells for myeloma and found that these cells were highly tumorigenic, self-renewing, and able to recapitulate symptomatic disease in immunodeficient mice. Similar studies were carried out with mantle cell lymphoma, and an aldehyde dehydrogenase (ALDH)+, CD19+, and CD5+ cell were characterized as the stem cells. This cell also showed differential sensitivity to chemotherapy agents as compared to the majority of lymphoma

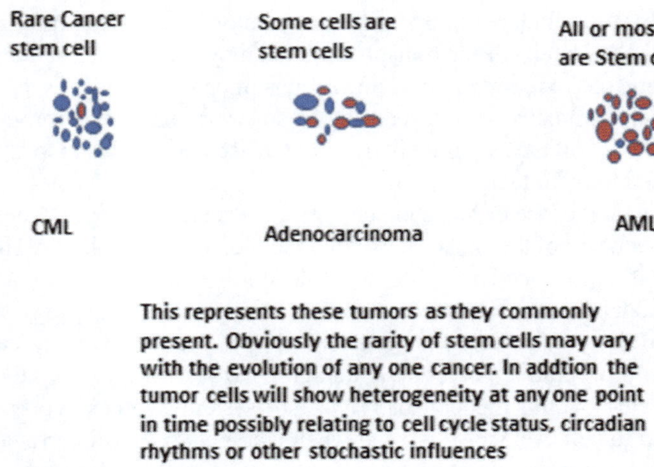

Fig. 1 Evolution of cancer stem cells. Chronic myelogenous leukemia is a disease in which a rare stem cell feeds into a differentiated cell compartment, while with acute myeloid leukemia, virtually all the cells act as stem cells. Many of the "solid tumors" have varying mixtures of stem cells and differentiated cell types

cells [41]. A putative stem cell for Hodgkin's lymphoma was described as an ALDH+, CD20+, and CD27+ clonotypic memory B cell [42]. This has led to a clinical trial combining rituximab, a chimeric anti-CD20 monoclonal antibody, and standard chemothrapy for Hodgkin's lymphoma.

Further work has suggested that CML stem cells selectively express CD25 and CD26 along with WT1 and PRAME [43]. Figure 1 illustrates the different evolutionary phases of tumor development. In this model, the role of the stem cell will change with evolutionary stage and other variables such as cell cycle status, circadian rhythms, or other stochastic influences.

The challenge going forward will be to define the existence of true cancer stem cells and whether differential sensitivities of these cells could offer unique therapeutic opportunities.

References

1. Furth J, Kahn MC (1937) The transmission of leukemia of mice with a single cell. Am J Cancer 31:276–282
2. Hamburger AW, Salmon SE (1977) Primary bioassay of human tumor stem cells. Science 197(4302):461–463
3. Salmon SE, Hamburger AW, Soehnlen B et al (1978) Quantitation of differential sensitivity of human-tumor stem cells to anticancer drugs. N Engl J Med 298(24):1321–1327
4. Hamburger AW, Salmon SE, Alberts DS (1980) Development of a bioassay for ovarian carcinoma colony-forming cells. Prog Clin Biol Res 48:63–73

5. Hamburger AW, Jones SE, Salmon SE (1980) Soft-agar cloning of cells from patients with lymphoma. Prog Clin Biol Res 48:43–52
6. Weisenthal LM, Lippman ME (1985) Clonogenic and nonclonogenic in vitro chemosensitivity assays. Cancer Treat Rep 69:615–632
7. Lapidot T, Sirard C, Vormoor J et al (1994) A cell intiating human acute myeloid leukemia after transplantation into SCID mice. Nature 367:645–648
8. Al-Hajj M, Wicha MS, Benito-Hernandez A, Morrison SJ et al (2003) Prospective identification of tumorigenic breast cancer cells. PNAS 100:3983–3988
9. Blair A, Hogge DE, Ailles LE et al (1997) Lack of expression of Thy-1 (CD90) on acute myeloid leukemia cells with long-term proliferative ability in vitro and in vivo. Blood 89:3104–3112
10. Blair A, Sutherland HJ (2000) Primitive acute myeloid leukemia cells with long-term proliferative ability of in vitro and in vivo lack surface expression of c-kit (CD117). Exp Hematol 28:660–671
11. Blair A, Hogge DE, Sutherland HJ (1998) Most acute myeloid leukemia progenitor cells with long-term proliferative ability in vitro and in vivo have the phenotype CD34+/CD71-/HLA-DR-. Blood 92:4325–4335
12. Jordan CT, Upchurch D, Szilvassy SJ et al (2000) The interleukin-3 receptor alpha chain is a unique markers for human acute myelogenous leukemia stem cells. Leukemia 14:1777–1784
13. Bonnet D, Dick JE (1997) Human acute myeloid leukemia is organized as a hierarchy that originates from a primitive hematopoietic cell. Nat Med 3:730–737
14. Ginestier C, Hur MH, Charafe-Jauffre E et al (2007) ALDH1 is a marker of normal and malignant human mammary stem cells and a predictor of poor clinical outcome. Cell Stem Cell 1:555–567
15. Singh SK, Hawkins C, Clarke ID et al (2004) Identification of human brain tumor initiating cells. Nature 432:396–401
16. Hemmati HD, Nakano I, Lazareff JA et al (2003) Cancerous stem cells can arise from pediatric brain tumors. Proc Natl Acad Sci U S A 100:15178–15183
17. Fang D, Nguyen TK, Leishear K et al (2005) A tumorigenic subpopulation with stem cell properties in melanomas. Cancer Res 65:9328–9337
18. Schatton T, Murphy GF, Frank NY et al (2008) Identification of cells initiating human melanomas. Nature 451(7176):345–349
19. O'brien CA, Pollert A, Gallinger S et al (2007) A human colon cancer cell capable of initiating tumour growth in immunodeficient mice. Nature 445:106–110
20. Ricci-Vitiani L, Lombardi DG, Pilozzi E et al (2007) Identification and expansion of human colon-cancer-initiating cells. Nature 445:111–115
21. Dalerba P, Dylla SJ, Park IK et al (2007) Phenotypic characterization of human colorectal cancer cells. Proc Natl Acad Sci U S A 104:10158–10163
22. Huang EH, Hynes MJ, Zhang T et al (2009) Aldehyde dehydrogenase 1 is a marker for normal and malignant human colonic stem cells (SC) and tracks CS overpopulation during colon tumorigenesis. Cancer Res 69:3382–3389
23. Ho MM, Ng AV, Lam S et al (2007) Side population in human lung cancer cell lines and tumors is enriched with stem-like cancer cells. Cancer Res 67:4827–4833
24. Eramo A, Lotti F, Sette G et al (2008) Identification and expansion of the tumorigenic lung cancer stem cell population. Cell Death Differ 15:504–514
25. Gibbs CP, Kukekov VG, Reith JD et al (2005) Stem-like cells in bone sarcomas: implications for tumorigenesis. Neoplasia 7:967–976
26. Prince ME, Sivanandan R, Kaczorowski A et al (2007) Identification of a subpopulation of cells with cancer stem cell properties in head and neck squamous cell carcinoma. Proc Natl Acad Sci U S A 104:973–978
27. Ma S, Cahan KW, Hu L et al (2007) Identification and characterization of tumorigenic liver cancer stem/progenitor cells. Gastroenterology 132:2542–2556
28. Yang ZF, Ho DW, Ng MN et al (2008) Significance of CD90+ cancer stem cells in human liver cancer. Cancer Cell 13:153166

29. Li C, Heidt DG, Dalerba P et al (2007) Identification of pancreatic cancer stem cells. Cancer Res 67:10301037
30. Hermann PC, Huber SL, Herrler T et al (2007) Distinct populations of cancer stem cells determine tumor growth and metastatic activity in human pancreatic cancer. Cell Stem Cell 1:313–323
31. Ebben JD, Treisman DM, Zorniak M et al (2010) The cancer stem cell paradigm: a new understanding of tumor development and treatment. Exper Opin Ther Targets 14:621–632
32. Shackleton M, Quintana E, Fearon ER et al (2009) Heterogeneity in cancer: cancer stem cells versus clonal evolution. Cell 138(5):822–829
33. Kelly PN, Dakic A, Adams JM et al (2007) Tumor growth need not be driven by rare cancer stem cells. Science 317:337
34. Somervaille TC, Cleary ML (2006) Identification and characterization of leukemia stem cells in murine MLL-AF9 acute myeloid leukemia. Cancer Cell Oct 10(4):257–268
35. Krivtsov AV, Twomey D, Feng Z et al (2006) Transformation from committed progenitor to leukaemia stem cell initiated by MLL-AF9. Nature 442(7104):818–822, Epub 2006 Jul 16
36. Quintana E, Shackleton M, Sabel MS et al (2008) Efficient tumour formation by single human melanoma cells. Nature 456(7222):593–598
37. Boiko AD, Razorenova OV, Van de Rijn M et al (2010) Human melanoma-initiating cells express neural crest nerve growth factor receptor CD271. Nature 466(7302):133–137
38. Quesenberry PJ, Dooner MS, Aliotta JM (2010) Stem cell plasticity revisited: the continuum marrow model and phenotypic changes mediated by microvesicles. Exp Hematol 38(7):581–592, Epub 2010 Apr 9 Review
39. Yaccoby S, Barlogie B, Epstein J (1998) Primary myeloma cells growing in SCID-hu mice. A model for studying the biology and treatment of myeloma and its manifestations. Blood 92:2908–2913
40. Matsui W, Wang Q, Barber JP et al (2008) Congenic multiple myeloma progenitors, stem cell properties, and drug resistance. Cancer Res 68:190–197
41. Brennan SK, Meade B, Wang Q et al (2010) Mantle cell lymphoma activation enhances Bortezomib sensitivity. Blood 116:4185–4191
42. Jones RJ, Gocke CD, Kasamon YL et al (2009) Circulating clonotypic B cells in classic Hodgkin lymphoma. Blood 113(23):5920–5926, Epub Feb 2
43. Gerber JM, Qin L, Kowalski J et al (2011) Characterization of chronic myeloid leukemia stem cells. Am J Hematol 86:31–37

B and T Cell Development

Loren D. Fast

Abstract Hematopoiesis is the ordered development of the different blood cell populations from stem cells. One early branch point in hematopoietic development is the lymphoid pathway which gives rise to B and T lymphocytes and NK cells. B and T lymphocytes express antigen-specific receptors that are generated by the genetic joining of segments randomly selected from multiple loci. The cells expressing the resulting antigen receptors are subjected to a selection process for receptors with appropriate binding properties. Following the selection process, the naïve cells enter the circulation and respond when they encounter antigen able to be bound by the receptor. Once stimulated, the cells mature into functional lymphocytes in a process that is dictated by the factors and signals that are present in the environment. While NK cells can develop in the thymus, NK cells do not express antigen-specific receptors, but instead express a variety of activating and inhibitory receptors. The integration of responses from these receptors determines if the NK cell will respond. The developmental process from stem cells into mature functional cells can be interrupted at any step by genetic mutations which cause uncontrolled proliferation. Thus, an understanding of the changes important for the development of leukemias and lymphomas facilitates generation of new treatments for these diseases and also enhances our understanding of lymphocyte differentiation pathways.

The Development and Differentiation of Lymphocytes

The responses of the immune system are divided into two categories: innate immune responses and adaptive immune responses. Innate immune responses occur rapidly in response to antigen but lack specificity and immunological memory. Immunological

L.D. Fast, Ph.D. (✉)
Hematology/Oncology, Rhode Island Hospital, 593 Eddy Street, Providence, RI 02903, USA
e-mail: Loren_Fast@brown.edu

P.J. Quesenberry and J.J. Castillo (eds.), *Non-Hodgkin Lymphoma: Prognostic Factors and Targets*, Cancer Drug Discovery and Development,
DOI 10.1007/978-1-4614-5851-7_2,

memory is the ability to mount a more rapid response upon subsequent encounter with the same antigen. Conversely, adaptive immune responses are antigen-specific and generate immunological memory but take more time to develop as they require the expansion of antigen-specific lymphocytes that are originally present in extremely low frequencies. Because first encounter with antigen both increases the number and functionality of antigen-specific adaptive immune system effector cells, immunological memory is established.

Lymphocytes, a subset of white blood cells, are important components of both innate and adaptive immune responses. There are three main types of lymphocytes: natural killer (NK) cells, B lymphocytes (B cells), and T lymphocytes (T cells). NK cells are large, granular lymphocytes that serve as the main effector cells of the innate immune system. Effector functions mediated by NK cells include secretion of cytokines and other soluble factors that regulate responses of number of subpopulations of immune cells and lysis of a variety of target cells. B cells and T cells are smaller lymphocytes essential to the adaptive immune response. These lymphocyte populations use similar mechanisms of random recombination to generate a highly diverse set of antigen-specific receptors that is key to the enablement of antigen-specific immune responses. These antigen-specific receptors are called immunoglobulins (or antibodies) on B cells and T cell receptors (TCR) on T cells.

B cells initially express membrane-bound immunoglobulin. Once activated, B cells secrete immunoglobulins which are able to trigger a variety of responses once they bind to antigen. T cells are also capable of providing help to other immune cells through the expression of activation antigens that serve as ligands for receptors on other lymphocytes and/or by the production of cytokines that regulate the immune responses of these immune cells. One subset of T lymphocytes is also able to mediate cytolytic activity when activated. This chapter will present an overview of these three populations of lymphocytes, including developmental pathways, mechanisms responsible for regulation and generation of function, and how dysregulated lymphocyte growth can result from oncogenic transformation and subsequently lead to development of leukemias and lymphomas.

Hematopoiesis

Hematopoiesis is the term used to describe the overall blood cell development process. This developmental pathway starts with hematopoietic stem cells (HSC), which are defined as cells able to both replicate themselves and generate progeny cells that can ultimately develop into more than ten different lineages. It was originally thought that receipt of specific signals directed the differentiation of HSC progeny to a particular pathway in a single step [1, 2]. Yet, recent studies suggest that the differentiation process is more progressive in nature, with cells gradually losing the ability to commit to certain lineages as they are placed in specific environments. Therefore, cells will eventually reach the point of being fully committed to a single lineage. Previous studies have shown that transferring cells from one environment to another will allow them to develop down alternative pathways if they are not yet fully committed to a particular pathway, demonstrating the environment to which differentiating cells are exposed plays an important role in differentiation. One method of distinguishing cells at different stages of hematopoiesis involves characterization of adhesion molecule and chemokine receptor cell surface expression. This pattern of cell surface marker expression is important because it directs cells to certain environments. An alternative approach is to study the expression of cell surface receptors that respond to signals in that environment and direct the expression of regulatory factors such as transcription factors. Transcription factors, which are proteins that bind to DNA and influence gene expression, are important because they are responsible for activating loci whose products drive cells toward certain pathways or away from alternative pathways. For B and T lymphocytes, it is also important to study the stages involved in the development of the clonal antigen-specific receptors.

The initial approach to identify HSC has been to sort cells based on their cell surface markers and then test the ability of the sorted cell populations to repopulate immunodeficient murine recipients [1]. This approach identified cells expressing the cell surface marker combination $Lin^{-}CD45^{lo}CD34^{+}CD38^{+}CD45RA^{-}CD90^{-}Ki67^{+}$ as the cell population that contained HSC. However, this approach is limited to the analysis of the expression of cell surface markers and cannot be used to measure the ability of these cells to respond to specific stimuli. Single-cell level analysis of HSC-containing populations indicated that responses to different cytokine stimuli were exceedingly heterogeneous [3]. It was also observed that adding combinations of different cytokines often generated greater responses than a single cytokine alone. This observation is consistent with concept of heterogeneous populations within these HSC populations.

Stochastic differences may also contribute to HSC heterogeneity. Sorting HSC-containing populations based on cell cycle stage suggested that HSC in different stages produced different types of cells [4, 5]. A related experiment used single-cell mass cytometry, which permits simultaneous analysis of 34 parameters by using antibodies labeled with transition element isotopes in chelated tags [6]. Analysis of the resulting multidimensional data segregated healthy human bone marrow cell populations into a number of different populations. Using this technology, analysis of HSC-containing populations indicated that even the Lin^{-} population is still quite heterogeneous and that the differentiation of HSC, as well as of more differentiated cells, actually represents a continuum along which cells increasingly develop more constrained differentiative outcomes as they progress. This data suggests that the development of cells down unique hematological pathways is not the result of discrete steps, but instead a gradual transition marked by the progressive loss of differentiation options.

From HSC, the next step in the development of T and B lymphocytes is the presence of multipotential progenitor cells (MPP), which are characterized as $Lin^{-}CD45^{lo}CD34^{+}CD38^{+}CD45RA^{-}CD90^{-}Ki67^{+}$. MPP have lost self-renewal potential but still retain the capacity to differentiate down multiple lineage pathways [6]. In mice, MPP further differentiate into lymphoid-primed MPP (LMPP), or alternatively, to common lymphoid precursors (CLP). Both LMPP and CLP are strongly biased toward lymphoid differentiation but have differing abilities to differentiate along other pathways (such as the myeloid pathway). The reason for the presence of these heterogeneous categories of lymphoid precursors in mice remains unclear. In humans, the cells that migrate to and populate the thymus are CLP ($CD10^{+}CD24^{-}CD34^{+}$) [7] . Directing these lymphoid precursors toward the B lymphocyte or T lymphocyte pathway appears to be based on the ability to repress alternative differentiative pathways. Signaling via Notch receptors is important for repressing the development of other pathways and generating T lymphocytes. Conversely, the silencing of the Notch1 receptor signaling by the Pax5 transcription factor, along with EBF1, appears to be important in the directing lymphoid precursors toward the B lymphocyte pathway [8].

B Lymphocytes

The development of B lymphocytes in the bone marrow was recently studied using single-cell mass cytometry multiparameter analysis. The results of this study identified a progression of B lymphocyte precursors which undergo gradual changes in cell surface marker expression. These different combinations of surface markers can be used to define the different precursor populations [6]. In B cell development, Pro-B cells first give rise to Pre-B1 cells, which then subsequently mature into Pre-B2 cells. Pre-B2 cells give rise to immature B cells, which in turn lead to mature- and IL3Rα^{+}-mature B cells. Some of the more dramatic phenotypic changes that occur as B cells differentiate include the loss of CD38 expression, increased expression of CD45RA and CD20, and, at the end of B cell differentiation in the bone marrow, a more modest increase of CD19 and CD123 (IL3Rα). While the genetic rearrangement needed to generate heavy and light immunoglobulin chains occurs early in the differentiation of B cells, the cytoplasmic expression of μ heavy chain, the first heavy chain produced, occurs in the pre-B cells. The μ heavy chain combines with two proteins called $\lambda5$ and VpreB to generate the pre-B cell receptor (BCR). A positive signal from the pre-BCR is needed to complete differentiation into an immature B cell expressing IgM (μ heavy chain plus light chain) on the cell surface [9].

Once the B cells leave the bone marrow, they express additional cell surface markers including CD21, CD22, and surface IgD. B cells continuously recirculate through secondary lymphoid organs and move to B cell follicles, which are concentrated areas of B cells [9, 10]. When B cells encounter antigen in the follicle, they move to the boundary between the B cell follicles and the T cell areas in order to interact with T cells. The costimulatory signal provided by CD40 ligand (CD154) expressed on activated CD4+ T cells binding to CD40 on B cells drives the initial proliferation of the antigen-bound B cell. Within days, the cytokines produced by activated CD4+ T cells dictate a switch from the μ heavy chain to the γ, ε, or α heavy chain constant region genes. This switch is mediated by the enzyme, activation-induced, cytidine deaminase (AID), which demethylates deoxycytidine residues in the targeted switch recombination sequences. The resulting deoxyuracil bases are then excised by a uracil DNA glycosylase (UNG). The excision of bases triggers the recombination process, which results in the downstream heavy chain assuming the position of the μ heavy chain gene. This is the process by which a B cell initially producing IgM converts to an IgG-, IgE-, or IgA-producing cell.

Activated B cells choose one of two paths after the initial antigen and costimulation-driven activation of the B cells [9, 10]. Some of the activated B cells migrate to extrafollicular areas in the secondary lymphoid organs where they rapidly expand and differentiate into antibody-secreting plasmablasts and plasma cells. These cells provide the earliest source of antigen-specific antibodies, which are an important component of the specificity mediated by the adaptive immune system. The remaining antigen-stimulated B cells stay in the follicles where they seed germinal centers. Germinal centers are locally defined environments within the secondary lymphoid organs where B cells are able to mature and undergo affinity maturation, a process that generates higher affinity antibodies [10]. The factors that dictate which path an activated B cell will take include the B cell's initial affinity for antigen and the level of T cell help that is generated.

Histologically, germinal centers have been shown to be composed of dark zone and light zone compartments [10]. The dark zone is located next to the T cell areas and contains a high density of large, proliferating B cells. These B cells have decreased surface immunoglobulin and are called centroblasts. The B cells in the light zone, known as centrocytes, are small, nonmitotic B cells expressing surface immunoglobulin. The light zone also has a network of follicular dendritic cells, which, while not derived from hematopoietic stem cells, express a number of Fc and complement receptors that allow them to trap antigens. The follicular dendritic cells can then present these antigens to B cells. In addition to the follicular dendritic cells, there is a minor population of follicular CD4+ T cells that provide signals for germinal center B cell survival.

The movement of the B cells to all of these different sites is controlled by the expression of specific chemokine markers and production of their ligands [10]. Chemokines are chemoattractant cytokines that are able to guide lymphocytes expressing appropriate receptors toward the cell sources producing the chemokines. CXCR5 is found on naïve and activated B cells and drives cells toward B cell follicles where cells producing the CXCR5 ligand, CXCL13, are located. Once B cells are activated, they upregulate expression of CCR7, whose ligands, CCL19 and CCL20, are produced by cells in the T cell area. Cells in the germinal center also express CXCR4, which recognizes the CXCL12 ligand.

Affinity maturation of B cells takes place within germinal centers [10]. When B cells proliferate in germinal centers, they exhibit high rates of mutation in the immunoglobulin variable region. This process is termed somatic hypermutation and occurs using the same enzymes that are used for switching heavy chains. AID demethylates deoxycytidine bases and the resulting deoxyuracil bases are removed by UNG. The polymerase that fills in the missing bases is error prone so wrong bases are often added randomly. The consequence of somatic hypermutation is that a number of immunoglobulin variants are generated. B cells expressing immunoglobulin variants that exhibit increased binding affinity to the immunizing antigen are induced to proliferate further. These expanded B cell clones then differentiate into either memory B cells or long-lived plasma cells that exit germinal centers and move to other sites in the body, such as the bone marrow. In contrast, the B cells in which the affinity maturation process induced immunoglobulin variants with decreased affinity toward the immunizing antigen undergo apoptosis. This selective process is the driving force for the increasing affinity of the antigen-specific antibodies that is observed.

Another consequence of B cell somatic hypermutation is the induction of DNA strand breaks. These mistakes appear to be the primary driving force for the development of a number of different types of B cell lymphomas. Many of the categories of B cell malignancies that have been identified are listed below [9, 11].

Malignancy	Source/origin	Markers
Acute lymphocytic leukemia	Bone marrow	CD10, CD19, CD24, TdT
Chronic myelocytic leukemia-lymphoid blast crisis	Bone marrow	CD10, CD19, CD24, TdT
Chronic lymphocytic leukemia	Blood	CD19, CD20, CD21, CD24, BCR, μ, CD5
Small lymphocytic lymphoma	Primary follicle	CD19, CD20, CD21, CD22, CD24, BCR, μδ
Mantle cell lymphoma	Primary follicle	CD19, CD20, CD21, CD22, CD24, BCR, μδ
Follicular lymphoma	Germinal center	CD10, CD19, CD20, CD24, BCR, μδ
Diffuse large B cell lymphoma	Germinal center	CD10, CD19, CD20, CD24, BCR, μδ
Burkitt lymphoma	Germinal center	CD10, CD19, CD20, CD24, BCR, μδ
Hodgkin lymphoma	Germinal center	CD10, CD19, CD20, CD24, BCR, μδ
Multiple myeloma	Post-germinal center	CD19, CD138
Waldenstrom macroglobulinemia	Post-germinal center	CD19, CD138
Marginal zone lymphoma	Post-germinal center	CD19, CD138
Hairy cell leukemia	Post-germinal center	CD19, CD138
Plasmablastic lymphoma	Post-germinal center	CD19, CD138

T Lymphocytes

While development of B lymphocytes occurs in the bone marrow, T lymphocyte development occurs primarily in the thymus. This means that T lymphocyte precursor cells must be able to migrate from the bone marrow through the blood to the thymus. Experimental data indicates that the interaction between the chemokine receptors, CCR9 and CCR7, expressed on precursor cells and the thymic-produced chemokines, CCL25 and CCL19-CCL21, is essential to the process of directing these cells toward the thymus. However, the expression of these receptors does not appear to play a role in the differentiation of the thymocytes [8].

Precursor cells that settle in the thymus develop along the T lymphocyte pathway because of signals generated by the Notch1 transcription factor and the cytokine, IL-7. The role of these different signals in thymopoiesis appears to vary somewhat between mice and humans. These differences include different responses to varying levels of these respective factors, varying degrees of dependence on these two factors, and the stages at which T cell precursors respond to the factors. One of the primary roles of the signals induced by these factors is to repress the ability of early T cell precursors to differentiate along alternative pathways. However, when these early thymocytes are removed from the repressive environment of the thymus, they have been shown to still retain the ability to develop into B lymphocytes, myeloid cells, dendritic cells, and NK cells in the presence of the appropriate factors. However, as demonstrated in mice, commitment to the erythroid and megakaryocyte lineages cannot be achieved once T cell precursors arrive in the thymus, as these pathways are permanently repressed prior to the thymic arrival. Once reaching the thymus, studies suggest that the ability of T cell precursors to differentiate into B lymphocytes is rapidly inhibited, followed by somewhat later inhibition of the myeloid and dendritic cell pathways, and the NK cell pathway is the latest pathway to be repressed. Analysis of human T lymphocyte precursors indicates that these cells have already lost myeloid differentiation capacity at the time of thymic arrival.

The differentiation stages of murine thymocytes are described as follows: DN1/ETP, DN2a, DN2b, DN3a, DN3b, and lastly $\alpha\beta$ T cells [8]. These stages are defined according to the expression levels of certain cell markers, including c-kit, CD44, CD25, and the β-chain of the T cell receptor. The β-chain of the T cell receptor is first expressed in stages DN3a and DN3b and is therefore an important marker of these stages. In humans, thymocyte differentiation starts with $CD10^+CD24^-CD34^+$ cells that mature in a stepwise fashion by first acquiring CD7 and secondly acquiring CD1a [7]. Human TCR β-chain rearrangements are initially detected in $CD4^-CD8^-CD34^+CD1\alpha^+$ cells. Cells then begin to express CD4 but not CD8 and then subsequently express both CD8α and CD8β in addition to CD4. A number of studies have suggested that TCR β-chain rearrangements can occur at any of these stages. The TCR β-chain then associates with a surrogate α-chain which forms a pre-TCR. Triggering this pre-TCR results in the expansion of the $CD4^+CD8^+$ double positive cells and initiation of α-chain TCR rearrangements [12]. The process of α-chain TCR rearrangement continues sequentially on both chromosomes until (1) an α-chain is formed that is able to properly associate with the previously formed β-chain and (2) the TCR complex is able to bind to a self-major histocompatibility complex (MHC) molecule/peptide complex and transduce a signal. Receiving this positive signal allows a T cell to continue differentiating, while no signal results in death of the cell. Too strong an interaction between the TCR and self-MHC molecule/peptide complex also causes a cell to undergo activation-induced apoptosis (negative selection) eliminating the cell. Presumably, this negative selection process removes autoreactive T cells that could contribute to autoimmunity if they were allowed to complete differentiation and be released to the periphery.

Once the naïve $CD4^+$ and $CD8^+$ T lymphocytes leave the thymus, they circulate throughout the body in the blood or reside temporarily in lymphoid organs (such the spleen or lymph nodes). Expression of the selectin ligand, CD62L, and lack of expression of the adhesion molecule, VLA-4, direct the migration of naïve T cells to lymph nodes. Naïve T lymphocytes are unable to migrate to tissues because they have not yet been activated. Activation is achieved once T cells encounter antigen on antigen-presenting cells (APCs), such as dendritic cells, in the spleen or lymph nodes. T lymphocytes need to receive several different signals to become sufficiently activated and undergo proliferation and differentiation. Required APC signals to T cells include presentation of antigenic peptides by MHC molecules, presentation of costimulatory ligands such as CD80/86 on the APC cell surface, and production of inflammatory cytokines such as type I IFN and IL-12.

The effector responses of $CD4^+$ T lymphocytes, known as "T-helper cells," primarily consist of the production of cytokines. $CD4^+$ T lymphocytes can produce a wide variety of cytokines, but usually do not produce them all at once. Instead, $CD4^+$ T cells produce a discrete set of cytokines that is determined by the combination of cytokines already present in the environment when T cell activation occurs. $CD4^+$ T cells are divided into categories based on the cytokines they produce: T-helper 1 (Th1) cells, T-helper 2 (Th2) cells, T-helper 3 (Th3) cells, and T-helper 17 (Th17 cells). The cytokines produced by these subsets determine their mechanism of action. Th1 cytokines include IFN-γ, IL-2, and TNF-α, which are important in the generation of immune responses to intracellular pathogens, such as viruses. Th2 cytokines include IL-4, IL-5, IL-10, and IL-13. These are important in mounting responses to extracellular pathogens, such as worms. The presence of IFN-γ or IL-4 at the initiation of the immune response is crucial in determining whether an immune response will be skewed toward Th1 or Th2. IFN-γ promotes the production of Th1 cytokines and inhibits the production of Th2 cytokines. In contrast, the early presence of IL-4 directs the production of Th2 cytokines and inhibits Th1 cytokines. The early presence of TGF-β directs $CD4^+$ cells to produce Th3 cytokines, TGF-β and IL-10, which facilitate the production of IgA in mucosal tissues. When both TGF-β and IL-6 are present early in the immune response, $CD4^+$ T cells are directed toward the Th17 phenotype resulting in the production of IL-17 and are often found in inflammatory conditions.

$CD8^+$ T lymphocytes, often defined as cytolytic T lymphocytes (CTLs), play a major role in the Th1 response against intracellular pathogens but have also been shown to produce a variety of different cytokines. While $CD8^+$ T cells can produce Th1 cytokines when activated, the primary method these cells use to eliminate intracellular pathogens is by lysing the pathogen-infected cells. The lysis of these infected cells is accomplished through exocytosis of cytolytic granules. Main components of these granules include serine proteases called granzymes and perforin, a protein that forms holes in the cell membrane [13]. Perforin facilitates entry of granzymes into the cell cytoplasm where they are able to induce programmed cell death (apoptosis) in the target cell.

Naïve CD8$^+$ T cells do not contain cytolytic granules. Once CD8$^+$ T cells receive sufficient activating signals, they begin producing granzymes and perforin and packaging these proteins into granules. When an activated and armed CD8$^+$ T cell encounters a cell expressing the same antigen as that which triggered its initial activation, cytolytic granules are mobilized to the point of contact and triggered to exocytose stored contents into the extracellular environment next to the target cell. Once clearance of an infectious pathogen has been accomplished, activated CD8 T cells are reduced in number via a process called activation-induced cell death. Yet, even after this contraction, the number of memory CD8 T cells specific for the pathogen remains elevated. High levels of granzyme A have been observed in these resting memory CD8 T cell populations [14, 15]. With additional encounters with antigens, the process of repeated activation and return to rest results in even higher resting levels of cytolytic effector molecules. Initially, resting memory CD8 cells express granzyme A plus low levels of granzyme B or perforin. With more cycles of activation, these cells begin to express high levels of both granzyme A and granzyme B and low levels of perforin. Eventually, high resting levels of perforin are also established. These end-stage CD8$^+$ cells also are marked by the expression of NK cell markers, particularly CD57. As CD8$^+$ T cells progress through these different stages, it has been found that they express an increasing number of these NK markers, which can alter how they respond to specific antigens.

Five granzymes can be found in human cytolytic granules: A, B, H, K, and M [13]. These are produced and present in varying amounts depending on cell type. Out of these five types, granzymes A and B have been most extensively studied. Granzyme B induces target cell apoptosis through cleavage of caspases that trigger the apoptotic pathway. While granzyme A may also induce apoptosis via an alternative pathway, it also contributes to inflammation by cleaving, and thereby activating, assemblies of proteins called inflammasomes [16]. Inflammasome activation triggers the cleavage of IL-1β and IL-18 pro forms, which in turn leads to the production of active cytokines that induce inflammatory responses.

Natural Killer Cells

Natural killer (NK) cells are important effector cells in the innate response to antigenic stimulation [17]. These cells produce cytokines and also mediate cytolytic activity. The development of NK cells primarily occurs in the bone marrow, although it can occur at other sites as well. Transcription factors that appear to be important for NK cell maturation include IRF-2, Gata3, Tbx21, and Dlx. At an immature stage, NK cells require a common γ-chain and the IL-2Rβ-chain (both components of the IL-2 and IL-15 receptor), along with the associated signaling molecules. Knockout mice studies demonstrated that expression of IL-15 or the IL-15Rα-chain is essential for the development and maintenance of NK cells, as absence of either one of these molecules prevents NK cell development. In humans, no individuals exhibiting loss of IL-15 or IL-15R have been reported, but information can still be gained from studying individuals with mutations in other proteins involved in these pathways. Such studies have indicated that, like in mice, IL-15 is the key regulator of NK cell development in humans.

Although the phenotype of NK cell precursors has not been identified in humans, $CD3^-CD161^+CD56^-$ cells can be induced in vitro from Lin^-CD34^+ cells. When these precursor cells are further stimulated with IL-2 and IL-12, CD56 expression and natural cytotoxicity are acquired. NK cells also undergo a selection process that results in them expressing a varying number of inhibitory receptors depending on recognition of MHC molecules expressed in the environment during their development [18]. These inhibitory receptors are important in maintaining self-tolerance. If NK cell receptors interact with self-MHC on another cell, the kill signal will be inhibited and the self-cell will remain intact. However, if a self-MHC complex is not present, NK cell cytotoxic potential will be released. This system allows NK cells to target foreign antigens and also pathogen-infected syngeneic cells (which often downregulate expression of self-MHC).

NK cells can also develop in sites other than bone marrow, including the lymph node, thymus, and intestine [17]. In the thymus, the differentiation pathway to NK cells is the last alternative pathway lost before final commitment to T lymphocyte lineage. This has raised the question of how NK-cell-inducing signals within the thymus overcome the dominant push to become T cells. NK cells in the thymus have been found to express intracellular CD3ε proteins, a phenotype not observed in the peripheral NK cells. There is evidence that NK cells can also develop in the lymph nodes and intestines. The contribution of these non-bone marrow sites to the overall number of NK cells has not been determined. Unlike NK cells that develop in the bone marrow, many NK cells that develop in non-bone marrow sites are $CD56^{high}CD16^{low}$. The ratio observed is 10:1 $CD56^{high}CD16^{low}$:$CD56^{low}CD16^{high}$ NK cells in the lymph node and intestine, whereas the ratio of these two populations of NK cells is 1:10 in the peripheral blood and spleen. These two populations of NK cells have different primary effector functions. The $CD56^{high}CD16^{low}$ NK cells are primarily cytokine secretors, while the $CD56^{low}CD16^{high}$ NK cells are primarily cytolytic effector cells.

Mature NK cells leaving the bone marrow are fully armed with cytolytic granules containing granzymes and perforin. Activation of NK cells to carry out cytolytic activity is usually the result of receiving more activating signals than inhibitory signals. The balance tips toward an activating response in situations where there is a lack of self-MHC molecules. This happens when the target cells are allogeneic or have lost expression of MHC molecules because the cell has been infected or because of oncogenic transformation. Activation can also occur when an NK cell receives strong activating signals. The strongest activating signal, which is able to override all inhibitory signals, is triggered by the binding interaction between an Fc receptor and antibody-coated cells or antigen.

A number of different leukemias and lymphomas have been identified as malignant transformation of cells at all of the different stages of T cell and NK cell differentiation [11]. The transformation of the more differentiated T cell stages is reflected by the identification of a heterogenous group of T cell and NK lymphomas.

T cell lymphomas have been divided into the cutaneous T cell lymphomas and peripheral T cell lymphomas categories [19–21]. Peripheral T cell lymphomas are a heterogenous group of lymphomas that are often derived from cytolytic cells, including NK cells. These lymphomas occur with a relatively low frequency (<1 case/100,000). They are further divided into subcategories based on clinical features including nodal, extranodal, and leukemic. The nodal group of lymphomas includes peripheral T cell lymphomas not otherwise specified, anaplastic large cell lymphoma, and angioimmunoblastic T cell lymphoma. The extranodal group contains a number of less common types, including hepatosplenic $\gamma\delta$ T cell lymphoma, enteropathy-associated T cell lymphoma (associated with celiac disease), intestinal T and NK cell lymphomas, nasal-type NK^-/T^- lymphoma, and panniculitis-like T cell lymphoma.

The leukemia group includes the adult T cell lymphoma (ATL) associated with human T-lymphotropic virus type 1 (HTLV-1). The geographic distribution of the ATL is similar to where the HTLV-1 virus is endemic, which includes Japan and the Caribbean. T cell chronic large granular lymphocyte leukemia, aggressive NK cell leukemia, and T cell prolymphocytic leukemia also are included in the leukemic subcategory.

The cutaneous T cell lymphomas are primarily comprised of mycosis fungoides and the leukemic variant, Sezary syndrome [20]. Mycosis fungoides is a lymphoma primarily comprised of mature, skin-homing CD4+ clonal cells producing the Th2 cytokines IL-4, IL-5, and IL-10. They usually present as patches, plaques, tumors, or generalized erythema of the skin. These malignant cells can also be found in the lymph nodes and peripheral blood. These cells lack expression of T cell markers such as CD7 and CD26 but usually express clonal TCR. Gene expression profiling of STAT4, GATA3, Plastin-T, CD1d, and TRAIL has been found to be 90% accurate in predicating Sezary syndrome.

An understanding of the developmental and differentiation pathways of lymphocyte subpopulations including B lymphocytes, T lymphocytes, and NK cells is important for categorizing the different types of malignant transformed lymphocytes. This understanding will facilitate study of the different types of lymphomas and the mechanisms responsible for their development and provide a basis for the development of novel and better therapeutic protocols.

References

1. Ema H, Morita Y, Yamazaki S et al (2006) Adult mouse hematopoietic stem cells: purification and single-cell assays. Nat Protoc 1:2979–2987
2. Seita J, Weissman IL (2010) Hematopoietic stem cell: self-renewal versus differentiation. Wiley Interdiscip Rev Syst Biol Med 2:640–653
3. Gibbs KD Jr, Gilbert PM, Sachs K et al (2011) Single-cell phospho-specific flow cytometric analysis demonstrates biochemical and functional heterogeneity in human hematopoietic stem and progenitor compartments. Blood 117:4226–4233
4. Dooner GJ, Colvin GA, Dooner MS et al (2008) Gene expression fluctuations in murine hematopoietic stem cells with cell cycle progression. J Cell Physiol 214:786–795

5. Quesenberry PJ, Colvin G, Dooner G et al (2007) The stem cell continuum: cell cycle, injury, and phenotype lability. Ann N Y Acad Sci 1106:20–29
6. Bendall SC, Simonds EF, Qiu P et al (2011) Single-cell mass cytometry of differential immune and drug responses across a human hematopoietic continuum. Science 332:687–696
7. Vicente R, Swainson L, Marty-Gres S et al (2010) Molecular and cellular basis of T cell lineage commitment. Semin Immunol 22:270–275
8. Rothenberg EV (2011) T cell lineage commitment: identity and renunciation. J Immunol 186:6649–6655
9. LeBien TW, Tedder TF (2008) B lymphocytes: how they develop and function. Blood 112:1570–1580
10. Gatto D, Brink R (2010) The germinal center reaction. J Allergy Clin Immunol 126:898–907, quiz 8–9
11. Campo E, Swerdlow SH, Harris NL et al (2011) The 2008 WHO classification of lymphoid neoplasms and beyond: evolving concepts and practical applications. Blood 117:5019–5032
12. Gascoigne NR, Palmer E (2011) Signaling in thymic selection. Curr Opin Immunol 23:207–212
13. Lieberman J (2003) The ABCs of granule-mediated cytotoxicity: New weapons in the arsenal. Nat Rev Immunol 3:361–382
14. Takata H, Takiguchi M (2006) Three memory subsets of human CD8+ T cells differently expressing three cytolytic effector molecules. J Immunol 177:4330–4340
15. Chattopadhyay P, Betts M, Price D et al (2009) The cytolytic enzymes granzyme A, granzyme B, and perforin: expression patterns, cell distribution, and their relationship to cell maturity and bright CD57 expression. J Leukoc BIol 85:88–97
16. Lamkanfi M, Dixit VM (2011) Modulation of inflammasome pathways by bacterial and viral pathogens. J Immunol 187:597–602
17. Huntington N, Mention J-J, Vosshenrich C et al (2010) Dissecting Human NK cell development and differentiation. In: Zimmer J (ed) Natural killer cells. Springer, Heidelberg, pp 39–61
18. Pegram HJ, Andrews DM, Smyth MJ et al (2011) Activating and inhibitory receptors of natural killer cells. Immunol Cell Biol 89:216–224
19. Zeerleder S, Hack C, Caliezi C et al (2005) Activated cytotoxic T cells and NK cells in severe sepsis and septic shock and their role in multiple organ dysfunction. Clin Immunol 116:158–165
20. Kim EJ, Lin J, Junkins-Hopkins JM et al (2006) Mycosis fungoides and sezary syndrome: an update. Curr Oncol Rep 8:376–386
21. Foss FM, Zinzani PL, Vose JM et al (2011) Peripheral T-cell lymphoma. Blood 117:6756–6767

HIV Lymphomagenesis

Liron Pantanowitz and Antonino Carbone

Abstract Patients with human immunodeficiency virus (HIV) infection are at increased risk of developing non-Hodgkin lymphoma (NHL) and Hodgkin lymphoma. Only certain NHL subtypes are AIDS-defining conditions. Risk factors for developing AIDS-related lymphomas (ARLs) include HIV-specific factors (e.g., CD4+ count and HIV viral load) and general factors (e.g., EBV and/or HHV8 coinfection). ARLs comprise a heterogeneous group that are divided by the World Health Organization (WHO) into lymphomas also occurring in immunocompetent patients (e.g., Burkitt lymphoma), lymphomas occurring more specifically in HIV-infected patients (e.g., primary effusion lymphoma), and those lymphomas that also occur in other immunodeficiency states (e.g., polymorphic B-cell lymphomas). While the pathogenesis of ARL is still incompletely understood, research to date indicates that immune deregulation leading to loss of control of viruses such as EBV and HHV8, accompanied by genetic alterations and cytokine production, plays an important role in HIV lymphomagenesis. This chapter provides a contemporary overview of ARL and highlights the mechanisms involved in their pathogenesis.

Introduction

Both non-Hodgkin lymphoma (NHL) and Hodgkin lymphoma are conditions likely to be encountered in patients with human immunodeficiency virus (HIV) infection. The high frequency of NHL among HIV-positive patients was acknowledged by the

L. Pantanowitz (✉)
Department of Pathology, University of Pittsburgh Medical Center Shadyside Hospital, 5150 Centre Avenue, Suite 201, Pittsburgh, PA 15232, USA
e-mail: pantanowitzl@upmc.edu

A. Carbone
Department of Pathology and Laboratory Medicine, Istituto Nazionale Tumori, Milan, Italy

P.J. Quesenberry and J.J. Castillo (eds.), *Non-Hodgkin Lymphoma: Prognostic Factors and Targets*, Cancer Drug Discovery and Development, DOI 10.1007/978-1-4614-5851-7_3,

inclusion of specific types of high-grade NHL in the US Centers for Disease Control and Prevention (CDC) revised case definition of AIDS [20]. Hodgkin lymphoma, however, is a non-AIDS-defining cancer (NADC). The proportion of individuals with NHL presenting as the initial acquired immune deficiency syndrome (AIDS)-defining illness increased as the incidence of other AIDS-defining conditions (e.g., *Pneumocystis jirovecii* pneumonia and Kaposi sarcoma) declined following the introduction of highly active antiretroviral therapy (HAART). While almost all AIDS-related lymphomas (ARLs) are of B-cell origin, cases of HIV-related T-cell NHL may still be observed. ARLs comprise a heterogeneous group including Burkitt lymphoma, diffuse large B-cell lymphoma (DLBCL), plasmablastic lymphoma, primary effusion lymphoma (PEL), and polymorphic lymphoproliferative disorders. While these ARLs may differ in their clinical presentation (e.g., varying anatomic distribution) and molecular mechanism of lymphomagenesis, they share several similarities including an aggressive clinical course with frequent extranodal disease, plasmacellular differentiation, and an association with the gamma herpesviruses Epstein-Barr virus (EBV) and/or Kaposi sarcoma-associated herpesvirus/human herpesvirus-8 (KSHV/HHV8). Patients with ARL have traditionally tolerated chemotherapy poorly. However, their response rates and survival appear to be improving owing to advances in supportive care and effective HAART. This chapter focuses specifically on the lymphomagenesis of HIV-related lymphomas.

Overview of AIDS-Related Lymphomas

Classification

ARLs are divided by the World Health Organization (WHO) into three main categories [73]:

- Lymphomas also occurring in immunocompetent patients, for example, Burkitt lymphoma, DLBCL, extranodal marginal zone B-cell lymphoma of mucosa-associated lymphoid tissue type (MALT), peripheral T-cell lymphoma (PTCL), and classical Hodgkin lymphoma
- Lymphomas occurring more specifically in HIV-infected patients, for example, PEL, plasmablastic lymphoma, and lymphoma arising in HHV8-associated multicentric Castleman disease
- Lymphomas also occurring in other immunodeficiency states, for example, polymorphic B-cell lymphomas

ARLs have also been classified according to their location (systemic NHL, primary central nervous system lymphoma or PCNSL, and primary effusion or body cavity lymphoma) or categorized based upon clinical behavior (indolent, aggressive, and highly aggressive). Systemic NHL accounts for most ARL, whereas PCNSL represents approximately 15% and PEL <1% of cases [1, 28, 59]. Effusion lymphomas in the setting of HIV infection can be further subtyped into primary or

Table 1 Effusion lymphomas associated with HIV infection

Secondary	**To systemic lymphomas**
	HHV8 negative
	Various histotypes
Primary	**Primary effusion lymphoma**
	HHV8+
	c-*MYC* negative
	Immunoblastic/anaplastic morphology
	Extranodal large cell lymphoma
	(HHV8-unrelated PEL-like lymphoma)
	HHV8-
	c-*MYC* negative
	Centroblastic/immunoblastic morphology
	Extranodal Burkitt lymphoma
	HHV8-
	c-*MYC*+
	Burkitt morphology

secondary lymphomas (Table 1). The majority (70–90%) of ARLs are highly aggressive, most of which are due to the immunoblastic variant of DLBCL and Burkitt lymphoma. The aggressive lymphomas consist predominately of the other variants of DLBCL. Indolent lymphomas in HIV + persons are uncommon and comprise >10% of ARLs.

Epidemiology

In the pre-HAART era, NHL represented the second most common cancer associated with AIDS after Kaposi sarcoma [1]. In the HAART era (post-1996), the proportion of NHL cases associated with AIDS has since modestly declined. A meta-analysis involving 23 cohort studies that included 47,936 HIV-infected patients found a decline in the incidence of ARL from 1992–1996 (0.62% per year) to 1997–1999 (0.36% per year) [53]. In particular, there has been a marked decline in the incidence of PCNSL due to the impact of HAART. The change in incidence restricted to only some NHL subtypes suggests that there may be differential involvement of immune function in tumor development [76]. Despite the beneficial effect of HAART on the survival of HIV-infected patients, NHL continues to be a major source of morbidity and mortality. Compared with the general population, the relative risk for ARL shows a 400-fold increase for highly aggressive lymphomas, 110-fold increase for aggressive lymphomas, and more than 15-fold increase for indolent lymphomas [31]. Interestingly, those infected with HIV have a 650-fold increased risk of developing DLBCL and 260-fold risk of having Burkitt lymphoma [28].

Clinical–Pathologic Features

ARL is distributed relatively homogeneously throughout the spectrum of HIV-risk groups [1, 12]. While ARL usually manifests late in HIV infection, these lymphomas can arise at any CD4 T-lymphocyte cell count. For example, Burkitt lymphoma tends to occur at relatively higher CD4+ cell counts (>200 cells/mm^3), whereas PCNSL and PEL are more often associated with advanced stages of immune deficiency (CD4 <50 cells/mm^3) and hence are more likely to be associated with opportunistic infections [82]. Patients with ARL are more likely to have advanced stages of lymphoma at presentation, present with B symptoms (fevers, night sweats, and weight loss), and develop extranodal disease. Common sites of extranodal ARL include the CNS, gastrointestinal tract (stomach, anorectum), bone marrow, body cavities, Waldeyer's ring, and jaw, and with Burkitt lymphoma, several (10–20%) patients may have leptomeningeal involvement at diagnosis. Adverse prognostic factors include a low CD4 count (<100 cells/mm^3), age >35 years, intravenous drug use, poor performance status including International Prognostic Index (IPI), elevated lactate dehydrogenase (LDH), advanced lymphoma stage at diagnosis, prior AIDS diagnosis, and poor control of HIV viral replication through the use of HAART [1, 80].

Several of the more aggressive ARL exhibit plasmacellular differentiation. They exhibit plasmacytoid morphology and demonstrate immunophenotypic and molecular attributes in keeping with plasma cell differentiation. Hence, their pathologic diagnosis is frequently problematic. ARLs that share similar plasmacellular features include Burkitt lymphoma with plasmacytoid differentiation, immunoblastic variant of DLBCL, plasmablastic lymphoma, PEL, and polymorphic lymphoproliferative disorder ("polyclonal" lymphoma). A combination of clinical, morphologic, virologic, immunophenotypic, and molecular findings is usually required to adequately differentiate between these various ARLs (Table 2) [55].

Burkitt Lymphoma

Burkitt lymphoma accounts for up to 30% of HIV-associated lymphomas. As noted before, these lymphomas typically develop in the setting of mild immunodeficiency (CD4 count >200 cells/mm^3). Patients with HIV infection may develop classical Burkitt lymphoma, less frequently atypical Burkitt lymphoma, and occasionally Burkitt lymphoma with plasmacytoid differentiation, which is relatively unique to patients with AIDS [73]. These lymphomas frequently involve bone marrow, peripheral blood, leptomeninges, and the face and may also manifest with lymphadenopathy. A high proliferation index is typical, with >90% of cells staining positive for Ki-67 (Mib-1). Lymphoma cells are medium-sized, non-cleaved lymphocytes that have a deeply basophilic cytoplasm, lipid vacuoles, and several nucleoli (Fig. 1). In the plasmacytoid variant, lymphoma cells have a more basophilic cytoplasm with an eccentric nucleus and single central nucleolus. Burkitt cells are positive for

Table 2 Comparison of AIDS-related lymphomas with plasmacellular differentiation

Lymphoma type	Plasmacytoid Burkitt lymphoma	DLBCL immunoblastic lymphoma	Plasmablastic lymphoma	Classic PEL	Solid PEL	Polyclonal lymphoma	Plasmacytoma
CD4+ T-cell count (cells/mm^3)	Normal to low (>200)	Very low (<100)	Low	Very low (<100)	Low (<200)	Low (<200)	Normal to low
Common presentation	Mainly extranodal	Nodal and extranodal (including CNS)	Nodal and extranodal	Effusions	Extracavitary	Nodal and extranodal	Bone (solitary) and extramedullary
Tumor cell size	Intermediate	Large	Small to large	Large	Large	Variable	Small to intermediate
CD45 (LCA)	Positive	Positive	Positive (may be lost)	Positive	Positive	Positive	Positive
CD20	Positive	Positive (may be lost)	Positive (may be lost)	Rare positive	Positive (may be lost)	Positive	Rare positive
BCL-6	Positive	Occasional positive	Rare positive	Rare positive	Negative	Rare positive	Negative
Other positive markers	CD10	CD10 CD30 CD5 rare	CD10 CD31 CD56	CD30 CD71 CD31 EMA	CD30 EMA	CD43	Rare CD10 CD31 CD56 EMA
CD138	Negative	Negative	Positive	Positive	Positive	Not reported	Positive
CD38	Weak positive	Negative	Positive	Positive	Positive	Not reported	Positive
MUM1	Negative	Occasional positive	Positive	Positive	Not reported	Not reported	Positive
Proliferation index (Ki-67)	Very high (>90%)	High (<90%)	High (75–95%)	High (>80%)	High	Variable	Low
Paraprotein	Absent	Absent	Absent	Absent	Absent	Absent	Present (25%)
EBV	Positive (60%)	Positive (100%)	Positive (80%)	Positive (90%)	Positive (90%)	Positive	Negative
HHV8	Negative	Some positive	Controversial positive	Positive	Positive	Some positive	Controversial positive
Genetic features	MYC activation, p53 inactivation	p53 mutation & MYC rearrangement (minority)	MYC activation, p53 overexpression	Rare chromosome abnormalities	Occasional p53 positive cells	p53 mutation (minority)	MUM1/IRF4 activation

Plasmacytoma is included here for comparison purposes. Adapted from [12]

PEL primary effusion lymphoma, *LCA* leukocyte common antigen, *EMA* epithelial membrane antigen

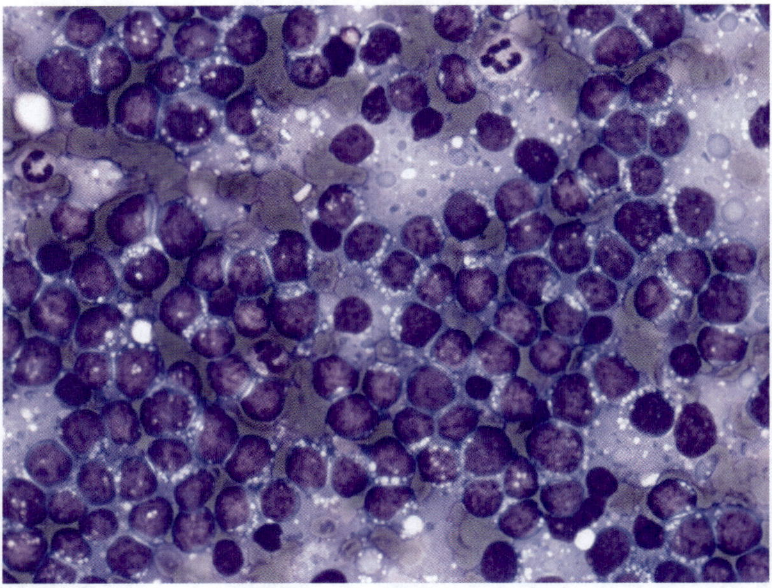

Fig. 1 Burkitt lymphoma of an intra-abdominal tumor showing characteristic tumor cells with non-cleaved nuclei and deeply basophilic cytoplasm with peripheral vacuoles (DQ stain; high magnification)

B-cell-associated antigens (CD19, CD20), CD10, and BCL-6, in keeping with a germinal center stage of differentiation. Frequently, there is also CD38 coexpression and monotypic cytoplasmic immunoglobulin present, although cases with absent immunoglobulins may be seen. All cases have c-*MYC* activation and p53 inactivation. EBV genomes can be demonstrated in 30% of classical, 30–50% of atypical, and 50–70% of plasmacytoid Burkitt lymphomas [73]. No association has been found between Burkitt lymphoma and HHV8 [72].

Diffuse Large B-Cell Lymphoma

There are several morphologic variants of DLBCL, not otherwise specified (NOS). These include:

- Centroblastic variant comprised of centroblasts with multiple nucleoli (Fig. 2)
- Immunoblastic variant, also called immunoblastic lymphoma (IBL), which by convention must contain ≥90% immunoblasts (which have single, central, prominent nucleoli)
- Anaplastic variant with large bizarre tumor cells

Centroblastic lymphoma represents 25–30% of ARL, whereas IBL constitutes 10% of ARL [73]. IBL tends to present in patients with more advanced HIV disease

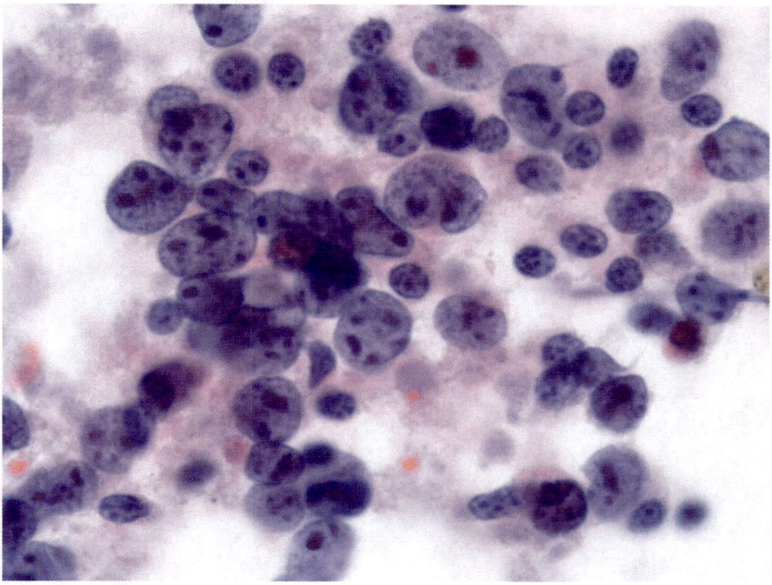

Fig. 2 Diffuse large B-cell lymphoma of the salivary gland showing tumor cells with centroblastic morphology (Pap stain; high magnification)

(CD4 count <100 cells/mm^3) than centroblastic lymphomas. Primary DLBCL of the CNS (so-called PCNSL) associated with HIV infection is usually of the immunoblastic type. HIV-associated DLBCL tends to be high grade and demonstrates a high proliferation index (but <90%), and is often associated with necrosis. IBL is the variant that most commonly exhibits plasmacytoid features. While immunoblasts typically express pan-B-cell markers (CD20, CD22, CD79a), these markers may be absent in some cases. Some lymphoma cells may also coexpress BCL-2, CD5, CD10, and CD30. Whereas rearrangements of BCL-6 are detected in around 20% of centroblastic lymphomas, IBL is characterized by an absence of BCL-6 rearrangements. EBV is positive in 30% of centroblastic lymphomas (LMP-1 negative), but is associated with 90% of IBL (LMP-1 positive) [73]. HHV8 has been shown to be associated with some (40%) cases of IBL in HIV-infected patients that lack effusions and do not have evidence of prior Castleman disease [37, 41].

Plasmablastic Lymphoma

This unique ARL was first described in the jaws and oral cavity of HIV-infected persons [7, 35, 74]. These lymphomas have subsequently been reported in many other extranodal sites including the lung, mediastinum, esophagus, anorectum, orbit, nose and paranasal sinuses, skin, testes, bone, breast, and also within long-standing sacrococcygeal cysts of HIV-positive individuals. Nodal involvement has

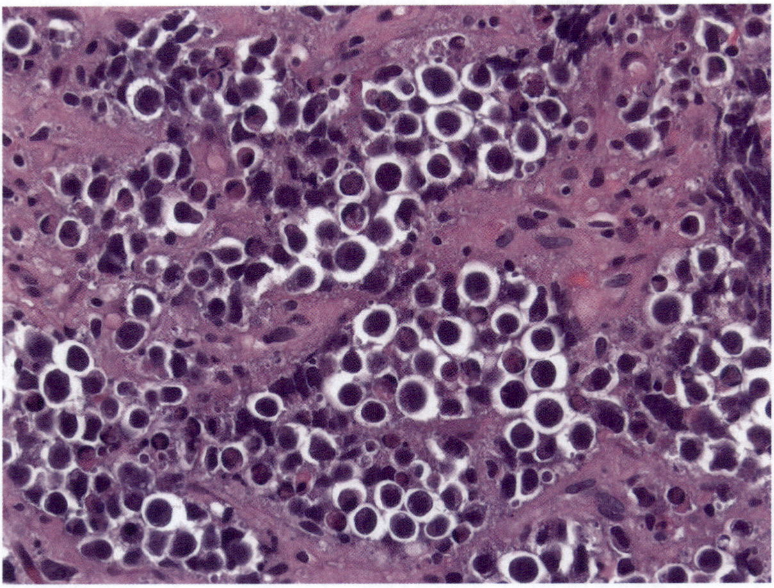

Fig. 3 Plasmablastic lymphoma of the retroperitoneum showing numerous plasmablasts (H&E stain; high magnification)

been reported, but is uncommon. This lymphoma arises mainly in young adult HIV-infected males [18]. Like Burkitt lymphoma, these lymphomas are rapidly growing destructive tumors that exhibit a proliferation index that ranges from >60% to 95%. Rarely, they may evolve into plasmablastic leukemia. They consist of plasmablasts (Fig. 3) which have abundant basophilic cytoplasm, eccentrically placed nuclei, and occasional perinuclear clearing. Plasmablastic lymphomas have been subdivided into two morphologic subgroups [25, 69]:

- Plasmablastic lymphoma of the oral mucosa type that is comprised of a monomorphic population of plasmablasts/immunoblasts with no or minimal plasmacytic differentiation
- Plasmablastic lymphoma with plasmacytic differentiation which is composed predominantly of plasmablasts/immunoblasts, but in addition exhibits more differentiation to mature plasma cells

Plasmablasts typically are negative for CD45, CD20, and/or PAX5, may be immunoreactive for the B-cell marker CD79a, and demonstrate strong immunoreactivity for plasma cell markers (VS38c, CD38, IRF4/MUM-1, or CD138) [79]. Cytoplasmic immunoglobulins (mainly IgG) are expressed in 50–70% of cases, and EMA, CD56, CD30, and CD31 are also frequently positive. AIDS-related plasmablastic lymphoma has virtually an identical tumor suppressor gene expression profile to myeloma [85]. They may also show structural alterations of the MYC locus. EBV appears to be highly associated (60–75% of cases) with plasmablastic lymphoma.

The presence of HHV8 in plasmablastic lymphomas is unlikely, but remains controversial based on some early reports [11]. The demonstration of HHV8 infection by LNA immunohistochemistry in a plasmablastic lymphoma has been suggested by some authors to rather indicate that it is a solid form of PEL [60]. The association of plasmablastic lymphoma with HHV8 would certainly help explain why some of these lymphomas develop from HHV8-related Castleman disease [40]. In such cases, HHV8-positive plasmablasts present in Castleman disease have been shown to coalesce into microscopic aggregates and sheets. These collections of plasmablasts all have similar (lambda) light-chain restriction and are referred to as microlymphomas [32, 38]. Microlymphomas may arise within the mantle, and less often in the germinal center of lymphoid follicles. Large sheets of plasmablasts are thought to represent frank lymphoma. Of interest, the new WHO classification now includes large B-cell lymphoma arising in HHV8-associated multicentric Castleman disease (also called HHV8-positive plasmablastic lymphoma) as a unique entity [54]. This new lymphoma corresponds to a naïve IgM-producing plasma cell without immunoglobulin somatic hypermutation.

Classic Primary Effusion Lymphoma

PEL, previously referred to as body cavity-based lymphoma, is a rare lymphoma that accounts for only a small proportion of ARL [23, 63]. This lymphoma has a unique tropism for serous cavities of the body. The classic variant of PEL is characterized by lymphomatous effusions of the pleural, peritoneal, and/or pericardial cavities (Fig. 4). Rare cases have been documented with PEL involving synovial joints and the subarachnoid space. By definition, there is usually no tumor mass, lymphadenopathy, or organomegaly present. However, although PEL tends to remain localized to the body cavity of origin, tissue extension of lymphoma into the pleura, lung, chest wall, peritoneum, omentum, and gastrointestinal tract may rarely occur. PEL tends to occur as a late manifestation of HIV, which may partly explain why these lymphomas have such a poor prognosis (3–5 month median survival) [78]. PEL cells are typically large and pleomorphic with immunoblast-like or anaplastic cytomorphology. Lymphoma cells are CD45 positive, have an indeterminate phenotype (i.e., most cases lack B- and T-cell-associated antigens or have a null lymphocyte immunophenotype), have no cytoplasmic or surface immunoglobulin, are positive for CD30 (75% of cases), and coexpress plasma cell antigens (CD38, CD138, VS38c, and MUM-1). While PEL is of B-cell origin, cases with an aberrant T-cell phenotype may occur [4, 75]. BCL-6 is usually absent. Almost all PEL cells are HHV8 positive, and they are also frequently (70%) coinfected with EBV [50]. HHV8, rather than EBV, is the driving force in these tumors. Rearrangement of the immunoglobulin heavy chain gene and occasionally also the T-cell receptor gene can be demonstrated. Gene expression profiling of PEL has shown a profile distinct from other lymphomas, but one that appears to be shared by multiple myeloma cell lines [57].

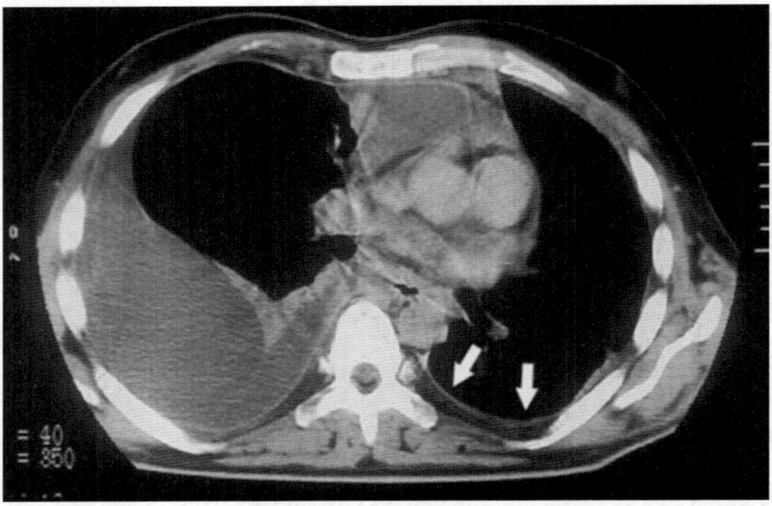

Fig. 4 CT scan showing primary effusion lymphoma (PEL) involving the pleural cavities. In this particular case, there was tissue infiltration of lymphoma cells causing focal thickening of the posterior pleura (*arrows*)

Extracavitary (Solid) Primary Effusion Lymphoma

Solid (tissue-based) HHV8-positive lymphomas are an uncommon lymphoma seen primarily in HIV-positive individuals [22, 27, 68]. Solid PEL involves mainly extranodal solid tissues such as the lower gastrointestinal tract, lung, or skin and may infrequently also present with nodal involvement [13, 29, 56, 65]. Like other HHV8-associated lymphomas, solid PEL is often associated with Kaposi sarcoma or multicentric Castleman disease. In rare cases, secondary distant (noncontiguous) lymphomatous effusions may develop. Apart from their clinical presentation, these lymphomas are virtually identical morphologically, immunophenotypically, and genetically to classic PEL. However, patients who developed solid PEL appear to have a slightly better survival (median 11 months) compared to those with classic PEL.

Polymorphic Lymphoproliferative Disorder

Published cases of an AIDS-associated lymphoid proliferation resembling post-transplant lymphoproliferative disorder (PTLD) have previously been described [61, 64]. These "polyclonal" lymphomas represent less than 5% of ARL. They may be nodal based or arise in extranodal sites including the lung, parotid gland, perineum, and skin. Like PTLD, these proliferations are composed of a polymorphous population of lymphocytes exhibiting a variable degree of plasmacellular differentiation. The infiltrates range from small cells with plasmacytoid features to immunoblasts and even cases with large CD30+ bizarre cells. Admixed mature plasma cells are frequently present. Polymerase chain reaction (PCR) for clonality often reveals only a faint band representing a monoclonal subpopulation of lymphocytes. Most of the cells express a B-cell marker (CD20), with a subset coexpressing kappa or lambda light chains. In addition, several of these cases are often positive for both EBV and HHV8. Like PTLD, these lymphoid proliferations generally lack genetic lesions involving tumor suppressor genes or oncogenes. When clonal rearrangement and cytogenetic abnormalities (e.g., c-*MYC*, BCL-6, and p53 gene mutations) arise, they are usually indicative of transformation to DLBCL.

Low-Grade Non-Hodgkin Lymphoma

Indolent lymphomas in the setting of HIV are uncommon. Such lymphomas have not been considered to be an ARL as their incidence is not significantly increased with the AIDS epidemic. Among 10 HIV+patients with low-grade NHL identified from a single institution, cases were diagnosed with follicular lymphoma, small lymphocytic lymphoma (CLL/SLL), and MALT [58]. Unlike ARL, the median survival for these patients is comparable to that reported in their HIV-negative counterparts.

Mature T-Cell Non-Hodgkin Lymphoma

Despite the fact that most ARL are of a B-cell phenotype, several cutaneous and peripheral T-cell lymphoma (PTCL) subtypes have been documented in HIV-positive persons [19]. The risk of developing PTCL in HIV-positive individuals is 15 times higher than the general population. Also, there appears to be a slightly greater proportion of PTCL in Asian and Latin American populations, probably related to an increased prevalence of viral infections such as EBV and human T-lymphotropic virus type 1 (HTLV-1) and/or genetic predisposition. PTCL-NOS and anaplastic large cell lymphoma (ALCL) are the most common HIV-associated PTCL subtypes to be reported in HIV+persons. Lymphomas such as ALCL manifest almost exclusively with extranodal involvement (Fig. 5) and typically exhibit a very aggressive clinical course [70]. ALCL is characterized by the expression of CD30 in anaplastic lymphoma cells. HIV-associated ALCL cells rarely express anaplastic lymphoma kinase (ALK). EBV infection is associated with around one-third of cases.

Hodgkin Lymphoma

Hodgkin lymphoma is presently the most common non-AIDS-defining cancer. Several studies have shown an increased risk of Hodgkin lymphoma in patients with AIDS [26, 44]. Although some studies have linked Hodgkin lymphoma to advancing

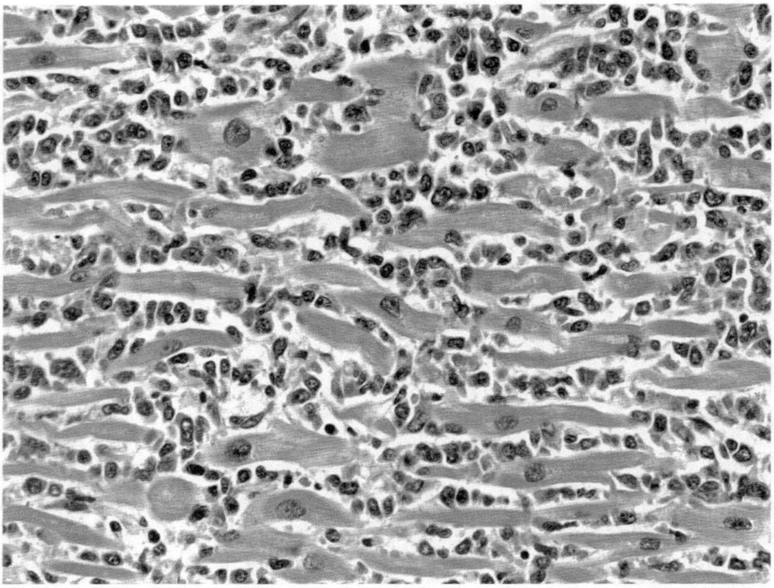

Fig. 5 Anaplastic large T-cell lymphoma (ALCL) showing large atypical lymphoma cells infiltrating through cardiac muscle diagnosed at postmortem (H&E stain; high magnification)

HIV-related immunosuppression [43], the exact relationship with CD4 count is unclear. In two large cohort studies, researchers found that there was a higher risk of Hodgkin lymphoma in HIV+persons treated with HAART compared to those who were not treated [24, 51]. Among these HAART-treated individuals, the relative risk compared with the general population appeared higher for Hodgkin lymphoma than for non-Hodgkin lymphoma. These patients typically have B symptoms and widely disseminated extranodal disease. Mixed cellularity and lymphocyte depleted are the two unfavorable subtypes most often seen in HIV+patients. CD4 and CD8 immunostaining of background T-cells usually shows an inverted CD4/CD8 ratio [83]. Almost all Hodgkin lymphomas in HIV+individuals are also EBV positive. The median survival in this population has been reported to be 12–18 months.

Risk Factors

The relative risk of developing ARL compared with the general population is addressed in section Epidemiology above, which shows that lymphoma risk varies by histologic subtype. Risk factors for developing ARL include HIV-specific factors (e.g., CD4 count, HIV viral load, and HAART) and general risk factors (e.g., EBV and/or HHV8 coinfection, B-cell dysfunction, and genetics). The risk of ARL appears to be highest in men and increases with age, chronic HIV infection, with the degree of immunosuppression and immune system dysfunction. This explains why several NHLs are seen mainly in patients with advanced HIV infection, with low CD4 counts (e.g., below 100/mm^3), and those with a history of a low CD4 count nadir [45]. In one study, investigators showed that HIV+patients with a CD4 count of 350–499 cells/mm^3 were twice as likely to develop NHL than individuals with a CD4 count >500 cells/mm^3 [49]. A high HIV viral load is also a risk factor for ARL, where the risk rises significantly for patients with plasma HIV RNA levels above 100,000 copies/ml [49]. Decreasing HIV viremia, along with concomitant improvement in CD4 cell counts, explains why the overall incidence of NHL has declined with the widespread use of HAART, which includes non-nucleoside reverse-transcriptase inhibitors (NNRTIs) and/or protease inhibitors (PIs). Genetics also seem to play a role in the risk for developing ARL. For example, HIV-seropositive patients who have a favorable ("protective") CCR5-32 deletion have been found to be threefold less likely to develop ARL [34]. In comparison, a polymorphism in the gene that encodes for the CXCR-4 chemokine receptor is associated with a two- to fourfold increase in the risk of developing ARL [30].

Lymphomagenesis

Several review articles have addressed the topic of HIV lymphomagenesis [9, 10, 12, 17]. While the pathogenesis of B-NHL in the setting of HIV infection is still incompletely understood, immune deregulation leading to loss of control of viruses such as EBV and HHV8, accompanied by genetic alterations and possibly impaired T-cell immunosurveillance, is believed to play an important role. In order to understand the pathogenesis of ARL, one needs to first appreciate the normal maturation of naive B cells (CD45+, CD20+) after passing through a germinal center. When naive B cells (BCL-6-, MUM1-, CD138-) enter the germinal center, they become centroblasts (BCL-6+, MUM1-, CD138-) that subsequently mature into centrocytes (BCL-6+, MUM1-, CD138-) as they undergo immunoglobulin class switching, somatic hypermutation of the immunoglobulin variable genes, and mutations of the proto-oncogene BCL-6. B cells that exit the germinal center begin to differentiate into memory B cells or plasma cells (BCL-6-, MUM1+, CD138+). As BCL-6 (regulates the germinal center cell reaction) and PAX5 (regulates B-cell transcription programs), expression declines; the synthesis of other markers indicative of plasmacellular differentiation including multiple myeloma oncogene-1 (MUM1 or interferon regulatory factor 4), VS38c, CD38, and CD138 (syndecan-1) increases. There is a simultaneous change from surface to cytoplasmic immunoglobulin expression, a reduction in CD45 (leukocyte common antigen or LCA), and CD20 expression in plasma cells.

Various ARLs may arise from transformed B cells at the pre-germinal center, follicular center, or post-germinal center stage during this differentiation process (Fig. 6). Burkitt lymphoma and DLBCL develop from follicular center B cells, while plasmablastic lymphoma and most cases of PEL arise from post-germinal

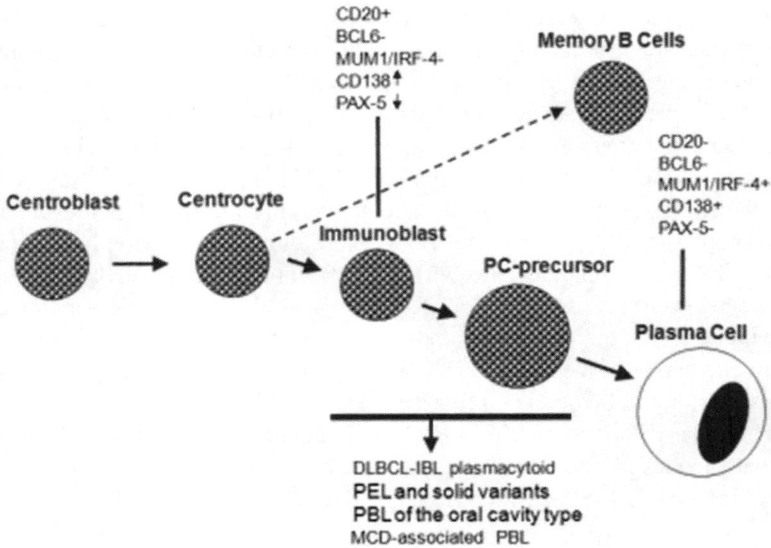

Fig. 6 Schematic showing the development of AIDS-related lymphomas with plasmablastic differentiation. *DLBCL* diffuse large B-cell lymphoma, *IBL* immunoblastic lymphoma, *MCD* multicentric Castleman disease, *PBL* plasmablastic lymphoma, *PC* plasma cell, *PEL* primary effusion lymphoma

center B cells. The expression of BCL-6, MUM1, and CD138 in these lymphomas corresponds to the stage from which they are thought to develop [6, 8]. Superimposed on this model are molecular events (e.g., MYC activation and p53 inactivation), aberrant somatic hypermutation resulting in mutations of one or more proto-oncogenes (e.g., c-*MYC*, PAX-5, PIM1, RhoH/TTF), and coinfection with EBV and HHV8. Moreover, cytokines (e.g., IL-6 and IL-10) and HAART likely further modify lymphomagenesis. HAART not only improves immune perturbations that may contribute to B-cell proliferation but also has other beneficial effects (e.g., enhances the responsiveness of EBV-specific cytotoxic T-cell lymphocytes and increases EBV-specific antibodies).

HIV Infection

Early in the AIDS epidemic, investigators presumed that HIV was a transforming retrovirus directly responsible for the development of ARL. However, we now know that HIV in fact does not infect lymphoma cells. The Tat (transactivator of transcription) protein of HIV, however, may be taken up by B lymphocytes, leading to deregulation of the oncosuppressor protein products of the pRb2/p130 gene [33]. Tat markedly increases the level of transcription of the HIV dsDNA and also plays a direct role in the HIV disease process (e.g., augments angiogenic activity in tumors). While HIV genomic sequences are rarely identified within lymphoma cells, tumor-associated macrophages have been found to harbor retroviral insertions [77]. Some authors have accordingly incorporated this information into a model of HIV lymphomagenesis in which the clonal proliferation of infected macrophages elaborates inflammatory cytokines that promote B-cell proliferation, with the eventual evolution to a monoclonal process [62]. Furthermore, HIV viral proteins likely also promote B-cell proliferation through T-cell gene alterations.

Immune Dysregulation

Proliferating viral-infected B-cells are controlled by cytotoxic T-cell (CTL) responses. However, disturbance of this equilibrium, which can occur in immunocompromised situations, may result in uncontrolled lymphoproliferation and the subsequent development of NHL [71]. HIV lymphomagenesis may also be related in part to impaired dendritic cell function and the resulting functional disorganization of lymph nodes that occurs with HIV infection [3].

Gamma Herpesviruses

Epstein-Barr virus (EBV) and Kaposi sarcoma herpesvirus/human herpesvirus 8 (KSHV/HHV8) are both members of the gamma herpesvirus subfamily. The 172 kbp EBV genome encodes approximately 100 genes, 10 of which are expressed during latency including six nuclear proteins (EBNAs 1, 2, 3A, 3B, 3C, and LP), two latent membrane proteins (LMP-1 and 2), and two EBV-encoded RNAs (EBERs 1 and 2). HHV8, a rhadinovirus, has a 165-kb genome with more than 80 open reading frames (ORF). HHV8 genes encode numerous proteins that are homologous to cell-signaling and regulatory-pathway proteins, such as viral interleukin-6 (vIL-6). While in latency, HHV8 exists as circular episomal DNA and expresses limited gene products, including LANA-1 (or LNA-1). As with all herpesviruses, the life cycle of these two viruses includes both latent and lytic phases. These viruses establish persistent latent infection in lymphocytes which contributes to the transformation process and helps drive cell proliferation and escape from immune attack [36, 66, 81]. Latency is characterized by persistence of the viral genome, restricted virus expression of latent gene products that alter cell growth and proliferation, and retained potential for reactivation to lytic replication. The frequency of EBV and HHV8 positivity in various ARLs is shown in Table 2. The relationship of HIV-associated lymphomas with EBV and HHV8 is further elaborated in Table 3.

Table 3 Relationship of HIV-associated lymphomas with EBV- and HHV8-associated lymphoproliferative disorders

EBV-associated B-cell lymphoproliferative disorders		HHV8-associated lymphoproliferative disorders
BL (both sporadic and epidemic)		PEL—in the absence of tumor masses
Classic Hodgkin's lymphoma		"Solid" lymphomas with serous effusions
Posttransplant lymphoproliferative disorders		Prior to the development of PEL
HIV-associated lymphomas	HIV-associated lymphomas	Following resolution of PEL
Immunodeficiency-associated BL-plasmacytoid		"Solid" lymphomas without serous effusions
Primary central nervous system lymphoma		Extracavitary (extranodal) tissue based
Diffuse large B-cell lymphoma, immunoblastic		Extracavitary (lymph node) tissue based
KSHV/HHV8-positive PEL and its solid variant		MCD-associated plasmablastic lymphomas
Plasmablastic lymphoma		Germinotropic lymphoproliferative disorder
Other histotypes (rare)[a]		Lymphomas with controversial association with KSHV/HHV8

EBV Epstein-Barr virus, *HHV8* human herpesvirus 8, *BL* Burkitt lymphoma, *PEL* primary effusion lymphoma, *MCD* multicentric Castleman disease

[a]Other histotypes include the following: lymphomatoid granulomatosis, pyothorax-associated lymphoma, senile EBV-associated B-cell lymphoproliferative disorders

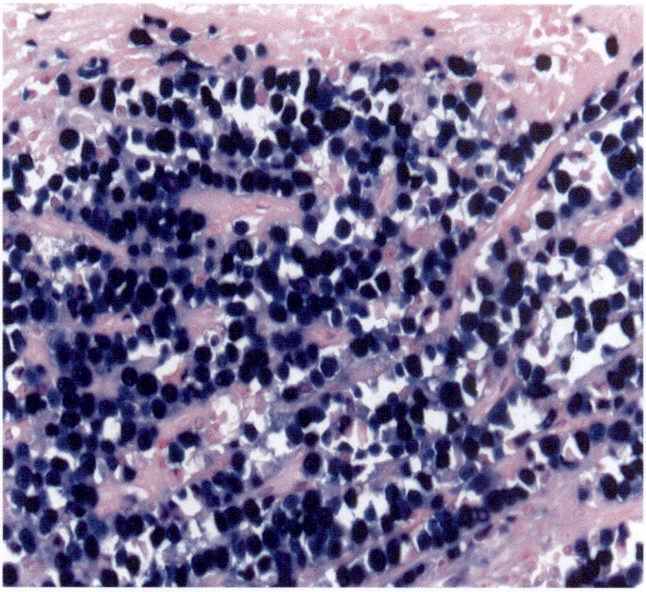

Fig. 7 Diffuse large B-cell lymphoma (DLBCL) of the anus showing strong Epstein-Barr Virus-encoded RNA (EBER) positivity in tumor cells (in situ hybridization; high magnification)

EBV Coinfection

Many HIV+patients are coinfected with EBV. Of interest, EBV-positive B lymphocytes occur more frequently in the CNS of HIV-infected individuals than in HIV-negative persons [2], which may account for the fact that almost all cases of PCNSL are associated with EBV infection. In many of the ARL, EBV directly infects lymphoma cells (Fig. 7) [67]. Defective T-cell immunity associated with HIV infection is partly responsible for the high frequency of EBV-infected B cells in patients with AIDS. The risk of developing an ARL appears to correlate with the decrease in EBV-specific cytotoxic lymphocytes [5], and not with the EBV viral load in peripheral blood mononuclear cells, as is the case in transplant recipients [84]. HIV immunosuppression with EBV coinfection favors the expansion of B-cell clones that when coupled with genetic alterations may transform into lymphoma.

HHV8 Coinfection

In 1995, HHV8 DNA sequences were identified within lymphoma cells of PEL [21]. Detecting evidence of viral infection by HHV8 in neoplastic cells (e.g., LNA-1 immunohistochemistry) is often essential for the diagnosis of PEL. Subsequently, the spectrum of HHV8-associated lymphomas has been expanded to include cases of extracavitary (solid) lymphomas without serous effusions and multicentric Castleman disease-associated plasmablastic lymphoma [14, 16]. While the exact mechanisms of HHV8-related oncogenesis are still under active investigation, researches have shown that this virus owns an elaborate set of tools aimed at overcoming antiviral responses and promoting tumorigenesis [39]. In PEL cells, the HHV8 genome exists as mono- or oligoclonal episomes, where most of the infected cells have been shown to express a latent pattern of gene expression. Latent gene products believed to play significant roles in lymphomagenesis include LNA-1 (ORF73), viral cyclin (v-*Cyc*, ORF72), and viral FLICE inhibitory protein (v-*FLIP*, ORF71). LNA-1 is required for the segregation and maintenance of viral DNA during replication, but may also impair apoptosis by binding to and inhibiting the human tumor suppressor genes TP53 and RB. Other potential genes that may be involved in lymphomagenesis are the viral interleukin-6 (IL6) and BCL-2 homologues, as well as a viral G-protein-coupled receptor (v-*GPCR*). Many of these viral genes are homologous to cellular oncogenes that modulate the cell cycle, apoptosis, and signal transduction or promote oncogenesis by other mechanisms. For example, signaling via v-*GPCR* upregulates vascular endothelial growth factor (VEGF) expression, which in turn induces angiogenesis.

Gene Dysregulation

ARLs contain several genetic abnormalities, some of which are peculiar to this group of lymphomas. DLBCL in AIDS, for example, has several genotypic differences compared with DLBCL in immunocompetent individuals; these include greater (20%) c-*MYC* translocations and absent BCL-2 activation [46]. Aberrant somatic hypermutation activity noted in DLBCL of HIV-negative patients has also been reported in many ARL including Burkitt lymphoma, PCNSL, and PEL [48].

BCL-6 Expression

The B-cell lymphoma 6 (BCL-6) gene, located at band 3q27, is a strong repressor of transcription for many proteins, including itself (autoregulation). BCL-6 is normally expressed in mature germinal center B cells, but not in differentiated plasma cells or memory B cells. Downregulation is necessary for normal B cells to exit the germinal center. BCL-6 overexpression in B-cell lymphomas prevents tumor cells from undergoing apoptosis, as a result of damaged DNA, and also blocks these cells from differentiating and exiting the germinal center. Overexpression of BCL-6 also downregulates several other genes such as p53. This explains why mutations in the p53 gene of DLBCL are seen almost exclusively in cases without BCL-6 translocations. Over 70% of all ARL have been shown to contain mutations resulting in deregulation of BCL-6 [47]. However, only 20% of AIDS-related DLBCL have BCL-6 mutations compared to 40% of DLBCL seen in HIV-negative hosts.

ARLs with BCL-6 overexpression exhibit a better prognosis than those with a post-germinal center (BCL-6 negative) origin [52].

c-*MYC* Expression

c-*MYC* overexpression is important in the pathogenesis of AIDS-related Burkitt lymphoma, as well as certain subtypes of high-grade DLBCL (20% of cases) and plasmablastic lymphomas in which it signifies a poor prognosis. c-*MYC* translocations in AIDS-related DLBCL occur more commonly than in DLBCL of HIV-negative patients [46]. The breakpoints within the c-*MYC* gene also differ between AIDS-related and endemic Burkitt lymphoma [42]. However, almost all tumor cells in cases of AIDS-related Burkitt lymphoma still have a reciprocal chromosomal translocation that places the c-*MYC* gene adjacent to the immunoglobulin loci. This in turn causes loss of regulation and constitutive expression of c-*MYC*.

p53 Mutation

Normal activation of p53 is important for cell cycle arrest, apoptosis, senescence, and differentiation. Downregulation of p53 expression or expression of mutant p53 products results largely in deregulation of apoptosis. In general, the presence of a p53 mutation is associated with poor overall survival. Limited studies have specifically explored p53 in ARL, even though many (60%) cases of AIDS-related Burkitt-like lymphoma appear to harbor mutations of this tumor suppressor gene [12].

Conclusion

ARLs encompass a heterogeneous group of lymphomas. Their heterogeneity likely reflects the various pathologic mechanisms important in lymphomagenesis including HIV-induced immunosuppression, chronic antigenic stimulation, genetic abnormalities, cytokine release and dysregulation, dendritic cell impairment, and coinfection with the herpesviruses EBV and HHV8. However, many of these ARL also have similarities such as plasmacellular differentiation, which may make them difficult to differentiate and therefore appropriately manage. In general, ARLs tend to be aggressive lymphomas with a propensity to present with advanced clinical disease, bulky tumors, high tumor burden, and involvement of extranodal sites. Enormous research efforts have allowed us to better understand the mechanisms involved in HIV lymphomagenesis, and as a result, several plausible pathogenesis models have been proposed. Although this chapter dealt mainly with the pathogenesis of B-cell AIDS-related NHL, the literature addressing mechanisms underlying other HIV-related lymphomas such as Hodgkin lymphoma is emerging [15]. Elucidating the exact role of HIV lymphomagenesis will hopefully provide us with potential therapeutic targets in the near future.

References

1. Aboulafia DM, Pantanowitz L, Dezube BJ (2004) AIDS-related non-Hodgkin's lymphoma: still a problem in the era of highly active antiretroviral therapy. AIDS Reader 14:605–617
2. Anthony IC, Crawford DH, Bell JE (2003) B lymphocytes in the normal brain: contrasts with HIV-associated lymphoid infiltrates and lymphomas. Brain 126:1058–67
3. Biancotto A, Grivel JC, Iglehart SJ et al (2007) Abnormal activation and cytokine spectra in lymph nodes of people chronically infected with HIV-1. Blood 109:4272–4279
4. Brimo F, Michel RP, Khetani K, Auger M (2007) Primary effusion lymphoma: a series of 4 cases and review of the literature with emphasis on cytomorphologic and immunocytochemical differential diagnosis. Cancer 111:224–233
5. Carbone A, Tirelli U, Gloghini A, Volpe R, Boiocchi M (1993) Human immunodeficiency virus-associated systemic lymphomas may be subdivided into two main groups according to Epstein-Barr viral latent gene expression. J Clin Oncol 11:1674–81
6. Carbone A, Gaidano G, Gloghini A et al (1998) Differential expression of BCL-6, CD138/syndecan-1, and Epstein-Barr virus-encoded latent membrane protein-1 identifies distinct histogenetic subsets of acquired immunodeficiency syndrome-related non-Hodgkin's lymphomas. Blood 91:747–755
7. Carbone A, Gaidano G, Gloghini A, Ferlito A, Rinaldo A, Stein H (1999) AIDS-related plasmablastic lymphomas of the oral cavity and jaws: a diagnostic dilemma. Ann Otol Rhinol Laryngol 108:95–99
8. Carbone A, Gloghini A, Larocca LM et al (2001) Expression profile of MUM1/ IRF4, BCL-6, and CD138/syndecan-1 defines novel histogenetic subsets of human immunodeficiency virus-related lymphomas. Blood 97:744–751
9. Carbone A (2002) AIDS-related non-Hodgkin's lymphomas: from pathology and molecular pathogenesis to treatment. Hum Pathol 33:392–404
10. Carbone A (2003) Emerging pathways in the development of AIDS-related lymphomas. Lancet Oncol 4:22–9
11. Carbone A, Gloghini A, Gaidano G (2004) Is plasmablastic lymphoma of the oral cavity an HHV-8-associated disease? Am J Surg Pathol 28:1538–1540
12. Carbone A, Gloghini A (2005) AIDS-related lymphomas: from pathogenesis to pathology. Br J Haematol 130:662–670
13. Carbone A, Gloghini A, Vaccher E et al (2005) Kaposi's sarcoma-associated herpesvirus/human herpesvirus type 8-positive solid lymphomas: a tissue-based variant of primary effusion lymphoma. J Mol Diagn 7:17–27
14. Carbone A, Gloghini A (2007) HHV-8-associated lymphoma: state-of-the-art review. Acta Haematol 117:129–131
15. Carbone A, Cabras A, Gloghini A (2007) HIV-associated Hodgkin's lymphoma. Antiapoptotic pathways and mechanisms for immune escape by tumor cells in the setting of improved immunity. Int J Biol Markers 22:161–163
16. Carbone A, Gloghini A (2008) KSHV/HHV8-associated lymphomas. Br J Haematol 140:13–24
17. Carbone A, Cesarman E, Spina M, Gloghini A, Schulz TF (2009) HIV-associated lymphomas and gamma-herpesviruses. Blood 113:1213–1224
18. Castillo J, Pantanowitz L, Dezube BJ (2008) HIV-associated plasmablastic lymphoma: lessons learned from 112 published cases. Am J Hematol 83:804–809
19. Castillo J, Perez K, Milani C, Dezube BJ, Pantanowitz L (2009) Peripheral T-cell lymphomas in HIV-infected individuals: a comprehensive review. J HIV Ther 14:34–40
20. Centers for Disease Control (1985) Revision of the case definition of acquired immunodeficiencies syndrome for national reporting. United States. MMWR 34:373
21. Cesarman E, Chang Y, Moore PS, Said JW, Knowles DM (1995) Kaposi's sarcoma-associated herpesvirus-like DNA sequences are present in AIDS-related body cavity-based lymphoma. NEJM 332:1186–1191

22. Chadburn A, Hyjek E, Mathew S, Cesarman E, Said J, Knowles DM (2004) KSHV-positive solid lymphomas represent an extra-cavitary variant of primary effusion lymphoma. Am J Surg Pathol 28:1401–1416
23. Chen YB, Rahemtullah A, Hochberg E (2007) Primary effusion lymphoma. Oncologist 12:569–576
24. Clifford GM, Rickenbach M, Lise M et al (2009) Hodgkin lymphoma in the Swiss HIV Cohort Study. Blood 113:5737–5742
25. Colomo L, Loong F, Rives S et al (2004) Diffuse large B-cell lymphomas with plasmablastic differentiation represent a heterogeneous group of disease entities. Am J Surg Pathol 28:736–747
26. Corti M, Villafane MF, Trione N, Narbaitz M (2005) Hodgkin lymphoma associated with human immunodeficiency virus type-1 infection: epidemiologic, clinic and histopathologic findings in 18 patients (article in Spanish). Med Clin (Barc) 124:116–117
27. Costes V, Faumont N, Cesarman E et al (2002) Human herpesvirus-8-associated lymphoma of the bowel in human immunodeficiency virus-positive patients without history of primary effusion lymphoma. Hum Pathol 33:846–849
28. Cote TR, Biggar RJ, Rosenberg PS et al (1997) Non-Hodgkin's lymphoma among people with AIDS: incidence, presentation and public health burden. AIDS/Cancer Study Group. Int J Cancer 73:645–650
29. Coupland SE, Charlotte F, Mansour G, Maloum K, Hummel M, Stein H (2005) HHV-8 associated T-cell lymphoma in a lymph node with concurrent peritoneal effusion in an HIV-positive man. Am J Surg Pathol 29:647–652
30. D'Apuzzo M, Rolink A, Loetscher M, Hoxie JA, Clark-Lewis I, Melchers F, Baggiolini M, Moser B (1997) The chemokine SDF-1, stromal cell-derived factor 1, attracts early stage B cell precursors via the chemokine receptor CXCR4. Eur J Immunol 27:1788–93
31. Dal Maso L, Franceschi S (2003) Epidemiology of non-Hodgkin lymphomas and other haemolymphopoietic neoplasms in people with AIDS. Lancet Oncol 4:110–119
32. Dargent JL, Lespagnard L, Sirtaine N, Cantinieaux B, Li R, Hermans P (2007) Plasmablastic microlymphoma occurring in human herpesvirus 8 (HHV-8)-positive multicentric Castleman's disease and featuring a follicular growth pattern. APMIS 115:869–874
33. De Falco G, Bellan C, Lazzi S, Claudio P, La Sala D, Cinti C, Tosi P, Giordano A, Leoncini L (2003) Interaction between HIV-1 Tat and pRb2/p130: a possible mechanism in the pathogenesis of AIDS-related neoplasms. Oncogene 18:6214–9
34. Dean M, Jacobson LP, McFarlane G et al (1999) Reduced risk of AIDS lymphoma in individuals heterozygous for the CCR5-delta32 mutation. Cancer Res 59:3561–3564
35. Delecluse HJ, Anagnostopoulos I, Dallenbach F et al (1997) Plasmablastic lymphomas of the oral cavity: a new entity associated with the human immunodeficiency virus infection. Blood 89:1413–1420
36. Delecluse HJ, Feederle R, O'Sullivan B, Taniere P (2007) Epstein Barr virus-associated tumours: an update for the attention of the working pathologist. J Clin Pathol 60:1358–1364
37. Deloose ST, Smit LA, Pals FT, Kersten MJ, van Noesel CJ, Pals ST (2005) High incidence of Kaposi sarcoma-associated herpesvirus infection in HIV-related solid immunoblastic/plasmablastic diffuse large B-cell lymphoma. Leukemia 19:851–855
38. Du MQ, Liu H, Diss TC et al (2001) Kaposi sarcoma-associated herpesvirus infects monotypic (IgM lambda) but polyclonal naive B cells in Castleman disease and associated lymphoproliferative disorders. Blood 97:2130–2136
39. Du MQ, Bacon CM, Isaacson PG (2007) Kaposi sarcoma-associated herpesvirus/human herpesvirus 8 and lymphoproliferative disorders. J Clin Pathol 60:1350–1357
40. Dupin N, Diss TL, Kellam P et al (2000) HHV-8 is associated with a plasmablastic variant of Castleman disease that is linked to HHV-8-positive plasmablastic lymphoma. Blood 95:1406–1412

41. Engels EA, Pittaluga S, Whitby D et al (2003) Immunoblastic lymphoma in persons with AIDS-associated Kaposi's sarcoma: a role for Kaposi's sarcoma-associated herpesvirus. Mod Pathol 16:424–429
42. Ferry JA (2006) Burkitt's lymphoma: clinicopathologic features and differential diagnosis. Oncologist 11:375–383
43. Frisch M, Biggar RJ, Engels EA et al (2001) Association of cancer with AIDS-related immunosuppression in adults. JAMA 285:1736–1745
44. Engels EA, Goedert JJ (2005) Human immunodeficiency virus/acquired immunodeficiency syndrome and cancer: past, present, and future. J Natl Cancer Inst 97:407–409
45. Engels EA, Pfeiffer RM, Landgren O, Moore RD (2010) Immunologic and virologic predictors of AIDS-related non-hodgkin lymphoma in the highly active antiretroviral therapy era. J Acquir Immune Defic Syndr 54:78–84
46. Gaidano G, Dalla-Favera R (1995) Molecular pathogenesis of AIDS-related lymphomas. Adv Cancer Res 67:113–153
47. Gaidano G, Capello D, Carbone A (2000) The molecular basis of acquired immunodeficiency syndrome-related lymphomagenesis. Semin Oncol 27:431–41
48. Gaidano G, Pasqualucci L, Capello D et al (2003) Aberrant somatic hypermutation in multiple subtypes of AIDS-associated non-Hodgkin lymphoma. Blood 102:1833–1841
49. Guiguet M, Boué F, Cadranel J, Lang JM, Rosenthal E, Costagliola D, Clinical Epidemiology Group of the FHDH-ANRS CO4 cohort (2009) Effect of immunodeficiency, HIV viral load, and antiretroviral therapy on the risk of individual malignancies (FHDH-ANRS CO4): a prospective cohort study. Lancet Oncol 10:1152–9
50. Hamoudi R, Diss TC, Oksenhendler E et al (2004) Distinct cellular origins of primary effusion lymphoma with and without EBV infection. Leuk Res 28:333–338
51. Herida M, Mary-Krause M, Kaphan R et al (2003) Incidence of non-AIDS-defining cancers before and during the highly active antiretroviral therapy era in a cohort of human immunodeficiency virus-infected patients. J Clin Oncol 21:3447–3453
52. Hoffmann C, Tiemann M, Schrader C et al (2005) AIDS-related B-cell lymphoma (ARL): correlation of prognosis with differentiation profiles assessed by immunophenotyping. Blood 106:1762–1769
53. International Collaboration on HIV and Cancer (2000) Highly active antiretroviral therapy and incidence of cancer in human immunodeficiency virus-infected adults. J Natl Cancer Inst 92:1823–1830
54. Isaacson PG, Campo E, Harris NL (2008) Large B-cell lymphoma arising in HHV8-associated multicentric Castleman disease. In: Swerdlow SH, Campo E, Harries NL et al (eds) WHO classification of tumours of haematopoeitic and lymphoid tissues, 4th edn. IARC Press, Lyon, pp 258–259
55. Jaffar SA, Pihan G, Dezube BJ, Pantanowitz L (2005) Differentiating HIV-associated lymphomas that exhibit plasmacellular differentiation. HIV AIDS Rev 4:43–49
56. Katano H, Suda T, Morishita Y et al (2000) Human herpesvirus 8-associated solid lymphomas that occur in AIDS patients take anaplastic large cell morphology. Mod Pathol 13:77–85
57. Klein U, Gloghini A, Gaidano G et al (2002) Gene expression profile analysis of AIDS-related primary effusion lymphoma (PEL) suggests a plasmablastic derivation and identifies PEL-specific transcripts. Mod Pathol 15:1273–1278
58. Levine AM, Sadighi S, Espina B, Tulpule A, Nathwani B (2002) Characteristics of indolent non-Hodgkin's lymphoma in patients infected with type 1 human immunodeficiency virus infection. Cancer 94:1500–1506
59. Mantina H, Wiggill TM, Carmona S, Perner Y, Stevens WS (2010) Characterization of lymphomas in a high prevalence HIV setting. J Acquir Immune Defic Syndr 53:656–60
60. Mate JL, Navarro JT, Ariza A et al (2004) Oral solid form of primary effusion lymphoma mimicking plasmablastic lymphoma. Hum Pathol 35:632–635
61. McGrath MS, Shiramizu B, Meeker TC et al (1991) AIDS-associated polyclonal lymphoma: identification of a new HIV-associated disease process. J Acquir Immune Defic Syndr 4:408–415

62. McGrath MD, Herndier B (2000) Clonal HIV in the pathogenesis of AIDS-related lymphoma: sequential pathogenesis. In: Goedert JJ (ed) Infectious causes of cancer: targets for intervention. Humana Press, Totowa, NJ, pp 231–242
63. Nador RG, Cesarman E, Chadburn A et al (1996) Primary effusion lymphoma: a distinct clinicopathologic entity associated with the Kaposi's sarcoma-associated herpes virus. Blood 88:645–656
64. Nador RG, Chadburn A, Gundappa G, Cesarman E, Said JW, Knowles DM (2003) Human immunodeficiency virus (HIV)-associated polymorphic lymphoproliferative disorders. Am J Surg Pathol 27:293–302
65. Navarro JT, Ribera JM, Junca J, Milla F (2003) Anorectal lymphoma without effusion associated with human herpesvirus-8 and type 1 Epstein-Barr virus in an HIV-infected patient. Hum Pathol 34:630
66. Ng SB, Khoury JD (2009) Epstein-Barr virus in lymphoproliferative processes: an update for the diagnostic pathologist. Adv Anat Pathol 16:40–55
67. Ometto L, Menin C, Masiero S et al (1997) Molecular profile of Epstein-Barr virus in human immunodeficiency virus type 1-related lymphadenopathies and lymphomas. Blood 90:313–22
68. Pantanowitz L, Wu Z, Dezube BJ, Pihan G (2005) Human Herpesvirus 8 (HHV8)-associated extracavitary-based lymphoma of the anorectum. Clin Lymphoma 6:49–152
69. Pantanowitz L, Dezube BJ (2007) Editorial comment: plasmablastic lymphoma—a diagnostic and therapeutic puzzle. AIDS Read 17:448–449
70. Perez K, Castillo J, Dezube BJ, Pantanowitz L (2010) Human immunodeficiency virus-associated anaplastic large cell lymphoma. Leuk Lymphoma 51:430–438
71. Pietersma F, Piriou E, van Baarle D (2008) Immune surveillance of EBV-infected B cells and the development of non-Hodgkin lymphomas in immunocompromised patients. Leuk Lymphoma 49:1028–41
72. Queiroga EM, Gualco G, Chioato L, Harrington WJ, Araujo I, Weiss LM, Bacchi CE (2008) Viral studies in burkitt lymphoma: association with Epstein-Barr virus but not HHV-8. Am J Clin Pathol 130:186–192
73. Raphael M, Said J, Borisch B, Cesarman E, Harris NL (2008) Lymphomas associated with HIV infection. In: Swerdlow SH, Campo E, Harries NL et al (eds) WHO classification of tumours of haematopoeitic and lymphoid tissues, 4th edn. IARC Press, Lyon, pp 340–342
74. Rafaniello Raviele P, Pruneri G, Maiorano E (2009) Plasmablastic lymphoma: a review. Oral Dis 15:38–45
75. Said JW, Shintaku IP, Asou H et al (1999) Herpesvirus 8 inclusions in primary effusion lymphoma: report of a unique case with T-cell phenotype. Arch Path Lab Med 123:257–260
76. Scadden DT (2003) AIDS-related malignancies. Annu Rev Med 54:285–303
77. Shiramizu B, Herndier B, McGrath M (1994) Identification of a common clonal HIV integration site in HIV-associated lymphomas. Cancer Res 54:2069–2072
78. Simonelli C, Spina M, Cinelli R et al (2003) Clinical Features and outcome of primary effusion lymphoma in HIV-infected patients: a single-institution study. J Clin Oncol 21:3948–3954
79. Stein H, Harris NL, Campo E (2008) Plasmablastic lymphoma. In: Swerdlow SH, Campo E, Harries NL et al (eds) WHO classification of tumours of haematopoeitic and lymphoid tissues, 4th edn. IARC Press, Lyon, pp 256–257
80. Straus DJ, Juang J, Testa MA, Levine AM, Kaplan LD (1998) Prognostic factors in the treatment of HIV-associated non-Hodgkin's lymphoma: Analysis of AIDS Clinical Trials Group protocol 142: Low-dose versus standard dose m-BACOD plus GM-CSF. J Clin Oncol 16:3601–3606
81. Swaminathan S (2003) Molecular biology of Epstein-Barr virus and Kaposi's sarcoma-associated herpesvirus. Semin Hematol 40:107–115
82. Teruya-Feldstein J (2005) Diffuse large B-cell lymphomas with plasmablastic differentiation. Curr Oncol Rep 7:357–363

83. Thompson LD, Fisher SI, Chu WS et al (2004) HIV-associated Hodgkin lymphoma: a clinicopathologic and immunophenotypic study of 45 cases. Am J Clin Pathol 121:727–738
84. Van Baarle D, Wolthers KC, Hovenkamp E et al (2002) Absolute level of Epstein-Barr virus DNA in human immunodeficiency virus type 1 infection is not predictive of AIDS-related non-Hodgkin lymphoma. J Infect Dis 186:405–409
85. Vega F, Chang CC, Medeiros LJ et al (2005) Plasmablastic lymphomas and plasmablastic plasma cell myelomas have nearly identical immunophenotypic profiles. Mod Pathol 18:806–815

Epstein-Barr Virus Lymphomagenesis and Therapeutic Targets

Huilan Rao and Roberto N. Miranda

Abstract The pathogenic role of the Epstein-Barr virus (EBV) has been suggested because it is consistently found in some lymphoproliferative disorders. More than 90% of the population is exposed to the virus, usually during childhood, and after initial exposure, the virus survives for the lifetime of individuals as an episome, and expresses a limited set of proteins depending on the immune status of the host. The variable expression of viral proteins is known as latency pattern with minimal expression of viral products in immunocompetent hosts, but expression of numerous viral products in the immunocompromised host. Thus, the more virus products that are expressed, the more targets for an immune reaction. Since it is acknowledged that the neoplastic process including lymphoproliferative disorders result from a multistep chain of events, multiple pathways are affected, and in particular in EBV-positive lymphoproliferations, EBV products interact with abnormally activated pathways in the context of the immune response of the host. In this review we analyze the structure of the virus and its interaction in the immunocompetent as well as in the immunocompromised host, and discuss the possible roles of EBV products in various lymphoproliferative disorders. Finally, we discuss the potential role of expressed EBV viral proteins and activation of pathogenic pathways in the setting of specific diagnostic categories with the identification of potential molecular targets.

H. Rao
Department of Pathology, Cancer Center, Sun Yat-sen University,
Guangzhou 510060, China
e-mail: raohl@sysucc.org.cn

R.N. Miranda (✉)
Department of Hematopathology, M.D. Anderson Cancer Center,
1515 Holcombe Blvd., Houston, TX 77030, USA
e-mail: roberto.miranda@mdanderson.org

P.J. Quesenberry and J.J. Castillo (eds.), *Non-Hodgkin Lymphoma: Prognostic Factors and Targets*, Cancer Drug Discovery and Development,
DOI 10.1007/978-1-4614-5851-7_4, © Springer Science+Business Media New York 2013

Epstein-Barr Virus Structure, Expressed Genes, and Pathogenesis

Epstein-Barr virus (EBV) or human herpes virus 4 is a ubiquitous virus that infects more than 90% of the human population and usually establishes a persistent latent infection in the host. Primary infection occurs via salivary contact in infancy and is usually asymptomatic, however when primary infection occurs in adolescents or young adults it may manifest as infectious mononucleosis. After primary infection, the virus usually remains in an asymptomatic latent state within resting memory B-cells for the lifetime of the host. Cytotoxic T-cells, both CD8+ and CD4+, and natural killer (NK) cells are in charge to recognize and eliminate the virus-infected cells [1]. When infected B-cells evade or suppress the T-cell immune response, or the host's cellular immune system fails to control EBV-induced B-cell proliferations, the infected B-cells can transform into neoplastic cells and eventually manifest as a lymphoproliferative disorder. EBV-associated lymphoproliferative disorders encompass a heterogeneous group of disorders, including chronic active EBV infection, B-cell lymphoma, T/NK-cell lymphoma or leukemia, classical Hodgkin lymphoma, as well as immunodeficiency and posttransplant lymphoproliferative disorders.

EBV infection occurs through the binding of the major viral envelope glycoprotein gp350 to the CD21 receptor on the surface of B cells and through the binding of glycoprotein gp42 to human leukocyte antigen (HLA) as a coreceptor [2]. The viral genome is linear and becomes circular by fusion of either end of the genome, and the virus persists within cells as an episome. EBV virus expresses genes in two distinct programs known as the lytic cycle and the latent cycle [3, 4]. During the lytic cycle, there is production of infectious virus and expression of viral genes that encode proteins involved in DNA replication and in assembly of viral particles. In contrast, during the latent cycle only a limited number of viral genes are expressed, and these include six nuclear proteins, referred to as *EBV nuclear antigens* (EBNA 1, 2, 3A, 3B, 3C, and EBNA-LP), and three latent membrane proteins (LMP 1, 2A and 2B), which are associated with transforming activity [5]. There are two nontranslated RNA molecules known as the EBV-encoded RNAs designated as EBER1 and EBER2. In addition, there are EBV microRNAs (miRNAs), which are encoded in two regions: BHRF1 (Bam HI fragment H rightward open reading frame 1) and BART (Bam HI-A region rightward transcript). miRNAs are the only known functional products of the BARTs transcripts [6]. BHRF1 miRNAs have been found highly expressed in immortalized lymphoblastoid cell lines (LCL), whereas BARTs miRNAs have been found in all EBV-infected cell lines as well as in biopsies of lymphoma cases [6].

There are four types of latent infection, designated as latency 0, I, II, and III, that reflect the extent of viral protein expression allowed by the host in vivo. Latency 0 refers to infection of cells where most viral genes are not expressed and therefore cells are not recognized or targeted by EBV-specific T lymphocytes; this stage is also called "in vivo latency" [1, 7]. EBV resides in memory B cells, which constitute a long-term reservoir for EBV. Thus, in the absence of production of viral proteins or antigens, there is no EBV-specific T cells neither is there an immune response

Table 1 Latency patterns of infection with Epstein-Barr virus and associated lymphoproliferative disorders

Latency type	Viral gene expressed					Lymphomas and cells affected
	EBERs	BARTs	EBNA1	EBNA2/3A, 3B, 3C/LP	LMP1/2	
0	+	+	–	–	–	Memory B-cells
I	+	+	+	–	–	Memory B-cells, BL
II	+	+	+	–	+	GCB, CHL, PTCL, AITL, NK/T
III	+	+	+	+	+	LCL, PTLD, AIDS-related lymphoma, EBV+ DLBCL of the elderly

AIDS acquired immunodeficiency syndrome, *AITL* angioimmunoblastic T-cell lymphoma, *BART* EBV microRNA, *BL* Burkitt lymphoma, *CHL* classical Hodgkin lymphoma, *DLBCL* diffuse large B-cell lymphoma, *EBER* Epstein-Barr virus encoded RNA, *GCB* germinal center B-cells, *LCL* lymphoblastoid cell lines, *NK/T* NK/T-cell lymphoma, *PTCL* peripheral T-cell lymphoma

against EBV. Activation of EBV-infected memory B cells can lead to their differentiation into plasma cells, a process that might switch-on the lytic cycle of EBV and produce viral particles [8]. Three latency patterns are associated with different types of lymphoid proliferations (Table 1). In latency type I there is selective expression of EBNA-1 and LMP-2A, and this pattern is found typically in Burkitt lymphoma (BL). In latency type II, there is expression of EBNA-1, LMP-1, LMP-2A, and LMP-2B, and this pattern is found in classical Hodgkin lymphoma (HL), primary effusion lymphoma, angioimmmunoblastic T-cell lymphoma (AITL), peripheral T-cell lymphoma (PTCL) and NK/T cell lymphoma or leukemia. In latency type III there is expression of all nine latent cycle EBV antigens, and this pattern is typically found in posttransplant lymphoproliferative disorders (PTLD) and in AIDS-related lymphoma. Because there are more viral proteins expressed in latency type II and III infections, respective EBV-associated lymphoproliferations are more immunogenic than diseases associated with a latency type I.

EBV-Related Lymphoproliferative Disorders

Burkitt Lymphoma

Burkitt lymphoma (BL) is a highly aggressive B-cell lymphoma that was initially described in children around equatorial Africa [9]. There are three clinical variants of BL: endemic, sporadic, and human immunodeficiency virus (HIV)-associated.

The EBV genome is present in almost all cases of endemic BL and there is strong epidemiological link with endemic malaria. In sporadic BL, EBV is identified in 15–30% of cases, while it is more common in HIV-associated BL.

The neoplastic cells of BL express B-cell lineage and B-cell germinal center cell markers CD10 and Bcl6. At the molecular level, the neoplastic cells undergo somatic hypermutation (SHM) and class-switch recombination (CSR) supporting the notion that they derive from germinal center cells. It is suspected that SHM and CSR predispose GC cells to chromosome translocations or mutations in non-Ig genes [10]. Virtually all BL cases carry one of three characteristic chromosomal translocations between the *MYC* gene in chromosome 8 and one of the immunoglobulin genes on chromosomes 2, 14, or 22 [1]. The role of *MYC* deregulation as the key factor in the pathogenesis of BL is compelling [11–13]. Most cases of BL show DNA breakpoints in rearranged VJ regions or in S regions of the immunoglobulin heavy chain (IgH) loci, thus it is generally accepted that the chromosomal translocations are mediated by aberrant SHM or CSR, which require the intervention of DNA-modifying enzymes known as activation-induced deaminase (AID). Most *MYC*/Ig breakpoints in EBV-positive endemic BL appear to originate from aberrant SHM. On the other hand, the translocations in sporadic cases mostly involve the Ig switch regions of the IgH locus [14]. EBV may be accounted for the difference in *MYC* breakpoints between EBV-positive BL and EBV-negative BL [15].

Genes downstream of *MYC* regulate cell cycle progression, cell growth, apoptosis, and senescence. Deregulated expression of MYC induces p53 response and triggers apoptosis [16, 17].

EBV has a latency type I pattern, with expression of EBNA1 and LMP2A. Since EBNA1 is the only viral gene product in all latency patterns, it is suspected that EBNA1 promotes lymphomagenesis in EBV+ processes. Although Kang et al. [18] suggested that EBNA1 is limited to maintenance of the viral genome, other researchers showed that EBNA1 may activate the catalytic subunit p91 of the NADPH oxidase2 (NOX2) at the transcriptional level. Thus EBNA1 generates reactive oxygen species that may contribute to DNA damage and genomic instability [19]. Furthermore, other researchers reported that EBNA1 binds to the deubiquitinating enzyme HAUSP/USP7 and together sequester p53, contributing to p53 degradation [20].

LMP2A expression was recently confirmed in endemic BL using a sensitive RT-PCR assay [13, 21]. LMP2A contains a 119 amino terminal cytoplasmic domain that includes eight tyrosine residues, two of which form an immunoreceptor tyrosine-based activation motif (ITAM) [22]. Experimental data using EBV LCLs in vitro and LMP2A-transgenic mice indicate that the cytoplasmic tail of LMP2A mimic signals used by the B-cell receptor (BCR) and promotes B-cell development. In effect, LMP2A constitutively phosphorylates Lyn and Syk, with Lyn binding to tyrosine 112 and Syk binding to the ITAM motif of LMP2A. Additional studies using LMP2A-transgenic mice demonstrate that LMP2A constitutively phosphorylates and activates many of the proteins induced by BCR, such as Lyn, Syk, BLNK, BTK, Ras, P13K, NF-κB, and MAP kinases [23–26]. LMP2A also increases the levels of anti-apoptotic Bcl family members and protect B cells from apoptosis [13].

Chemotherapy is the standard of care for immunocompetent patients with EBV-associated BL; however it is expected that targeting EBV therapy may contribute to better outcomes, or the use of EBV vaccines may decrease the incidence of endemic BL.

Diffuse Large B-Cell Lymphoma of the Elderly

EBV-positive diffuse large B-cell lymphoma (EBV+ DLBCL) of the elderly, also known as age-related EBV+ lymphoproliferative disorder, accounts for 8–10% of DLBCL cases [27]. Neoplastic cells are B-lymphocytes that lack germinal center cell markers CD10 and Bcl6, consistent with post GC B-cells. The neoplastic cells most often display an EBV type III latency, positive for EBV protein products including LMP1 and EBNA-2, although some cases express latency II, and lack EBNA expression [28, 29] The variable presence of EBNA2 expression is attributed to the variable degrees of immune surveillance in aging individuals.

EBV infection and waning immunity that is part of the aging process, where a decrease in T-cell response occurs, naturally appear to be the main driving mechanisms [30]. Decrease in T-cell function leads to EBV reactivation that manifests with the expression of proteins such as LMP1 that leads to upregulation of anti-apoptotic proteins Bcl-2, MCL-1, and A20 [31, 32].

The prognosis of EBV-positive DLBCL of the elderly is worse than EBV-negative DLBCL, partially compounded by a high median age of patients between 70 and 75 years, who are often unable to tolerate aggressive therapeutic regimens, thus an optimal regimen has not been established for EBV-positive DLBCL of the elderly. The development of adoptive immunotherapy with cytotoxic T cells (CTLs) directed against EBV latency antigens has the potential of improving the outcome of this group of patients.

Classical Hodgkin Lymphoma

Classical Hodgkin lymphoma (CHL) is clinically distinct from non-Hodgkin lymphoma and histologically is characterized by an exuberant inflammatory background and only rare or few neoplastic cells. The neoplastic cells are large mononuclear or multinucleated known as Hodgkin Reed-Sternberg (HRS) cells. CHL comprises four histological subtypes [33] and the prevalence of EBV varies with the histological subtype. The prevalence is highest (~75%) in mixed cellularity HL, and lowest (10~40%) in nodular sclerosis HL [34]. It is also notorious that the prevalence of EBV in CHL varies with epidemiologic factors; EBV infection is more prevalent in developing countries and affects mostly childhood, and older adult age groups (age >50 years).

The neoplastic cells of CHL are monoclonal B cells at the germinal center stage of differentiation [35–37]. Analysis of the Ig variable (IgV) gene regions show evidence of somatic hypermutation, revealing a germinal center (GC) or post-GC origin [38].

EBV is believed to play a causal role in the pathogenesis of CHL. EBV is detected in HRS cells and the virus is clonal, indicating that infection occurred prior to neoplastic transformation [39, 40]. In EBV-positive CHL, the HRS cells demonstrate latency type II pattern, and express EBNA1, LMP1 and LMP2.

LMP1 is considered the major transforming protein of EBV. It has an integral membrane protein comprising 386 amino acids and consists of a short amino (N)-terminal cytoplasmic stretch, 6 trans-membrane (6TM) domains, and a long carboxyl (C)-terminal cytoplasmic region with no significant extracellular domain [41]. The 6TM domains regulate their own synthesis and degradation via the unfolded protein response (UPR) and autophagy. The carboxy terminal domain induces proliferation and survival of EBV-infected B cells in vitro and in vivo [42, 43]. LMP1 mimics CD40 and can substitute for the signaling of CD40 in B cells [41, 42, 44].

LMP1 activates the signaling pathways of nuclear factor-κB (NF-κB), activated protein 1 (AP1), and signal transducer and activator of transcription (STAT). Aberrant activation of NF-κB plays a determinant role in cell transformation, while tumor promotion is mediated by its anti-apoptotic functions. Evidence shows that NF-κB activation by LMP1 is critical for B cell transformation in vitro and in vivo [45, 46]. LMP1 can induce most of the phenotypic changes of neoplastic cells, including expression of surface antigens CD21, CD23, CD30, CD40, CD44, and Fas as well as cell adhesion molecules ICAM1, LFA1, and LFA3. LMP1 also upregulates expression of the anti-apoptotic proteins Bcl-2, A20, Bfl, and Mcl1 and stimulates production of cytokines interleukin (IL)-6 and IL-8 [47, 48]. HRS cells express constitutively CD30 that is a trans-membrane protein which belongs to the tumor necrosis factor (TNF) receptor family [49]. When stimulated by CD30 ligand, CD30 interacts with TNF receptor-associated factors TRAF2 and TRAF5, mediating signal transduction that leads to the activation of the NF-κB pathway. Another potential role of LMP1 is the downregulation of CD99. Loss of CD99 has been associated with generation of B cells with CHL immunophenotype.

LMP2A mimics the BCR and competes with BCR to bind tyrosine kinases, thereby modulating the activity of these tyrosine kinases. LMP2B is not essential for EBV-induced B-cell transformation in vitro [50].

Mechanisms and cell interactions of HRS in CHL are complex. In EBV+ CHL, most of the reactive T lymphocytes have a regulatory T-cell phenotype, and LMP1 may mediate their attraction through IL-10 secretion [51]. The presence of regulatory cells around HRS cells causes a profoundly immunosuppressive microenvironment, contributing to evade or suppress immune T-cell responses. Thus, the use of EBV-specific T-cells to deliver immunostimulatory cytokines may counteract immunoregulatory T-cells and contribute to eliminate HRS cells. Similarly, HRS cells positive for LMP1 and LMP2A can be targeted with adoptive transfer of

EBV-CTL (cytotoxic T cells) [52]. Clinical data showed that LMP2-specific CTLs augmented T-cell responses, migrated to tumor deposits, and caused regression of tumors in a subset of patients with CHL [53]. LMP1 is another potential target for CHL immunotherapy. LMP1 effect or function has been targeted directly, using single-chain antibodies or antisense RNA approaches, and indirectly, by the genetic or pharmacological interception of its downstream effects on NF-κB [54].

NK/T-Cell Lymphoproliferative Disorders

EBV-related NK/T-cell lymphoproliferative disorders (LPD) include aggressive NK-cell leukemia, EBV-positive T-cell lymphoproliferative disorders of childhood, angioimmunoblastic T-cell lymphoma (AITL), extranodal NK/T-cell lymphoma, nasal type, and peripheral T-cell lymphoma, not otherwise specified (PTCL, NOS).

EBV can infect CD4+ and CD8+ peripheral blood T-cells as well as NK-cells in a minority of patients with infectious mononucleosis. The mechanisms of access of EBV into T cells and NK cells in vivo are speculative. It has been shown that NK cells activated by EBV acquire CD21 by synaptic transfer from CD21+ B cells, and these ectopic receptors allow EBV binding to NK-cells. It is possible that NK cells in close contact with EBV-infected B cells may acquire EBV infection directly and then expand clonally [55].

Most EBV-associated T-cell lymphomas are thought to arise from chronic active EBV infection (CAEBV). CAEBV is considered as a progressive EBV infection from infected B-cells. Evidence suggests that CAEBV of NK/T-cells develops into NK/T cell lymphoma [56].

In EBV-positive T-cell LPD of childhood, there is a monoclonal proliferation of CD4+ or CD8+ cells with viral gene expression of EBNA1, LMP1 and LMP2, consistent with a latency type II pattern. In extranodal NK/T-cell lymphoma, nasal type, disease usually presents in the nasal or upper aerodigestive tract and most patients are of Asian origin.

The pathogenesis of EBV in NK/T-cell lymphoma may be similar to that of CHL, since both have a latency type II pattern of EBV infection. In this model, LMP1 mimics and activates NF-κB pathway, as previously discussed. Yang et al. [57] reported that increased IL-9 levels induced by the EBERs possess anti-apoptotic effects and promote T-cell proliferation and transformation. Further research is needed to determine how EBV infects NK/T cells and the pathogenic role of EBV.

Since LMP1 expression in EBV-associated NK/T cell lymphomas activates the NF-κB pathway, targeted therapies have been applied to inhibit NF-κB activation. Several targets that inhibit the NF-κB pathway have been identified [58]. For example, bortezomib, a proteasome inhibitor, leads to increased levels of I-κB kinase and inhibits activation of NF-κB. Dehydroxymethylepoxyquinomicin, another inhibitor of NF-κB, induces apoptosis of EBV-transformed B cells [48].

Immunodeficiency-Related Lymphoproliferative Disorders

Congenital Immunodeficiency-Related Lymphoproliferation

Congenital immunodeficiency also called primary immunodeficiency is present at the time of birth, and may occur as a result of defects in B- or T-lymphocytes, or both. X-linked lymphoproliferative disease (XLP) is an inherited syndrome characterized by extreme sensitivity to EBV infection that leads to severe infectious mononucleosis, acquired hypogammaglobulinemia, and/or malignant lymphoma [59]. The defective gene in XLP has been identified as src homology 2 domain protein 1A (SH2D1A) also known as signaling lymphocytic activation molecule (SLAM)-associated protein (SAP) gene [60]. SAP is a key regulator of normal immune function in T cells, NK cells, and in certain B-cell lines. Evidence both from knockout mice and from XLP patients show that SAP deficiency has multiple immunologic effects. These include significantly impaired Th2-like CD4+ T-cell responses, reflected as poor IL-10 production in in vitro assays of T-dependent B cell responses that associate with in vivo defective Ig class switching, affinity maturation of antibody responses, and memory B cell development [61]. Both functional cytotoxic T-cell defects and abnormal cytokine production as a result of SAP deficiency may explain the failure to control EBV infection and predisposition to B-cell lymphoma.

For some patients with primary immunodeficiency, there is promise with hematopoietic stem cell transplant (HSCT).

Lymphoproliferative Disorders Associated with Human Immunodeficiency Virus and Acquired Immunodeficiency Syndrome

There is an increased frequency of EBV infection in human immunodeficiency virus (HIV)/acquired immunodeficiency syndrome (AIDS)-associated lymphomas. AIDS patients have 10–20 times more EBV-infected B-cells than healthy counterparts and the risk of NHL is 60–200 times higher than persons noninfected with HIV [1]. EBV is detected in up to 60% of all HIV-related lymphomas, including nearly 100% of primary CNS lymphomas, 80% of DLBCL with immunoblastic features, 30–50% of BL, 70% of primary effusion lymphomas, and nearly 100% of CHL [62, 63]. The increased risk for EBV-related lymphoma among HIV-infected individuals appears related to multiple factors, including duration and degree of immunosuppression, induction of cytokines leading to B-cell proliferation, and coinfection with HHV8. HIV infection can act as chronic stimuli for the B-cell system, characterized by marked hyperplasia of germinal centers, which greatly increases the chances of *MYC* translocations. HIV also induces abnormal immune response and probably increases the number of EBV-infected B-cells that are at risk of being recruited into the germinal center reaction [48]. There is constitutive expression of LMP1 that supports an EBV-driven proliferation.

The use of highly active antiretroviral therapy (HAART) has resulted in a fall in the incidence of opportunistic infections and AIDS-related malignancies, including lymphoma. However, EBV-associated lymphoma still is one of the most frequent causes of death in HIV-infected patients. Therefore, there is a need in identifying viral targets and evaluate the potential benefit of molecular-targeted chemotherapy.

Iatrogenic Immunodeficiency-Associated Lymphoproliferative Disorders

The WHO classification includes the category of "Other iatrogenic immunodeficiency-associated lymphoproliferative disorders" that are lymphoid proliferations or lymphomas that arise in patients treated with immunosuppressive drugs for autoimmune diseases or conditions other than in the transplant setting. The most common subtype of lymphoma is DLBCL. The better-known agent is methotrexate (MTX), which is commonly used in patients with rheumatoid arthritis. MTX directly reactivates EBV with subsequent release of infectious virions [64]. Since patients with rheumatoid arthritis have impaired T-cell responses to EBV products [65], therapy with MTX results in higher EBV loads in their blood and immunodeficient conditions that predispose to EBV-driven lymphoma.

Posttransplant Lymphoproliferative Disorders

Posttransplant lymphoproliferative disorders (PTLD) constitute a heterogeneous group of lymphoproliferations that occur in the setting of allogeneic transplantation of solid organs (SOT) or hematopoietic stem cells (HSCT). In patients with PTLD, the incidence of EBV ranges from 73 to 100% [5]. Morphologically, PTLD can be subdivided into monomorphic, polymorphic, plasmacytic, or HL-like variants. Most PTLD are of B-cell origin, and 10–15% are of T-cell origin [66, 67].

Patients with PTLD have impaired anti-EBV cellular immunity because of iatrogenic immunosuppression, resulting in EBV-induced transformation of B-cells. In addition, the immunomodulation used to prevent graft-versus-host disease (GVHD) remove T-cells nonspecifically from the graft and increases the risk of PLTD [68].

The pathogenic mechanisms of EBV in PTLD are presumably similar to those in CHL. Because approximately 50% cases of PTLD are derived from aberrant GC B cells that lack a functional BCR, HRS cells escape apoptosis through alternative survival signals. It is considered that LMP1 and LMP2A replace survival signals induced by activated CD40 and BCR receptors and activate NF-κB signaling pathway, inducing proliferation of neoplastic cells. As already mentioned, the decreased cytotoxic T-cell surveillance also increases the susceptibility to EBV.

In the absence of effective T-cell surveillance, EBV+ lymphomas in immunodeficient individuals usually express a latency type III pattern. All the EBNA and LMP viral proteins are expressed together with various noncoding small RNAs (EBERs and miRNAs). EBNA3 family of proteins (EBNA3A, 3B, and 3C) are nuclear phosphoproteins that act as transcriptional regulators. Only EBNA3A and EBNA3B have been shown to be essential for B-cell transformation. A number of functional domains have been characterized for these proteins, including transactivation, repression, and nuclear localization domains, but their roles have not been elucidated. It has been noted that conserved regions of EBNA3A, 3B, 3C are capable of binding to RBP, while EBNA3A and 3C can bind to the ATPase/Helicase DP103 [69]. Krauer et al. [70] showed that EBNA-3 disrupt the DNA damage and replication at the G2/M checkpoint. EBNA3A and EBNA3C together have been found to interfere with the proapoptotic protein Bim [71]. EBNA3C appears to also have repressor functions potentially mediated via its interaction with a histone deacetylase [72]. In addition, studies have shown that EBNA3C is an immortalizing oncogene capable of cooperating with (Ha)-ras in cotransformation assays and is capable of overriding Rb-mediated pathways [73].

In latency III, EBNA2 acts as a transcription factor to induce expression of the viral LMP genes and many cell genes. EBNA2 interacts with a sequence-specific DNA-binding protein, Jκ-recombination-binding protein (RBP-Jκ) [3], to transcriptionally activate cellular genes such as CD21 and CD23 and key viral genes LMP1 and LMP2A [74, 75]. In addition, EBNA2 can modify chromatin structure through recruitment of SWI/SNF. EBNA-LP interacts with EBNA2 and is required for the efficient outgrowth of virus-transformed B cells in vitro. The transcriptional activation mediated by EBNA2/EBNA-LP is modulated by the EBNA3 family of proteins, repressing transactivation.

Therapeutic Targets of EBV

The association of EBV with various lymphoproliferative disorders suggests that EBV plays a pathogenic role. Various pathways linked with tumorigenesis are activated in these processes, and plausible mechanisms involving viral products have been identified. Thus, the identification of the molecular mechanisms associated with EBV tumor promotion and progression may contribute to identify molecular targets for immune attack, small molecules or interfering RNA. Other therapeutic options include adoptive immunotherapy, antiviral therapy, and therapies against EBV-driven signaling or transfer of antigens.

Adoptive transfer of EBV-specific cytotoxic T-cells (CTLs) has been proven effective in treating posttransplant EBV-associated lymphomas. The research in this field has moved quickly from animal experiments to the bedside [75]. EBV-specific CTL have been successfully infused in patients subjected to hematopoietic stem cell transplant (HSCT) and solid organ transplant (SOT), both with therapeutic and prophylactic purposes. In a study that included 108 HSCT recipients and 21 SOT recipients, patients received virus-specific CTL as a preemptive approach. No events of lymphoproliferation were reported at follow-up, except for one patient who received an infusion lacking a well-defined EBV-specific component [76]. The success of CTL therapy in PTLD has not been reproduced in CHL and BL probably due to cell mechanisms that evade EBV-specific immune responses. For example, HRS cells create a microenvironment that suppresses EBV-specific T-cell responses.

EBV-related lymphoproliferations have different latency patterns that reflect the interaction between the immune response of the host and the virus. Thus, the virus expresses as many proteins as the immune system of the host allows. As a rule, the most immunosuppressed the host is, the more viral particles are produced, and thus EBV+ neoplasms express more viral antigens. Of the viral antigens, EBNA1, LMP1, LMP2 are the targets more frequently challenged using CTL therapy. In particular, cytotoxic LMP1 or EBNA1-specific CD4+ T cells, have proven effective not only in vitro against LCLs and infected NK/T cells, but also against naturally expressed targets in NK/T cell lymphoma and CAEBV [77, 78]. These therapies need further refinement in generating such in vitro and in demonstrating their efficacy in vivo.

Antiviral therapy is another therapeutic approach. A phase I/II trial of arginine butyrate and ganciclovir in 15 patients with refractory EBV+ lymphoid malignancies was well tolerated, achieving good antitumor response in ten patients [79]. Cidofovir, another antiviral drug, downregulated LMP1 expression and decrease BCL-2 levels in lymphoma cells.

Anti-CD30 monoclonal antibody, which inhibits growth of CD30-expressing tumor cells has been used in patients with refractory CHL, independent of EBV status, achieving success [80]. Another study showed that the combination of MTX and irradiation significantly induced apoptosis and growth inhibition in two EBV-expressing NK/T-cell lines, via downregulation of NF-κB signaling. The NF-κB inhibition highlighted an efficacious therapeutic approach for patients with nasal T/NK-cell lymphoma and other EBV-related lymphomas.

Further experience and better delivery of molecular therapies may provide safe and efficacious therapeutic benefits for EBV-related lymphoproliferative disorders, which coupled with other therapies that target simultaneously other mechanisms of oncogenesis may contribute to better management of these disorders.

References

1. Roschewski M, Wilson WH (2012) EBV-associated lymphomas in adults. Best Pract Res Clin Haematol 25:75–89
2. Nemerow GR, Mold C, Schwend VK, Tollefson V, Cooper NR (1987) Identification of gp350 as the viral glycoprotein mediating attachment of Epstein-Barr virus (EBV) to the EBV/c3d receptor of B cells: sequence homology of gp350 and c3 complement fragment c3d. J Virol 61:1416–1420
3. Kieff E, Rickinson A (2001) Epstein-Barr virus. In: Knipe D, Howley P (eds) Fields virology, 4th edn. Lippincott, Philadelpia, PA, pp 2511–2573

4. Kieff E, Richardson AB (2007) Epstein-Barr virus and its replication. In: Knipe DM, Howley PM (eds) Fields virology, 5th edn. Lippincott, Williams and Wilkins, Philadelphia, PA, pp 2603–2654
5. Castillo JJ, Beltran BE, Miranda RN, Paydas S, Winer ES, Butera JN (2011) Epstein-Barr virus-positive diffuse large B-cell lymphoma of the elderly: what we know so far. Oncologist 16:87–96
6. Qiu J, Cosmopoulos K, Pegtel M et al (2011) A novel persistence associated EBV miRNA expression profile is disrupted in neoplasia. PLoS Pathog 7:e1002193
7. Bornkamm GW (2009) Epstein-Barr virus and its role in the pathogenesis of Burkitt's lymphoma: an unresolved issue. Semin Cancer Biol 19:351–365
8. Cader FZ, Kearns P, Young L, Murray P, Vockerodt M (2010) The contribution of the Epstein-Barr virus to the pathogenesis of childhood lymphomas. Cancer Treat Rev 36:348–353
9. Epstein MA, Achong BG, Barr YM (1964) Virus particles in cultured lymphoblasts from Burkitt's lymphoma. Lancet 1:702–703
10. Kuppers R (2005) Mechanisms of B-cell lymphoma pathogenesis. Nat Rev Cancer 5: 251–262
11. Scheller H, Tobollik S, Kutzera A et al (2010) c-Myc overexpression promotes a germinal center-like program in Burkitt's lymphoma. Oncogene 29:888–897
12. Allday MJ (2009) How does Epstein-Barr virus (EBV) complement the activation of Myc in the pathogenesis of Burkitt's lymphoma? Semin Cancer Biol 19:366–376
13. Bieging KT, Swanson-Mungerson M, Amick AC, Longnecker R (2010) Epstein-Barr virus in Burkitt's lymphoma: a role for latent membrane protein 2A. Cell Cycle 9:901–908
14. Guikema JE, de Boer C, Haralambieva E et al (2006) IGH switch breakpoints in Burkitt lymphoma: exclusive involvement of noncanonical class switch recombination. Genes Chromosomes Cancer 45:808–819
15. Bellan C, Lazzi S, Hummel M et al (2005) Immunoglobulin gene analysis reveals 2 distinct cells of origin for EBV-positive and EBV-negative Burkitt lymphomas. Blood 106: 1031–1036
16. Preudhomme C, Dervite I, Wattel E et al (1995) Clinical significance of p53 mutations in newly diagnosed Burkitt's lymphoma and acute lymphoblastic leukemia: a report of 48 cases. J Clin Oncol 13:812–820
17. Farrell PJ, Allan GJ, Shanahan F, Vousden KH, Crook T (1991) p53 is frequently mutated in Burkitt's lymphoma cell lines. EMBO J 10:2879–2887
18. Kang MS, Hung SC, Kieff E (2001) Epstein-Barr virus nuclear antigen 1 activates transcription from episomal but not integrated DNA and does not alter lymphocyte growth. Proc Natl Acad Sci U S A 98:15233–15238
19. Gruhne B, Sompallae R, Marescotti D, Kamranvar SA, Gastaldello S, Masucci MG (2009) The Epstein-Barr virus nuclear antigen-1 promotes genomic instability via induction of reactive oxygen species. Proc Natl Acad Sci U S A 106:2313–2318
20. Saridakis V, Sheng Y, Sarkari F et al (2005) Structure of the p53 binding domain of HAUSP/USP7 bound to Epstein-Barr nuclear antigen 1 implications for EBV-mediated immortalization. Mol Cell 18:25–36
21. Bell AI, Groves K, Kelly GL et al (2006) Analysis of Epstein-Barr virus latent gene expression in endemic Burkitt's lymphoma and nasopharyngeal carcinoma tumour cells by using quantitative real-time PCR assays. J Gen Virol 87:2885–2890
22. Fruehling S, Swart R, Dolwick KM, Kremmer E, Longnecker R (1998) Tyrosine 112 of latent membrane protein 2A is essential for protein tyrosine kinase loading and regulation of Epstein-Barr virus latency. J Virol 72:7796–7806
23. Swanson-Mungerson MA, Caldwell RG, Bultema R, Longnecker R (2005) Epstein-Barr virus LMP2A alters in vivo and in vitro models of B-cell anergy, but not deletion, in response to autoantigen. J Virol 79:7355–7362
24. Portis T, Longnecker R (2004) Epstein-Barr virus (EBV) LMP2A mediates B-lymphocyte survival through constitutive activation of the Ras/PI3K/Akt pathway. Oncogene 23:8619–8628

25. Merchant M, Longnecker R (2001) LMP2A survival and developmental signals are transmitted through Btk-dependent and Btk-independent pathways. Virology 291:46–54
26. Engels N, Merchant M, Pappu R, Chan AC, Longnecker R, Wienands J (2001) Epstein-Barr virus latent membrane protein 2A (LMP2A) employs the SLP-65 signaling module. J Exp Med 194:255–264
27. Wong HH, Wang J (2009) Epstein-Barr virus positive diffuse large B-cell lymphoma of the elderly. Leuk Lymphoma 50:335–340
28. Asano N, Yamamoto K, Tamaru J et al (2009) Age-related Epstein-Barr virus (EBV)-associated B-cell lymphoproliferative disorders: comparison with EBV-positive classic Hodgkin lymphoma in elderly patients. Blood 113:2629–2636
29. Oyama T, Ichimura K, Suzuki R et al (2003) Senile EBV+ B-cell lymphoproliferative disorders: a clinicopathologic study of 22 patients. Am J Surg Pathol 27:16–26
30. Lages CS, Suffia I, Velilla PA et al (2008) Functional regulatory T cells accumulate in aged hosts and promote chronic infectious disease reactivation. J Immunol 181:1835–1848
31. Park S, Lee J, Ko YH et al (2007) The impact of Epstein-Barr virus status on clinical outcome in diffuse large B-cell lymphoma. Blood 110:972–978
32. Kapatai G, Murray P (2007) Contribution of the Epstein Barr virus to the molecular pathogenesis of Hodgkin lymphoma. J Clin Pathol 60:1342–1349
33. Stein H, Delsol G, Pileri SA, Weiss LM, Poppema S, Jaffe ES (2008) Classic Hodgkin lymphoma, introduction. In: Swerdlow SH, Campo E, Harris NL, Jaffe ES, Pileri SA, Stein H, Thiele J, Vardiman JW (eds) WHO classification of tumors of haematopoietic and lymphoid tissues, 4th edn. IARC, Lyon, p 326
34. Hummel M, Anagnostopoulos I, Dallenbach F, Korbjuhn P, Dimmler C, Stein H (1992) EBV infection patterns in Hodgkin's disease and normal lymphoid tissue: expression and cellular localization of EBV gene products. Br J Haematol 82:689–694
35. Marafioti T, Hummel M, Foss HD et al (2000) Hodgkin and reed-sternberg cells represent an expansion of a single clone originating from a germinal center B-cell with functional immunoglobulin gene rearrangements but defective immunoglobulin transcription. Blood 95: 1443–1450
36. Kuppers R, Hajadi M, Plank L et al (1996) Molecular Ig gene analysis reveals that monocytoid B cells lymphoma is a malignancy of mature B cells carrying somatically mutated V region genes and suggests that rearrangement of the kappa-deleting element(resulting in deletion of the Ig kappa enhancers) abolishes somatic hypermutation in the human. Eur J Immunol 26:1794–1800
37. Kanzler H, Kuppers R, Hansmann ML et al (1996) Hodgkin and Reed-Sternberg cells in Hodgkin's disease represent the out growth of a dominant tumor clone derived from(crippled) germinal center B cells. J Exp Med 184:1495–1505
38. Kuppers R (2002) Molecular biology of Hodgkin's lymphoma. Adv Cancer Res 84:277–312
39. Farrell K, Jarrett RF (2011) The molecular pathogenesis of Hodgkin lymphoma. Histopathology 58:15–25
40. Gulley ML, Eagan PA, Quintanilla-Martinez L et al (1994) Epstein-Barr virus DNA is abundant and monoclonal in the Reed-Sternberg cells of Hodgkin's disease: association with mixed cellularity subtype and Hispanic American ethnicity. Blood 83:1595–1602
41. Lam N, Sugden B (2003) CD40 and its viral mimic, LMP1: similar means to different ends. Cell Signal 15:9–16
42. Graham JP, Arcipowski KM, Bishop GA (2010) Differential B-lymphocyte regulation by CD40 and its viral mimic, latent membrane protein 1. Immunol Rev 237:226–248
43. Rastelli J, Homig-Holzel C, Seagal J et al (2008) LMP1 signaling can replace CD40 signaling in B cells in vivo and has unique features of inducing class-switch recombination to IgG1. Blood 111:1448–1455
44. Pratt ZL, Zhang J, Sugden B (2012) The latent membrane protein 1 (LMP1) oncogene of Epstein-Barr virus can simultaneously induce and inhibit apoptosis in B cells. J Virol 86:4380–4393

45. He Z, Xin B, Yang X, Chan C, Cao L (2000) Nuclear factor-kappaB activation is involved in LMP1-mediated transformation and tumorigenesis of rat-1 fibroblasts. Cancer Res 60: 1845–1848
46. Cahir-McFarland ED, Carter K, Rosenwald A et al (2004) Role of NF-kappa B in cell survival and transcription of latent membrane protein 1-expressing or Epstein-Barr virus latency III-infected cells. J Virol 78:4108–4119
47. Lee IS, Kim SH, Song HG, Park SH (2003) The molecular basis for the generation of Hodgkin and Reed-Sternberg cells in Hodgkin's lymphoma. Into J Hematology 77:330–335
48. Cohen JI, Bollard CM, Khanna R, Pittaluga S (2008) Current understanding of the role of Epstein-Barr virus in lymphomagenesis and therapeutic approaches to EBV-associated lymphomas. Leuk Lymphoma 49(Suppl 1):27–34
49. Aizawa S, Nakano H, Ishida T et al (1997) Tumor necrosis factor receptor-associated factor (TRAF) 5 and TRAF2 are involved in CD30-mediated NFkappaB activation. J Biol Chem 272:2042–2045
50. Longnecker R (2000) Epstein-Barr virus latency: LMP2, a regulator or means for Epstein-Barr virus persistence? Adv Cancer Res 79:175–200
51. Marshall NA, Culligan DJ, Tighe J, Johnston PW, Barker RN, Vickers MA (2007) The relationships between Epstein-Barr virus latent membrane protein 1 and regulatory T cells in Hodgkin's lymphoma. Exp Hematology 35:596–604
52. Carbone A, Gloghini A, Dotti G (2008) EBV-associated lymphoproliferative disorders: classification and treatment. Oncologist 13:577–585
53. Bollard CM, Aguilar L, Straathof KC et al (2004) Cytotoxic T lymphocyte therapy for Epstein-Barr virus+ Hodgkin's disease. J Exp Med 200:1623–1633
54. Young LS, Rickinson AB (2004) Epstein-Barr virus: 40 years on. Nat Rev Cancer 4:757–768
55. Kimura H, Ito Y, Kawabe S et al (2012) EBV-associated T/NK-cell lymphoproliferative diseases in nonimmunocompromised hosts: prospective analysis of 108 cases. Blood 119:673–686
56. Cohen JI, Kimura H, Nakamura S, Ko YH, Jaffe ES (2009) Epstein-Barr virus-associated lymphoproliferative disease in non-immunocompromised hosts: a status report and summary of an international meeting, 8–9 September 2008. Ann Oncol 20:1472–1482
57. Yang L, Aozasa K, Oshimi K, Takada K (2004) Epstein-Barr virus (EBV)-encoded RNA promotes growth of EBV-infected T cells through interleukin-9 induction. Cancer Res 64: 5332–5337
58. Kim A, Lee JE, Jang WS et al (2012) A combination of methotrexate and irradiation promotes cell death in NK/T-cell lymphoma cells via down-regulation of NF-kappaB signaling. Leuk Res 36:350–357
59. Sharifi R, Sinclair JC, Gilmour KC et al (2004) SAP mediates specific cytotoxic T-cell functions in X-linked lymphoproliferative disease. Blood 103:3821–3827
60. Booth C, Gilmour KC, Veys P et al (2011) X-linked lymphoproliferative disease due to SAP/SH2D1A deficiency: a multicenter study on the manifestations, management and outcome of the disease. Blood 117:53–62
61. Hislop AD, Taylor GS, Sauce D, Rickinson AB (2007) Cellular responses to viral infection in humans: lessons from Epstein-Barr virus. Annu Rev Immunol 25:587–617
62. Raphael M, Said J, Borisch B, Cesarman E, Harris NL (2008) Lymphomas associated with HIV infection. In: Swerdlow SH, Campo E, Harris NL, Jaffe ES, Jaffe ES, Pileri SA, Stein H, Thiele J, Vardiman JW (eds) WHO classification of tumors of haematopoietic and lymphoid tissues, 4th edn. IARC, Lyon, pp 340–342
63. Bibas M, Antinori A (2009) EBV and HIV-related lymphoma. Mediterr J Hematology Infect Dis 1:e2009032
64. Feng WH, Cohen JI, Fischer S et al (2004) Reactivation of latent Epstein-Barr virus by methotrexate: a potential contributor to methotrexate-associated lymphomas. J Natl Cancer Inst 96:1691–1702
65. Balandraud N, Roudier J, Roudier C (2005) What are the links between Epstein-Barr virus, lymphoma, and tumor necrosis factor antagonism in rheumatoid arthritis? Semin Arthritis Rheum 34:31–33

66. Draoua HY, Tsao L, Mancini DM, Addonizio LJ, Bhagat G, Alobeid B (2004) T-cell post-transplantation lymphoproliferative disorders after cardiac transplantation: a single institutional experience. Br J Haematol 127:429–432
67. Hochberg D, Middeldorp JM, Catalina M, Sullivan JL, Luzuriaga K, Thorley-Lawson DA (2004) Demonstration of the Burkitt's lymphoma Epstein-Barr virus phenotype in dividing latently infected memory cells in vivo. Proc Natl Acad Sci U S A 101:239–244
68. Mautner J, Bornkamm GW (2012) The role of virus-specific CD4+ T cells in the control of Epstein-Barr virus infection. Eur J Cell Biol 91:31–35
69. Robertson ES, Lin J, Kieff E (1996) The amino-terminal domains of Epstein-Barr virus nuclear proteins 3A, 3B, and 3C interact with RBPJ(kappa). J Virol 70(5):3068–3074
70. Krauer KG, Burgess A, Buck M, Flanagan J, Sculley TB, Gabrielli B (2004) The EBNA-3 gene family proteins disrupt the G2/M checkpoint. Oncogene 23:1342–1353
71. Anderton E, Yee J, Smith P, Crook T, White RE, Allday MJ (2008) Two Epstein-Barr virus (EBV) oncoproteins cooperate to repress expression of the proapoptotic tumour-suppressor Bim: clues to the pathogenesis of Burkitt's lymphoma. Oncogene 27:421–433
72. Radkov SA, Touitou R, Brehm A et al (1999) Epstein-Barr virus nuclear antigen 3C interacts with histone deacetylase to repress transcription. J Virol 73:5688–5697
73. Parker GA, Touitou R, Allday MJ (2000) Epstein-Barr virus EBNA3C can disrupt multiple cell cycle checkpoints and induce nuclear division divorced from cytokinesis. Oncogene 19:700–709
74. Sjoblom A, Yang WW, Palmqvist L, Jansson A, Rymo L (1998) An ATF/CRE element mediates both EBNA2-dependent and EBNA2-independent activation of the Epstein-Barr virus LMP1 gene promoter. J Virol 72:1365–1376
75. Lucchesi W, Brady G, Dittrich-Breiholz O, Kracht M, Russ R, Farrell PJ (2008) Differential gene regulation by Epstein-Barr virus type 1 and type 2 EBNA2. J Virol 82:7456–7466
76. Gustafsson A, Levitsky V, Zou JZ et al (2000) Epstein-Barr virus (EBV) load in bone marrow transplant recipients at risk to develop posttransplant lymphoproliferative disease: prophylactic infusion of EBV-specific cytotoxic T cells. Blood 95:807–814
77. Demachi-Okamura A, Ito Y, Akatsuka Y et al (2008) Epstein-Barr virus nuclear antigen 1-specific CD4(+) T cells directly kill Epstein-Barr virus-carrying natural killer and T cells. Cancer Sci 99:1633–1642
78. Kobayashi H, Nagato T, Takahara N et al (2008) Induction of EBV-latent membrane protein 1-specific MHC class II-restricted T-cell responses against natural killer lymphoma cells. Cancer Res 68:901–908
79. Perrine SR, Hermine O, Small T et al (2007) A phase 1/2 trial of arginine butyrate and ganciclovir in patients with Epstein-Barr virus-associated lymphoid malignancies. Blood 109:2571–2578
80. Ansell SM, Horwitz SM, Engert A et al (2007) Phase I/II study of an anti-CD30 monoclonal antibody (MDX-060) in Hodgkin's lymphoma and anaplastic large-cell lymphoma. J Clin Oncol 25:2764–2769

Antigen-Driven Lymphomagenesis

Reve Shields and James N. Butera

Abstract Chronic antigenic stimulation has been postulated to play a central role in the pathophysiology of Non-Hodgkin lymphoma. Mucosa-associated lymphoid tissues or MALT lymphoma of the stomach and its association with Helicobacter pylori is one of the most well studied examples of this phenomenon. Furthermore, other infectious and noninfectious entities have been described to produce monoclonal lymphocyte proliferation with resultant malignant lymphoproliferative disorders. Among these are *Chlamydia psittaci*, hepatitis C virus infection, rheumatoid arthritis, systemic lupus erythematosus, Sjogren disorder, and Hashimoto thyroiditis. This review focuses on these entities and summarizes the available data which associates these conditions with the development of malignant lymphoma.

Introduction

Over the recent decades, several studies have linked certain persistent infections, autoimmune and chronic inflammatory conditions to an increased incidence of lymphomas. The magnitude of this risk is still unclear as risk varies considerably among these studies. There are several hypotheses on how chronic infections lead to the

R. Shields
Division of Hematology and Oncology, Rhode Island Hospital,
The Warren Alpert Medical School of Brown University, Providence, RI, USA

J.N. Butera (✉)
Division of Hematology and Oncology, Rhode Island Hospital,
The Warren Alpert Medical School of Brown University, Providence, RI, USA

Comprehensive Cancer Center, George Clinic at Rhode Island Hospital,
593 Eddy Street, Providence, RI 02903, USA
e-mail: jbutera@lifespan.org

P.J. Quesenberry and J.J. Castillo (eds.), *Non-Hodgkin Lymphoma: Prognostic Factors and Targets*, Cancer Drug Discovery and Development,
DOI 10.1007/978-1-4614-5851-7_5,

development of lymphoma. In the case of lymphotropic viruses such EBV, HTLV-1, and HHV-8, there is evidence of direct infection of these viruses with subsequent immortalization and transformation of B-cells in vitro through the expression of viral oncogenes [1, 2]. An alternative hypothesis has emerged where certain microbial species are able to escape the host's immune surveillance, establish a chronic infection, and acquire the ability to persist chronically in the host [3, 4]. These persistent infections trigger a sustained lymphoid proliferation due to the presence of chronic antigen stimulation. The microorganism responsible is not thought to be directly tumorigenic but can be viewed as a chronic source of antigens that create a milieu which promote lymphoid proliferation. Likewise, in patients with chronic autoimmune disease, there is a persistent inflammatory state due to auto-antigen stimulation creating an ideal microenvironment for lymphomagenesis.

The precise mechanism for "indirect" antigen-driven lymphomagenesis is still unclear and may vary among different disease states and infectious organism. Certain infectious organisms that have been linked to lymphoma through the process of indirect lymphomagenesis are *Helicobacter pylori*, *Chlamydia psittaci*, Hepatitis C virus, *Borrelia burgdorferi*, and *Campylobacter jejuni*. In this chapter, we will discuss the first three organisms in detail. The unifying pathologic entity is the presence of the antigen that drives lymphoproliferation. In Hepatitis C, the HCV envelope protein is a potential antigen responsible for B-cell lymphoproliferation while a specific antigen has not been elucidated in others [5]. Many autoantigens have also been identified in certain autoimmune disorders particularly Sjogren syndrome and autoimmune thyroiditis [6, 7]. Bacterial or viral antigens or autoantigens bind to the B-cell receptor and trigger lymphoproliferation. Chronic infection of the host produces inflammatory cytokines that create a local environment suitable to sustain B-cell proliferation [8]. In certain models, lymphoma progression is thought to be a stepwise process, which starts with oligoclonal lymphoproliferation. Immunoglobulin analysis of these lymphomas reveals a biased immunoglobulin V gene use and somatic hypermutation suggesting antigen selection [9–11]. Ongoing antigen stimulation amplifies B-cell proliferation and exposes these B-cell to the development of mutations [12]. B-cells that undergo somatic hypermutation and class-switching are generally genetically unstable and have an increased risk of transformation to lymphoma [13].

Chronic infection and inflammation lead to the formation of reactive oxygen species which can also create genetic defects and lead to tumorigenesis [12]. Initially, lymphoid proliferation is dependent on the presence of antigen; however, generation of these genetic defects can often lead to antigen independence and malignant transformation [14, 15]. Several studies have shown that elimination of the source of antigens through bacterial or viral eradication can in some cases lead to lymphoma regression and cure.

Advancement in the management of lymphomas is due to the progress in our understanding of the pathogenesis and etiology of this diverse malignancy. In this chapter we will talk about lymphomas that are infection driven. We will also discuss autoimmunity and inflammation and review the risk factors and current knowledge that associate these entities to lymphomas. Although much has been learned over the past decades to elucidate the steps in antigen-driven lymphomagenesis, there is still much to be learned. Discovery of these steps can lead to breakthroughs that can be exploited to eliminate the source of antigenicity, determine therapeutic targets, and halt the progression of lymphoma.

Helicobacter pylori

Marginal zone lymphomas are subdivided into three entities by the World Health Organization (WHO): nodal marginal zone lymphoma, splenic marginal zone lymphoma, and extranodal marginal zone lymphoma [16]. Extranodal marginal zone lymphoma of mucosa-associated lymphoid tissue (MALT lymphoma) is the third most common form of non-Hodgkin lymphoma (NHL) [17]. Gastric MALT lymphomas comprise about 50% of MALT lymphomas and typically have an indolent clinical course. Extranodal MALT lymphomas are different from splenic and marginal zone lymphomas as they typically occur in organs that normally lack lymphoid tissue such as the gastrointestinal tract, lung, liver, salivary glands, ocular adnexa, thyroid tissue, and skin. It has long been known that these lymphoid follicles accumulate in response to chronic antigenic stimulation from *Helicobacter pylori* (*H. pylori*) infection or autoimmune disease [18, 19].

H. pylori is a gram-negative bacterium that colonizes the human gastric mucosa in approximately 50% of the world population. Those that are infected develop a chronic gastritis that may remain largely asymptomatic. However, about 10% of the population develop peptic ulcer disease, 1% develop gastric adenocarcinoma and 0.01% develop MALT lymphoma [20]. A causative association between *H. pylori* infection with gastric MALT lymphoma was first provided by the presence of the bacteria in up to 90% of gastric MALT lymphoma specimens [21–23]. Supporting this association is that the incidence of gastric MALT lymphoma is highest in *H. pylori* endemic areas [3] and seroprevalence for *H. pylori* is much higher in patients with gastric MALT lymphoma [24, 25]. Hussel and colleagues have shown in vitro that when B-cells from gastric biopsies of MALT lymphoma patients were cultured with heat-killed *H. pylori*, lymphocyte proliferation occurred [23]. Furthermore, eradication of *H. pylori* bacteria with antibiotic therapy lead to complete long-term regression of the MALT lymphoma in 70–80% of cases and is considered to be the first line therapy for this lymphoma [26, 27].

H. pylori plays an important role in both clonal expansion and subsequent malignant transformation. Unlike EBV, HIV, HTLV-1, and HHV-8 viruses where these viruses directly infect and transform B-cells in vitro, *H. pylori* induce a chronic activation of the immune system and subsequent proliferation of lymphocytes and eventual transformation to MALT lymphoma [1, 2, 28]. Under healthy conditions, the stomach lacks MALT as the low pH prevents survival of bacteria and lymphocytes in the gastric wall [29]. The first step in the pathogenesis of MALT lymphoma is infection of *H. pylori* resulting in secretion of bacterial urease that neutralizes gastric pH [30]. These events result in lymphoid infiltration and subsequent development of MALT lymphoma [30]. In vitro experiments show that *H. pylori*-activated T-cells were found to stimulate the gastric MALT lymphoma cells and removal of these T-cells from the tumor cell suspension stopped tumor cell proliferation [24]. These CD4-positive T-cells isolated from gastric MALT lymphoma directly respond in vitro to proteins from *H. pylori* and provide proliferative signals to malignant B-cells in a T-cell-dependent manner [24, 25]. *H. pylori* infection has the ability to persist in the host tissues and have the ability to sustain lymphoid proliferation giving a selective advantage to these lymphoid clones that are dependent on antigen stimulation [3, 31]. Hence, eradication of *H. pylori* infection early in the course of the disease leads to the eradication of MALT lymphoma. In this model, *H. pylori* is not directly involved in lymphomagenesis but is a chronic source of antigens which fuels lymphoid proliferation and eventually, under precise circumstances, development to lymphoma [32].

Interestingly, the antigen is not a permanent prerequisite for malignant expansion or persistence. Persistent B-cell clonal expansion and exposure of these B-cells to chronic inflammation lead to genetic and molecular derangements that lead to antigen independence. Genetic abnormalities identified in MALT lymphoma include trisomies in chromosomes 3, 7, and 12; p53 mutations; p16 deletions; and recurrent chromosomal translocations including t(11;18)(q21,21), t(1;14)(p22,q32), t(14;18)(q32;q21), and t(3;14)(p14.1,q32) [33–41]. These recurrent chromosomal translocations are found exclusively in MALT lymphomas in frequencies of about 3–30% [35, 41–44]. The t(11;18)(q21,21), t(1;14)(p22,q32), and t(14;18)(q32;q21) translocations involve different oncogenes which all ultimately target the same nuclear factor kappa B (NF-κB) signaling pathway in lymphocytes [45–48]. The transcription of NF-κB signaling pathway regulates the expression of genes that are involved in cell proliferation, inflammatory cascade, and eventual apoptosis. Chronic antigen stimulation generated through the B-cell receptor is then bypassed by activation of the NF-κB pathway leading to antigen independence. Of note, the t(11;18) positive MALT lymphomas do not respond to *H. pylori* eradication and is associated with adverse clinical features and in general require a more aggressive treatment approach such as radiation when antibiotic therapy fails [49]. Most of the t(1;14)-associated MALT lymphoma are diagnosed at advanced stages and is unlikely to respond to *H. pylori* eradication [50]. The role of t(3;14) translocation which deregulates the FOXP1 gene is still unclear. Despite the recognition of these chromosomal translocations in MALT lymphoma, only a small proportion is positive for these translocations and there is more we need to know to advance our knowledge of MALT lymphomas.

Chlamydia psittaci

Ocular adnexal lymphomas (OAL) are a diverse group of lymphomas that account for approximately 1–2% of all (NHL) and 8% of extranodal lymphomas [51, 52]. About 35–50% of cases are of extranodal marginal zone lymphoma MALT type and is the most common histologic subtype of primary OAL [53–55] with higher frequencies of about 80–90% observed in Japan and Korea [56, 57]. Ninety-five percent of reported cases of OAL are B-cell neoplasms. Recently, Ferreri and colleagues [58] reported the presence of *C. psittaci* infection in 32 of 40 (80%) OAL specimens in an Italian cohort and of those that were positive 66% were of MALT type. Furthermore, Ferreri and colleagues [59] demonstrated that eradication of *C. psittaci* infection using antibiotic therapy caused a response in 6 out of 9 treated patients including 2 complete responses. However, several other studies have reported dissimilar results. In the United States, Rosado [60] and Vargas [61] in South Florida and New York State, respectively, reported absence of *C. psittaci* infection suggesting a geographical variation in the prevalence of *C. psittaci* infection.

C. psittaci is an obligate intracellular pathogen that is transmitted by inhalation, contact, or ingestion. Psittacosis is an infection caused by *C. psittaci* caused by exposure to droppings of infected birds, cats, and household animals. Half of patients with OAL have reported exposure to household animals [58]. Macrophages and monocytes are carriers of *C. psittaci*, which is transported to various organs causing local and systemic infections [62]. Clinical presentation of OAL is diverse and dependent upon the organ involved. The ocular adnexa involve the lacrimal apparatus, the extra ocular muscles, eyelids, eyelashes, eyebrows, and conjunctiva. The orbit is the most commonly involved (40%) followed by the conjunctiva (35–40%) and lacrimal gland (10–20%) [63–65]. The clinical presentation ranges from painless well-circumscribed to diffuse ill-defined erythematous lesions with a wide variety of symptoms such as blurry vision, lid erythema, exophthalmos, and proptosis. OAL has an indolent clinical course and 85–90% present as stage I disease. Radiation therapy is the treatment of choice for patients with localized disease with local control rates ranging from 86 to 100% and local recurrence rates from 0 to 15% [64, 66, 67]. There is limited data on the role of systemic chemotherapy; however, single agent chlorambucil and fludarabine has been reported as active agents against OAL [68].

C. psittaci is also linked to chronic infections of the conjunctiva which may display features of inclusion conjunctivitis. It also has the ability to persist in ocular tissues chronically and endure systemically over several years. Similar to the better-defined pathogenesis of *H. pylori* and gastric MALT lymphomas, OAL arises in tissues that are devoid of lymphoid tissue and persist in the setting of preexisting chronic inflammation [69]. Polymerase chain reaction analysis of immunoglobulin heavy-chain gene rearrangements shows somatic hypermutation in 66% of cases [70] and a clonal B-cell population in 55% of cases of OAL [71]. Coupland and colleagues have analyzed germ-line mutations in OAL patients and recognized that the most commonly involved genes are those implicated in the assembly of autoantibodies [70]. *C. psittaci* have a tendency to cause persistent infections due to its ability to inhibit apoptosis of infected cells and its ability for immune modulation [72, 73]. The pathogenesis of *C. psittaci* in lymphoma is not as clearly defined as compared to *H. pylori* in gastric MALT lymphoma. One mechanism is that *C. psittaci*, similar to gastric MALT, can potentially trigger both humoral and cell-mediated immune responses that may cross-react to self-antigens to break local tolerance.

Additional clonal expansion can lead to subsequent genetic mutations. Molecular cytogenetic studies in OAL reveal common abnormalities such as trisomy 13 and trisomy 18 [74, 75]. Chromosomal translocations, similar to gastric MALT are also found in OAML with t(14;18)(pq32,21) as the most common (7–11%) [75, 76] followed by t(11;18)(q21,q21) (0–10%) [34, 75]. Again, similar to gastric MALT, the oncogenic products of these mutations lead to ability to enhance activation of NF-κB pathway which activates several genes responsible for lymphocyte proliferation, survival, and apoptosis inhibition. There is evidence of geographic variations in the incidence of these cytogenetic abnormalities in OAL. How these genetic and molecular differences correlate with *C. psittaci* infection and how they affect prognosis and treatment still remain to be defined.

Hepatitis C Virus

Hepatitis C virus (HCV) is a major public health problem and is known to infect 3% of the world population, affecting about 170 million people worldwide. It is estimated that 80% of infected individuals will be unable to clear the virus. Most of these individuals will develop a chronic hepatitis with 30% ultimately developing cirrhosis and hepatocellular carcinoma [77]. HCV chronic infection is also associated with a variety of extrahepatic manifestations including autoimmune-related disorders and B-cell lymphoproliferative disorders [78]. The most common of which is essential mixed cryoglobulinemia (MC), which is a chronic benign immune complex-mediated systemic vasculitis with underlying B-cell proliferation that predisposes to overt B-cell malignancy [78–80]. Epidemiological studies report a higher frequency of HCV infection in B NHL than in any other hematologic diseases. In 1994, Ferri and colleagues reported a surprisingly high prevalence of HCV infection in patients with NHL in Italy, which is a highly endemic area for HCV [79]. Additional studies in United States [81] and Japan [82] reported similar results; although there may be some geographical variability, as the Netherlands [83, 84] and Canada [85] have reported otherwise. Most studies report different histologic subtypes: marginal zone lymphoma (most common), lymphoplasmacytic lymphoma, and diffuse large B-cell lymphoma [86]. The association of HCV infection and NHL is further supported by the observation that eradication of HCV by the use of interferon and ribavirin could induce complete remissions in patients with lymphomas [87].

The precise mechanism of how chronic HCV infection leads to cryoglobulinemia and the subsequent development of malignant B-cell lymphoma are not fully elucidated. One possibility is that HCV can stimulate B-cell proliferation by direct infection of lymphocytes, such as the case in liver hepatocytes [87]. Viral sequences have been found in B-cells and monocytes; however, recent studies suggest that there is no convincing evidence that viral replication occurs in these cells [87]. Other studies have also shown that malignant cells in HCV-associated NHL are uninfected [88]. Taken together, the hypothesis of direct infection by HCV makes it less likely. An alternative model has been proposed linking the role of HCV infection in lymphomagenesis through a process of chronic antigen stimulation. Multiple studies have demonstrated the presence of oligoclonal and monoclonal expansion in HCV-infected patients. Sequencing of immunoglobulin variable regions in MC type II and NHL with chronic HCV infection have revealed somatic hypermutation which is a trademark of antigenic stimulation [89].

The HCV virus is a positive stranded RNA virus belonging to the Flaviviridae family [90]. The HCV mature protein consists of the core protein, envelope proteins E1 and E2, and six structural proteins (NS1-5B). A possible candidate antigen in this model of antigen-driven lymphoproliferation is the HCV-E2 envelope glycoprotein. Several studies reveal anti-HCV E2 B-cell clones isolated from patients with HCV-associated NHL [91]. The HCV E2 glycoprotein has the ability to bind to the CD81 B-cell surface protein and lower the threshold for B-cell activation and subsequent proliferation [92, 93]. Furthermore, CD81 has been found to be upregulated in HCV infected patients and has a positive correlation with HCV viral load [94]. The other possible candidate for the source of the antigen is the HCV nonstructural protein (NS3) which has been known to promote oncogenic transformation [94] by its interaction with p53 to prevent apoptosis [95]. The HCV core protein has also been shown in vitro to promote immortalization of different cell lines as well as interfere with c-myc-induced apoptosis [95]. Other regulatory proteins, such as the B-lymphocyte stimulator (BlyS), are overexpressed in HCV-induced lymphoproliferation inducing expansion of B-cell clones and autoantibody production [96]. Other genetic events contribute to B-cell clonal expansion and immortalization such as bcl-2 overexpression. Studies of peripheral blood mononuclear cells in chronically infected patients with HCV have revealed high levels of bcl-2 overexpression with a much higher increase in patients with MC type II and NHL [97]. Furthermore, antiviral treatment and eradication of HCV lead to a decrease in bcl-2 translocation [97].

As described above, there are several essential steps that have been elucidated in the pathophysiology of HCV-induced clonal expansion. However, there are likely more steps that are involved in lymphomagenesis leading to a maladaptive response to antigen stimulation. More studies are needed as the identification of these steps can give us better therapeutic strategies and targets in the future.

Rheumatoid Arthritis

Several studies have documented an increased risk of rheumatoid arthritis (RA) and NHL [98–105]. The first published case reports of this association were in the 1940s–1970s [106, 107]. Between 1980 and 1990, several large studies have shown that the risk ratio of NHL in patients with RA is about 2 when compared to the general population. These studies were confirmed by a recent meta-analysis. Two possible explanations for this association were hypothesized: (1) chronic inflammation causes chronic antigenic stimulation and lymphomagenesis, and

(2) treatment-related immunosuppression favoring lymphoma development. Whether either or both are primarily responsible for the increased association between NHL and RA is still a subject of much debate [100, 101, 104]. Studies to date have been unsuccessful at separating the inherent risk of RA in the development of NHL from its treatment effects. In a recently published large Swedish study, there appears to be a strong correlation between RA inflammatory disease activity and the development of NHL [108]. In this trial a "high inflammatory activity" is defined as the entire period from onset of RA until the diagnosis, the number of tender and swollen joints, erythrocyte sedimentation rate, and physician's global assessments. A high inflammatory activity was seen in 23% of RA patients who had developed NHL and in only 1% of RA control patients. Interestingly, the authors also found an increased lymphoma risk as the inflammatory activity increased. This would suggest that the increased lymphoma risk seen in RA patients is, at least in part, related to its associated chronic inflammatory state.

The effect of disease-modifying antirheumatic drugs (DMARDs) on the development of NHL is the subject of much controversy. Part of this challenge is that patients who may have more active disease may be the same population who are treated often or treated more aggressively with antirheumatic therapy. As a result, separating the severity of RA and its treatment outcome has been challenging. Many DMARDs have been evaluated for their role in lymphomagenesis including methotrexate (MTX), antitumor necrosis factor (TNF) therapy, antimalarial agents, azathioprine, gold salts, sulfasalazine, and steroidal and nonsteroidal anti-inflammatory drugs [109–120]. These studies have revealed conflicting results although the bulk of the literature is centered on MTX and anti-TNF therapy.

Although initial studies suggest an association between RA and MTX use with NHL, two large studies have refuted this. Moder and colleagues found 39 hematologic malignancies among 16,263 RA patients, but found no association with MTX use [120]. Another study found no association with MTX use in 19,562 patients with RA [104]. This is difficult to reconcile with the many published case reports and case series of spontaneous remissions of NHL as a result of MTX cessation [121, 122]. In fact, the WHO has recognized the entity of "Methotrexate-associated lymphoproliferative disorder" (LPD) as a subcategory of "Immunodeficiency-associated LPD" [123]. A recent published review, which included 26 patients with autoimmune disorders, showed spontaneous complete remissions of their LPD after withdrawal of their MTX. In this study, 21 of the 26 patients had RA (80%) and 22 of the 26 had NHL. There was frequent extranodal disease present (32%) and EBV infection could be demonstrated in a high proportion (56%) of cases. Complete remissions occurred within 4 weeks of discontinuation of therapy in 88% of patients [122]. It may be possible, that a small subset of cases of NHL in RA patients is, in fact, induced by MTX. The high number of EBV-positive cases in this series questions the possibility that EBV infection may be an etiologic link between MTX and lymphomagenesis in RA patients. However, more detailed reviews on this subject found EBV to be present in 12% of RA patients who develop NHL [124]. It is likely that in a subset of RA patients, the interactions between DMARDs (particularly MTX) and EBV are essential in the pathogenesis of NHL. The association between anti-TNF therapy in RA and NHL has often been debated. While some studies have noted an association between the two, others have not. However, recently, a large analysis of 19,562 patients with RA did not show an increased risk of lymphoma [104].

When NHL occurs in patients with RA, it is not exclusive to one subtype. Most studies suggest a modest overrepresentation of diffuse large cell lymphoma (40–50%) in these patients although this has been refuted in one large case-control study where no bias was found in the representation of the different subtypes in NHL [110].

Systemic Lupus Erythematosus

Most of the literature on systemic lupus eryhtematosus (SLE) and NHL evolve around establishing an association between these two entities. Many published series have documented an association with SLE and NHL with a relative risk (RR) of 3–7 times the risk of the general population [125–128]. Although others seem to refute this relationship, a large-scale meta-analysis estimated a 2.7-fold increased RR of NHL in patients with SLE [129]. Although some studies have attempted to determine the impact of disease severity, immune suppression, and EBV infection on the risk of NHL in patients with SLE, this has not been as well studied compared to patients with RA [125, 130]. The mean duration of SLE at the time of diagnosis of NHL was 17.8 years. Renal disease or immune suppressants did not appear to confer an increased risk of NHL development [125]. As in the case with RA, the subtype of diffuse large B-cell lymphoma appears to be overrepresented [125–128].

Sjogren Syndrome

Sjogren syndrome (SS) is an autoimmune epithelitis histologically characterized as lymphocytic infiltration of the salivary and lacrimal glands. Clinical manifestations include dry mouth and eyes (*sicca*). Approximately one-half of these patients will develop a systemic disease. Primary SS can be separated into three categories according to the extent of organ damage and the course of the disease. Stage I disease accounts for 45% of patients where *sicca* is the only manifestation of the disease. Stage II patients (approximately 50%) experience lymphocytic organ damage which can involve the pulmonary, renal, hepatic, gastrointestinal, vascular, and dermatologic systems. Approximately 5% of stage III patients will develop lymphoma.

Risk estimates of NHL in SS range from a RR between 4 and 44-fold the risk of the general population [98, 125, 127–129, 131]. In one large cohort, which evaluated 676 patients with primary SS, a RR of 8.7 (95% CI, 4.3–15) of NHL was noted [132]. Similar to RA patients, characteristics associated with more severe disease such as parotid enlargement, hypocomplementemia, and palpable purpura, carry the highest risk of NHL [133–136]. Mixed monoclonal cryoglobulinemia, leg ulcers, low CD4 counts, and a low CD4/CD8 ratio have also been reported to be associated with a higher risk of NHL [132–137]. The median time to development of NHL in SS patients is 7.5 years [138, 139]. There is also an increased frequency of circulating monoclonal immunoglobulins, free light chains, increased levels of circulating CD5-positive B-cells and monoclonal cryoglobulinemia [140, 141] in patients with SS, which strongly suggests a lymphoproliferative process.

Benign myoepithlial sialadenitis (MESA) lesions are characteristic of SS. These are primarily composed of CD4-positive T-cell lymphocytes, monocytoid cells, and marginal zone B-cells. These cells surround and infiltrate salivary ducts and histologically show proliferation of ductal epithelial cells [142]. Although B-cells only represent a minority of the infiltrating cells, they are thought to undergo clonal expansion in the presence of this T-cell milieu. In fact, oligoclonal lymphocytes are frequently seen in the benign SS-associated MESA [143]. The monoclonal expansion seen on these B-cells is similar to the one seen in HCV and *H. pylori*-induced inflammatory changes. Furthermore, different clones of B-cells can arise at different sites in the same patient with SS [144].

The biological event implicated in the transition from a benign reactive polyclonal or oligoclonal process to monoclonal expansion and subsequently to malignant lymphoma is not well understood. Many believe that this is a multistep process. It is speculated that chronic stimulation by exoantigens or autoantigens plays a role in this process by driving the proliferation of specific B-cells. This process of lymphoproliferation increases the risk of their transformation to lymphoma. This process of malignant transformation typically arises from the affected exocrine glands of SS patients but may also arise from visceral organs and lymph nodes [144]. One study found eleven different B-cell clones in seven patients with MESA. In this same study, eight were derived from the same V1-69 VH gene segment and the remaining three were derived from a V3-7 VH gene segment. MESA clones show conservative amino acid sequence motifs in the third complementary determining regions (CDR3). The marked VH gene restriction together with the similar CDR3 sequences suggest that MESA clones are directed against and may bind to similar or the same common antigen [144]. Pisa and colleagues found t(14;18) translocations in five SS-associated lymphomas which are also found in relatively high frequency in *H. pylori*-associated MALT lymphoma [145]. It has also been shown that p53 abnormalities and antirheumatic factor producing B-cells may also play a role in some cases of SS-associated lymphomas [146, 147].

There is a wide spectrum of NHL subtypes in SS patients. These include follicular lymphoma, small lymphocytic, diffuse large B-cell lymphoma and lymphoplasmacytic lymphoma. However, the majority are MALT lymphomas or their nodal counterparts, nodal marginal zone lymphoma subtypes [6, 131, 139, 148]. In a large European multicentered, retrospective clinical study, it was noted that 54% of NHL in patients with SS typically present at stages I or II, with 54% of cases involving the salivary glands. Lymphadenopathy was present in 63% of cases and 18% were exclusively nodal disease [139].

There is an interesting relationship between SS- and HCV-associated B-cell lymphoma. Type II mixed cryoglobulinemia is associated with both SS-related and

HCV-related B-cell lymphoproliferative disorders. HCV can infect the salivary gland epithelium, produce chronic inflammatory salivary lesions and cause *sicca* symptoms similar to that seen in SS. Salivary gland lymphomas are associated with HCV infection. Similar immunologic, molecular, and pathogenic events have been reported in both SS-related and HCV-related lymphoproliferation [149–151].

Hashimoto Thyroiditis

Hashimoto thyroiditis (HT, a.k.a. *struma lymphomatosa*), first described by Hashimoto in 1912, is an autoimmune inflammation of the thyroid gland commonly affecting middle-aged women. Histological features of HT include a diffuse infiltration of lymphoid cells commonly associated with formation of lymphoid follicles [152]. HT is present in approximately 55–60% of patients with thyroid lymphoma [153–155]. This association has led investigators to postulate that chronic antigenic stimulation of HT plays an important role in the pathophysiology of these tumors. Clonal B-lymphocytes can be seen in 10–30% of patients with HT [156–158]. However, similar to SS, clonality does not equal malignancy. These patients who have known clonal B-lymphocytes on biopsy have been followed for many years and often do not develop thyroid lymphoma [152]. It has been observed that there is a sequence similarity between the clonal bands in patients with HT and the clonal bands demonstrated in their respective thyroid lymphoma. This is supportive of the argument that primary thyroid lymphoma may evolve from HT [154]. The most common subtype of thyroid lymphomas is DLBCL, which accounts for approximately 70% of all cases. However, 40% of these patients will have evidence of MALT lymphoma in the background tissue. Approximately 6–27% of thyroid lymphomas are of MALT type [159].

Conclusion

Much progress has been made in the understanding of the association between chronic inflammation from infection and the development of lymphoma. Suppression of infection and eradication of the antigen suggest that lymphoma progression can be halted. There have been significant advances in the characterization of molecular mechanisms involved in lymphomagenesis. How these mechanisms can be exploited is an area of interest and needs further research. An important endeavor in the upcoming years is the identification of other pathogens that may play a role in lymphoma development. Their discovery may lead to identification mechanisms that we can utilize to prevent and treat these lymphomas. Similarly, an association between autoimmune disorders and lymphoma has been established. Risk of lymphoma is mainly due to degree of inflammatory activity and severity of disease. There is still great controversy on whether lymphoma risk is due to the disease itself versus whether this is a consequence of treatment. We need to better identify these individuals at a high risk of lymphoma so we can adequately intervene and decrease this risk.

References

1. Boshoff C, Weiss R (2002) AIDS-related malignancies. Nat Rev Cancer 2(5):373–382
2. Okano M (2000) Haematological associations of Epstein-Barr virus infection. Baillieres Best Pract Res Clin Haematol 13(2):199–214
3. Morse HC 3rd et al (2001) Cells of the marginal zone-origins, function and neoplasia. Leuk Res 25(2):169–178
4. Derringer GA et al (2000) Malignant lymphoma of the thyroid gland: a clinicopathologic study of 108 cases. Am J Surg Pathol 24(5):623–639
5. Quinn ER et al (2001) The B-cell receptor of a hepatitis C virus (HCV)-associated non-Hodgkin lymphoma binds the viral E2 envelope protein, implicating HCV in lymphomagenesis. Blood 98(13):3745–3749
6. Royer B et al (1997) Lymphomas in patients with Sjogren's syndrome are marginal zone B-cell neoplasms, arise in diverse extranodal and nodal sites, and are not associated with viruses. Blood 90(2):766–775
7. Voulgarelis M, Moutsopoulos HM (2003) Lymphoproliferation in autoimmunity and Sjogren's syndrome. Curr Rheumatol Rep 5(4):317–323
8. Seto M (2004) Genetic and epigenetic factors involved in B-cell lymphomagenesis. Cancer Sci 95(9):704–710
9. Marasca R et al (2001) Immunoglobulin gene mutations and frequent use of VH1-69 and VH4-34 segments in hepatitis C virus-positive and hepatitis C virus-negative nodal marginal zone B-cell lymphoma. Am J Pathol 159(1):253–261
10. De Re V et al (2000) Sequence analysis of the immunoglobulin antigen receptor of hepatitis C virus-associated non-Hodgkin lymphomas suggests that the malignant cells are derived from the rheumatoid factor-producing cells that occur mainly in type II cryoglobulinemia. Blood 96(10):3578–3584
11. Du M et al (1996) Ongoing mutation in MALT lymphoma immunoglobulin gene suggests that antigen stimulation plays a role in the clonal expansion. Leukemia 10(7):1190–1197
12. Coussens LM, Werb Z (2002) Inflammation and cancer. Nature 420(6917):860–867
13. Goossens T, Klein U, Kuppers R (1998) Frequent occurrence of deletions and duplications during somatic hypermutation: implications for oncogene translocations and heavy chain disease. Proc Natl Acad Sci U S A 95(5):2463–2468
14. Yeh KH et al (2005) Nuclear expression of BCL10 or nuclear factor kappa B helps predict Helicobacter pylori-independent status of low-grade gastric mucosa-associated lymphoid tissue lymphomas with or without t(11;18)(q21;q21). Blood 106(3):1037–1041
15. Liu H et al (2002) T(11;18) is a marker for all stage gastric MALT lymphomas that will not respond to H. pylori eradication. Gastroenterology 122(5):1286–1294
16. Swerdlow SH (2008) International Agency for Research on Cancer and World Health Organization, WHO classification of tumours of haematopoietic and lymphoid tissues. 4th edn. World Health Organization classification of tumours. International Agency for Research on Cancer, Lyon, France, p. 439
17. (1997) A clinical evaluation of the International Lymphoma Study Group classification of non-Hodgkin's lymphoma. The Non-Hodgkin's Lymphoma Classification Project. Blood 89(11):3909–3918
18. Wotherspoon AC et al (1991) Helicobacter pylori-associated gastritis and primary B-cell gastric lymphoma. Lancet 338(8776):1175–1176

19. Bergman MP, D'Elios MM (2010) Cytotoxic T cells in H. pylori-related gastric autoimmunity and gastric lymphoma. J Biomed Biotechnol 2010:104918
20. Ferrand J et al (2008) Modulation of lymphocyte proliferation induced by gastric MALT lymphoma-associated Helicobacter pylori strains. Helicobacter 13(3):167–173
21. Parsonnet J et al (1994) Helicobacter pylori infection and gastric lymphoma. N Engl J Med 330(18):1267–1271
22. Doglioni C et al (1992) High incidence of primary gastric lymphoma in northeastern Italy. Lancet 339(8797):834–835
23. Hussell T et al (1993) The response of cells from low-grade B-cell gastric lymphomas of mucosa-associated lymphoid tissue to Helicobacter pylori. Lancet 342(8871):571–574
24. Hussell T et al (1996) Helicobacter pylori-specific tumour-infiltrating T cells provide contact dependent help for the growth of malignant B cells in low-grade gastric lymphoma of mucosa-associated lymphoid tissue. J Pathol 178(2):122–127
25. Greiner A et al (1997) Low-grade B cell lymphomas of mucosa-associated lymphoid tissue (MALT-type) require CD40-mediated signaling and Th2-type cytokines for in vitro growth and differentiation. Am J Pathol 150(5):1583–1593
26. Isaacson PG (1999) Mucosa-associated lymphoid tissue lymphoma. Semin Hematol 36(2):139–147
27. Thiede C et al (2000) Eradication of Helicobacter pylori and stability of remissions in low-grade gastric B-cell lymphomas of the mucosa-associated lymphoid tissue: results of an ongoing multicenter trial. Recent Results Cancer Res 156:125–133
28. Bazarbachi A et al (2004) New therapeutic approaches for adult T-cell leukaemia. Lancet Oncol 5(11):664–672
29. Sagaert X et al (2010) Gastric MALT lymphoma: a model of chronic inflammation-induced tumor development. Nat Rev Gastroenterol Hepatol 7(6):336–346
30. Zucca E et al (2003) Nongastric marginal zone B-cell lymphoma of mucosa-associated lymphoid tissue. Blood 101(7):2489–2495
31. Cavalli F et al. (2001) MALT lymphomas. Hematology Am Soc Hematol Educ Program 241–258
32. Suarez F et al (2006) Infection-associated lymphomas derived from marginal zone B cells: a model of antigen-driven lymphoproliferation. Blood 107(8):3034–3044
33. Streubel B et al (2005) T(3;14)(p14.1;q32) involving IGH and FOXP1 is a novel recurrent chromosomal aberration in MALT lymphoma. Leukemia 19(4):652–658
34. Murga Penas EM et al (2003) Translocations t(11;18)(q21;q21) and t(14;18)(q32;q21) are the main chromosomal abnormalities involving MLT/MALT1 in MALT lymphomas. Leukemia 17(11):2225–2229
35. Ott G et al (1997) The t(11;18)(q21;q21) chromosome translocation is a frequent and specific aberration in low-grade but not high-grade malignant non-Hodgkin's lymphomas of the mucosa-associated lymphoid tissue (MALT-) type. Cancer Res 57(18):3944–3948
36. Clark HM, Jones DB, Wright DH (1992) Cytogenetic and molecular studies of t(14;18) and t(14;19) in nodal and extranodal B-cell lymphoma. J Pathol 166(2):129–137
37. Du M et al (1995) The accumulation of p53 abnormalities is associated with progression of mucosa-associated lymphoid tissue lymphoma. Blood 86(12):4587–4593
38. Wotherspoon AC, Finn TM, Isaacson PG (1995) Trisomy 3 in low-grade B-cell lymphomas of mucosa-associated lymphoid tissue. Blood 85(8):2000–2004
39. Dierlamm J et al (1996) Trisomy 3 in marginal zone B-cell lymphoma: a study based on cytogenetic analysis and fluorescence in situ hybridization. Br J Haematol 93(1):242–249
40. Dierlamm J et al (1997) Characteristic pattern of chromosomal gains and losses in marginal zone B cell lymphoma detected by comparative genomic hybridization. Leukemia 11(5):747–758
41. Auer IA et al (1997) t(11;18)(q21;q21) is the most common translocation in MALT lymphomas. Ann Oncol 8(10):979–985
42. Dierlamm J et al (1996) Marginal zone B-cell lymphomas of different sites share similar cytogenetic and morphologic features. Blood 87(1):299–307

43. Suzuki H et al (1999) API1-MALT1-MLT is involved in mucosa-associated lymphoid tissue lymphoma with t(11;18)(q21;q21). Blood 94(9):3270–3271
44. Maes B et al (2000) The product of the t(11;18), an API2-MLT fusion, is an almost exclusive finding in marginal zone cell lymphoma of extranodal MALT-type. Ann Oncol 11(5):521–526
45. Lucas PC, McAllister-Lucas LM, Nunez G (2004) NF-kappaB signaling in lymphocytes: a new cast of characters. J Cell Sci 117(Pt 1):31–39
46. Hosokawa Y et al (2005) API2-MALT1 fusion protein induces transcriptional activation of the API2 gene through NF-kappaB binding elements: evidence for a positive feed-back loop pathway resulting in unremitting NF-kappaB activation. Biochem Biophys Res Commun 334(1):51–60
47. Lucas PC et al (2001) Bcl10 and MALT1, independent targets of chromosomal translocation in malt lymphoma, cooperate in a novel NF-kappa B signaling pathway. J Biol Chem 276(22):19012–19019
48. Hosokawa Y (2005) Anti-apoptotic action of API2-MALT1 fusion protein involved in t(11;18)(q21;q21) MALT lymphoma. Apoptosis 10(1):25–34
49. Liu H et al (2001) Resistance of t(11;18) positive gastric mucosa-associated lymphoid tissue lymphoma to Helicobacter pylori eradication therapy. Lancet 357(9249):39–40
50. Ye H et al (2006) Strong BCL10 nuclear expression identifies gastric MALT lymphomas that do not respond to H pylori eradication. Gut 55(1):137–138
51. Bairey O et al (1994) Orbital and adnexal involvement in systemic non-Hodgkin's lymphoma. Cancer 73(9):2395–2399
52. Freeman C, Berg JW, Cutler SJ (1972) Occurrence and prognosis of extranodal lymphomas. Cancer 29(1):252–260
53. Knowles DM et al (1990) Lymphoid hyperplasia and malignant lymphoma occurring in the ocular adnexa (orbit, conjunctiva, and eyelids): a prospective multiparametric analysis of 108 cases during 1977 to 1987. Hum Pathol 21(9):959–973
54. Meunier J et al (2004) Ophthalmologic and intraocular non-Hodgkin's lymphoma: a large single centre study of initial characteristics, natural history, and prognostic factors. Hematol Oncol 22(4):143–158
55. Sullivan TJ et al (2005) Lymphoproliferative disease of the ocular adnexa: a clinical and pathologic study with statistical analysis of 69 patients. Ophthal Plast Reconstr Surg 21(3):177–188
56. Cho EY et al (2003) Clinicopathologic analysis of ocular adnexal lymphomas: extranodal marginal zone b-cell lymphoma constitutes the vast majority of ocular lymphomas among Koreans and affects younger patients. Am J Hematol 73(2):87–96
57. Yoon JS et al (2007) Prognosis for patients in a Korean population with ocular adnexal lymphoproliferative lesions. Ophthal Plast Reconstr Surg 23(2):94–99
58. Ferreri AJ et al (2004) Evidence for an association between Chlamydia psittaci and ocular adnexal lymphomas. J Natl Cancer Inst 96(8):586–594
59. Ferreri AJ et al (2005) Regression of ocular adnexal lymphoma after Chlamydia psittaci-eradicating antibiotic therapy. J Clin Oncol 23(22):5067–5073
60. Rosado MF et al (2006) Ocular adnexal lymphoma: a clinicopathologic study of a large cohort of patients with no evidence for an association with Chlamydia psittaci. Blood 107(2):467–472
61. Vargas RL et al (2006) Is there an association between ocular adnexal lymphoma and infection with Chlamydia psittaci? The University of Rochester experience. Leuk Res 30(5):547–551
62. Ponzoni M et al (2008) Chlamydia infection and lymphomas: association beyond ocular adnexal lymphomas highlighted by multiple detection methods. Clin Cancer Res 14(18):5794–5800
63. Martinet S et al (2003) Outcome and prognostic factors in orbital lymphoma: a Rare Cancer Network study on 90 consecutive patients treated with radiotherapy. Int J Radiat Oncol Biol Phys 55(4):892–898
64. Uno T et al (2003) Radiotherapy for extranodal, marginal zone, B-cell lymphoma of mucosa-associated lymphoid tissue originating in the ocular adnexa: a multiinstitutional, retrospective review of 50 patients. Cancer 98(4):865–871

65. Fung CY et al (2003) Ocular adnexal lymphoma: clinical behavior of distinct World Health Organization classification subtypes. Int J Radiat Oncol Biol Phys 57(5):1382–1391
66. Bhatia S et al (2002) Curative radiotherapy for primary orbital lymphoma. Int J Radiat Oncol Biol Phys 54(3):818–823
67. Tsang RW et al (2003) Localized mucosa-associated lymphoid tissue lymphoma treated with radiation therapy has excellent clinical outcome. J Clin Oncol 21(22):4157–4164
68. Ben Simon GJ et al (2006) Oral chlorambucil for extranodal, marginal zone, B-cell lymphoma of mucosa-associated lymphoid tissue of the orbit. Ophthalmology 113(7):1209–1213
69. Hara Y et al (2001) Immunoglobulin heavy chain gene analysis of ocular adnexal extranodal marginal zone B-cell lymphoma. Invest Ophthalmol Vis Sci 42(11):2450–2457
70. Coupland SE et al (1999) Immunoglobulin VH gene expression among extranodal marginal zone B-cell lymphomas of the ocular adnexa. Invest Ophthalmol Vis Sci 40(3):555–562
71. Mannami T et al (2001) Clinical, histopathological, and immunogenetic analysis of ocular adnexal lymphoproliferative disorders: characterization of malt lymphoma and reactive lymphoid hyperplasia. Mod Pathol 14(7):641–649
72. Byrne GI, Ojcius DM (2004) Chlamydia and apoptosis: life and death decisions of an intracellular pathogen. Nat Rev Microbiol 2(10):802–808
73. Miyairi I, Byrne GI (2006) Chlamydia and programmed cell death. Curr Opin Microbiol 9(1):102–108
74. Tanimoto K et al (2006) Fluorescence in situ hybridization (FISH) analysis of primary ocular adnexal MALT lymphoma. BMC Cancer 6:249
75. Remstein ED et al (2002) Mucosa-associated lymphoid tissue lymphomas with t(11;18)(q21;q21) and mucosa-associated lymphoid tissue lymphomas with aneuploidy develop along different pathogenetic pathways. Am J Pathol 161(1):63–71
76. Ye H et al (2005) MALT lymphoma with t(14;18)(q32;q21)/IGH-MALT1 is characterized by strong cytoplasmic MALT1 and BCL10 expression. J Pathol 205(3):293–301
77. Haydon GH et al (1997) Association between chronic hepatitis C infection and hepatocellular carcinoma in a Scottish population. Gut 40(1):128–132
78. De Vita S et al (1995) Hepatitis C virus within a malignant lymphoma lesion in the course of type II mixed cryoglobulinemia. Blood 86(5):1887–1892
79. Ferri C et al (1994) Hepatitis C virus infection in patients with non-Hodgkin's lymphoma. Br J Haematol 88(2):392–394
80. Ferri C et al (1995) Etiopathogenetic role of hepatitis C virus in mixed cryoglobulinemia, chronic liver diseases and lymphomas. Clin Exp Rheumatol 13(Suppl 13):S135–S140
81. Zuckerman E, Zuckerman T (2002) Hepatitis C and B-cell lymphoma: the hemato-hepatologist linkage. Blood Rev 16(2):119–125
82. Izumi T et al (1996) B cell malignancy and hepatitis C virus infection. Leuk Res 20(5):445
83. Hanley J et al (1996) HCV and non-Hodgkin lymphoma. Lancet 347(9011):1339
84. Thalen DJ et al (1997) Absence of hepatitis C virus infection in non-Hodgkin's lymphoma. Br J Haematol 96(4):880–881
85. Shariff S et al (1999) Hepatitis C infection and B-cell non-Hodgkin's lymphoma in British Columbia: a cross-sectional analysis. Ann Oncol 10(8):961–964
86. Vallisa D et al (1999) Association between hepatitis C virus and non-Hodgkin's lymphoma, and effects of viral infection on histologic subtype and clinical course. Am J Med 106(5):556–560
87. Boisvert J et al (2001) Quantitative analysis of hepatitis C virus in peripheral blood and liver: replication detected only in liver. J Infect Dis 184(7):827–835
88. De Vita S et al (2002) Lack of HCV infection in malignant cells refutes the hypothesis of a direct transforming action of the virus in the pathogenesis of HCV-associated B-cell NHLs. Tumori 88(5):400–406
89. Ivanovski M et al (1998) Somatic hypermutation, clonal diversity, and preferential expression of the VH 51p1/VL kv325 immunoglobulin gene combination in hepatitis C virus-associated immunocytomas. Blood 91(7):2433–2442

90. Miller RH, Purcell RH (1990) Hepatitis C virus shares amino acid sequence similarity with pestiviruses and flaviviruses as well as members of two plant virus supergroups. Proc Natl Acad Sci U S A 87(6):2057–2061
91. Chan CH et al (2001) V(H)1-69 gene is preferentially used by hepatitis C virus-associated B cell lymphomas and by normal B cells responding to the E2 viral antigen. Blood 97(4):1023–1026
92. Pileri P et al (1998) Binding of hepatitis C virus to CD81. Science 282(5390):938–941
93. Levy S, Todd SC, Maecker HT (1998) CD81 (TAPA-1): a molecule involved in signal transduction and cell adhesion in the immune system. Annu Rev Immunol 16:89–109
94. Sakamuro D, Furukawa T, Takegami T (1995) Hepatitis C virus nonstructural protein NS3 transforms NIH 3T3 cells. J Virol 69(6):3893–3896
95. Ray RB, Meyer K, Ray R (1996) Suppression of apoptotic cell death by hepatitis C virus core protein. Virology 226(2):176–182
96. Trejo O et al (2003) Hematologic malignancies in patients with cryoglobulinemia: association with autoimmune and chronic viral diseases. Semin Arthritis Rheum 33(1):19–28
97. Zignego AL et al (2002) Prevalence of bcl-2 rearrangement in patients with hepatitis C virus-related mixed cryoglobulinemia with or without B-cell lymphomas. Ann Intern Med 137(7):571–580
98. Kauppi M, Pukkala E, Isomaki H (1997) Elevated incidence of hematologic malignancies in patients with Sjogren's syndrome compared with patients with rheumatoid arthritis (Finland). Cancer Causes Control 8(2):201–204
99. Thomas E et al (2000) Risk of malignancy among patients with rheumatic conditions. Int J Cancer 88(3):497–502
100. Mellemkjaer L et al (1996) Rheumatoid arthritis and cancer risk. Eur J Cancer 32A(10):1753–1757
101. Hakulinen T, Isomaki H, Knekt P (1985) Rheumatoid arthritis and cancer studies based on linking nationwide registries in Finland. Am J Med 78(1A):29–32
102. Franklin J et al (2006) Incidence of lymphoma in a large primary care derived cohort of cases of inflammatory polyarthritis. Ann Rheum Dis 65(5):617–622
103. Smedby KE et al (2006) Autoimmune and chronic inflammatory disorders and risk of non-Hodgkin lymphoma by subtype. J Natl Cancer Inst 98(1):51–60
104. Wolfe F, Michaud K (2007) The effect of methotrexate and anti-tumor necrosis factor therapy on the risk of lymphoma in rheumatoid arthritis in 19,562 patients during 89,710 person-years of observation. Arthritis Rheum 56(5):1433–1439
105. Askling J et al (2005) Haematopoietic malignancies in rheumatoid arthritis: lymphoma risk and characteristics after exposure to tumour necrosis factor antagonists. Ann Rheum Dis 64(10):1414–1420
106. Oleinick A (1967) Leukemia or lymphoma occurring subsequent to an autoimmune disease. Blood 29(1):144–153
107. Isomaki HA, Hakulinen T, Joutsenlahti U (1978) Excess risk of lymphomas, leukemia and myeloma in patients with rheumatoid arthritis. J Chronic Dis 31(11):691–696
108. Baecklund E et al (2006) Association of chronic inflammation, not its treatment, with increased lymphoma risk in rheumatoid arthritis. Arthritis Rheum 54(3):692–701
109. Cobeta-Garcia JC, Ruiz-Jimeno MT, Fontova-Garrofe R (1993) Non-Hodgkin's lymphoma, rheumatoid arthritis and methotrexate. J Rheumatol 20(1):200–202
110. Kamel OW et al (1999) A population based, case control study of non-Hodgkin's lymphoma in patients with rheumatoid arthritis. J Rheumatol 26(8):1676–1680
111. Morris CR, Morris AJ (1993) Localized lymphoma in a patient with rheumatoid arthritis treated with parenteral methotrexate. J Rheumatol 20(12):2172–2173
112. Kingsmore SF et al (1992) Association of methotrexate, rheumatoid arthritis and lymphoma: report of 2 cases and literature review. J Rheumatol 19(9):1462–1465
113. Klein HP (1992) Occurrence of highly malignant non-Hodgkin's lymphoma in correlation with Imurek therapy and later MTX therapy of chronic polyarthritis. Z Rheumatol 51(5):256–259

114. Ellman MH et al (1991) Lymphoma developing in a patient with rheumatoid arthritis taking low dose weekly methotrexate. J Rheumatol 18(11):1741–1743
115. Georgescu L, Paget SA (1999) Lymphoma in patients with rheumatoid arthritis: what is the evidence of a link with methotrexate? Drug Saf 20(6):475–487
116. Georgescu L et al (1997) Lymphoma in patients with rheumatoid arthritis: association with the disease state or methotrexate treatment. Semin Arthritis Rheum 26(6):794–804
117. Usman AR, Yunus MB (1996) Non-Hodgkin's lymphoma in patients with rheumatoid arthritis treated with low dose methotrexate. J Rheumatol 23(6):1095–1097
118. Shiroky JB et al (1991) Complications of immunosuppression associated with weekly low dose methotrexate. J Rheumatol 18(8):1172–1175
119. Mariette X et al (2002) Lymphomas in rheumatoid arthritis patients treated with methotrexate: a 3-year prospective study in France. Blood 99(11):3909–3915
120. Moder KG et al (1995) Hematologic malignancies and the use of methotrexate in rheumatoid arthritis: a retrospective study. Am J Med 99(3):276–281
121. Salloum E et al (1996) Spontaneous regression of lymphoproliferative disorders in patients treated with methotrexate for rheumatoid arthritis and other rheumatic diseases. J Clin Oncol 14(6):1943–1949
122. Rizzi R et al (2009) Spontaneous remission of "methotrexate-associated lymphoproliferative disorders" after discontinuation of immunosuppressive treatment for autoimmune disease. Review of the literature. Med Oncol 26(1):1–9
123. Harris NL, SS (2001) Methotrexate-associated lymphoproliferative disorders. In: Jaffe ES, Harris NL, Stein H, Vardinam JW (eds) World Health Organization classification of tumours. Pathology and genetics: tumours of haematopoietic and lymphoid tissues. 1st edn. IARC Press, Lyon, France, p 270–271
124. Starkebaum G (2001) Rheumatoid arthritis, methotrexate, and lymphoma: risk substitution, or cat and mouse with Epstein-Barr virus? J Rheumatol 28(12):2573–2575
125. Smedby KE, Baecklund E, Askling J (2006) Malignant lymphomas in autoimmunity and inflammation: a review of risks, risk factors, and lymphoma characteristics. Cancer Epidemiol Biomarkers Prev 15(11):2069–2077
126. Chen YJ et al (2010) Malignancy in systemic lupus erythematosus: a nationwide cohort study in Taiwan. Am J Med 123(12):1150 e1–1150 e6
127. Ekstrom Smedby K et al (2008) Autoimmune disorders and risk of non-Hodgkin lymphoma subtypes: a pooled analysis within the InterLymph Consortium. Blood 111(8):4029–4038
128. Zintzaras E, Voulgarelis M, Moutsopoulos HM (2005) The risk of lymphoma development in autoimmune diseases: a meta-analysis. Arch Intern Med 165(20):2337–2344
129. King JK, Costenbader KH (2007) Characteristics of patients with systemic lupus erythematosus (SLE) and non-Hodgkin's lymphoma (NHL). Clin Rheumatol 26(9):1491–1494
130. Sugai S, Masaki Y, Dong L (2004) Lymphoproliferative disorders in patients with Sjogren's syndrome. Autoimmun Rev 3(Suppl 1):S67–S69
131. Zulman J, Jaffe R, Talal N (1978) Evidence that the malignant lymphoma of Sjogren's syndrome is a monoclonal B-cell neoplasm. N Engl J Med 299(22):1215–1220
132. Voulgarelis M, Moutsopoulos HM (2001) Malignant lymphoma in primary Sjogren's syndrome. Isr Med Assoc J 3(10):761–766
133. Ioannidis JP, Vassiliou VA, Moutsopoulos HM (2002) Long-term risk of mortality and lymphoproliferative disease and predictive classification of primary Sjogren's syndrome. Arthritis Rheum 46(3):741–747
134. Engels EA et al (2005) Immune-related conditions and immune-modulating medications as risk factors for non-Hodgkin's lymphoma: a case-control study. Am J Epidemiol 162(12):1153–1161
135. Vitali C et al (2002) Classification criteria for Sjogren's syndrome: a revised version of the European criteria proposed by the American-European Consensus Group. Ann Rheum Dis 61(6):554–558
136. Ramos-Casals M et al (2005) Hypocomplementaemia as an immunological marker of morbidity and mortality in patients with primary Sjogren's syndrome. Rheumatology (Oxford) 44(1):89–94

137. Theander E et al (2006) Lymphoma and other malignancies in primary Sjogren's syndrome: a cohort study on cancer incidence and lymphoma predictors. Ann Rheum Dis 65(6):796–803
138. Kassan SS et al (1978) Increased risk of lymphoma in sicca syndrome. Ann Intern Med 89(6):888–892
139. Voulgarelis M et al (1999) Malignant lymphoma in primary Sjogren's syndrome: a multicenter, retrospective, clinical study by the European Concerted Action on Sjogren's Syndrome. Arthritis Rheum 42(8):1765–1772
140. Valesini G et al (1997) Differential risk of non-Hodgkin's lymphoma in Italian patients with primary Sjogren's syndrome. J Rheumatol 24(12):2376–2380
141. Youinou P et al (1988) CD5-expressing B lymphocytes in the blood and salivary glands of patients with primary Sjogren's syndrome. J Autoimmun 1(2):185–194
142. Gasparotto D et al (2003) Extrasalivary lymphoma development in Sjogren's syndrome: clonal evolution from parotid gland lymphoproliferation and role of local triggering. Arthritis Rheum 48(11):3181–3186
143. Dong L et al (2007) Clonality analysis of lymphoproliferative disorders in patients with Sjogren's syndrome. Clin Exp Immunol 150(2):279–284
144. Bahler DW, Swerdlow SH (1998) Clonal salivary gland infiltrates associated with myoepithelial sialadenitis (Sjogren's syndrome) begin as nonmalignant antigen-selected expansions. Blood 91(6):1864–1872
145. Pisa EK et al (1991) High frequency of t(14;18) translocation in salivary gland lymphomas from Sjogren's syndrome patients. J Exp Med 174(5):1245–1250
146. Tapinos NI, Polihronis M, Moutsopoulos HM (1999) Lymphoma development in Sjogren's syndrome: novel p53 mutations. Arthritis Rheum 42(7):1466–1472
147. Martin T et al (2000) Salivary gland lymphomas in patients with Sjogren's syndrome may frequently develop from rheumatoid factor B cells. Arthritis Rheum 43(4):908–916
148. Mariette X (1999) Lymphomas in patients with Sjogren's syndrome: review of the literature and physiopathologic hypothesis. Leuk Lymphoma 33(1–2):93–99
149. De Re V et al (2002) Salivary gland B cell lymphoproliferative disorders in Sjogren's syndrome present a restricted use of antigen receptor gene segments similar to those used by hepatitis C virus-associated non-Hodgkins's lymphomas. Eur J Immunol 32(3):903–910
150. Ramos-Casals M et al (2004) Triple association between hepatitis C virus infection, systemic autoimmune diseases, and B cell lymphoma. J Rheumatol 31(3):495–499
151. Mariette X (2001) Lymphomas complicating Sjogren's syndrome and hepatitis C virus infection may share a common pathogenesis: chronic stimulation of rheumatoid factor B cells. Ann Rheum Dis 60(11):1007–1010
152. Aozasa K (1990) Hashimoto's thyroiditis as a risk factor of thyroid lymphoma. Acta Pathol Jpn 40(7):459–468
153. Kapadia SB et al (1982) Malignant lymphoma of the thyroid gland: a clinicopathologic study. Head Neck Surg 4(4):270–280
154. Moshynska OV, Saxena A (2008) Clonal relationship between Hashimoto thyroiditis and thyroid lymphoma. J Clin Pathol 61(4):438–444
155. Hwang YC et al (2009) Clinical characteristics of primary thyroid lymphoma in Koreans. Endocr J 56(3):399–405
156. Hyjek E, Isaacson PG (1988) Primary B cell lymphoma of the thyroid and its relationship to Hashimoto's thyroiditis. Hum Pathol 19(11):1315–1326
157. Saxena A et al (2004) Clonal B cell populations in a minority of patients with Hashimoto's thyroiditis. J Clin Pathol 57(12):1258–1263
158. Huo Z et al (2006) Gene rearrangement studies in Hashimoto's thyroiditis and primary lymphoma of thyroid. Zhonghua Bing Li Xue Za Zhi 35(6):344–347
159. Widder S, Pasieka JL (2004) Primary thyroid lymphomas. Curr Treat Options Oncol 5(4):307–313

Preclinical Modeling in Lymphoid Malignancies

Richa Dawar and Francisco J. Hernandez-Ilizaliturri

Abstract Non-Hodgkin's lymphoma (NHL) is one of the most common cancers in the United States, accounting for about 4% of all cancers. In spite of aggressive chemotherapy and management, a majority of the patients relapse, making refractory NHL one of the dreaded nightmares for oncologists. Laboratory studies conducted on tumor cell lines, primary tumor cells isolated from cancer patients, and murine models contribute significantly to development of cancer therapeutics. The heterogeneity of the disease, limited availability of the biopsies, and variability of the disease in patients have necessitated the development of animal models to evaluate potential drug therapies. Moreover, the preclinical models also help us to understand the pathogenesis of the disease and the role of immune system in lymphoma. As we enter into an era of targeted therapeutics, these models provide new platforms for designing new anti-lymphoma drugs. In this chapter, we summarize the various tumor cell lines and murine models including tumor xenografts, syngeneic models, genetically engineered mice, and humanized mice used to study the initiation and growth of lymphoma, lymphoma microenvironment, and efficacy of new therapies. Later in the chapter, we also discuss the advantages and disadvantages of each model and explain how each of them aid in understanding of the pathogenesis of lymphoma and interactions between tumors and host environment.

R. Dawar, M.D.
Department of Medical Oncology, Roswell Park Cancer Institute, Buffalo, NY 14263, USA

F.J. Hernandez-Ilizaliturri, M.D. (✉)
Department of Medical Oncology, Roswell Park Cancer Institute, Buffalo, NY 14263, USA

Department of Medical Immunology, Roswell Park Cancer Institute, Elm and Carlton Streets, Buffalo, NY 14263, USA
e-mail: francisco.hernandez@roswellpark.org

P.J. Quesenberry and J.J. Castillo (eds.), *Non-Hodgkin Lymphoma: Prognostic Factors and Targets*, Cancer Drug Discovery and Development,
DOI 10.1007/978-1-4614-5851-7_6,

Introduction

Non-Hodgkin's lymphoma (NHL) is one of the most common types of cancer diagnosed in the United States, and its incidence has been increasing over the past 30 years. According to latest published cancer statistics (2012), approximately 79,190 lymphoma new cases will be diagnosed, and 20,130 lymphoma patients are expected to die from their disease despite currently available treatment [1]. Lymphoma is a heterogeneous group of malignancies with diverse biology, clinical behavior, and prognosis. The management of NHL, involving intense chemotherapy and stem cell transplant, is often associated with significant short- or long-term treatment-related toxicities. Although some aggressive forms of NHL can be cured by currently available treatment strategies, a significant number of patients relapse after a variable period of remission or exhibit primary refractory disease to upfront or salvage treatments. The management of relapsed/refractory lymphomas continues to be a challenge for the practicing oncologist.

In general, the clinical outcome of lymphoma patients has improved over the last decades as a result of several factors that include (1) the better understanding of the pathogenesis and biology of lymphoid malignancies, (2) the advanced technology resulting in a more precise diagnosis (i.e., immunophenotyping, cytogenetic or gene expression profiling studies) and staging (i.e., functional imaging), (3) the identification and validation of clinically based score indices or biomarkers capable of predicting clinical outcomes and/or response to therapy, and (4) the development and incorporation of novel and effective agents in the management of lymphoid malignancies (i.e., monoclonal antibodies).

Laboratory studies conducted on cell lines, lymphoma mouse models, and tumor cells isolated from cancer patients are contributing significantly not only in deciphering the pathogenesis of lymphoid malignancies but also in identifying prognostic markers of clinical outcome and therapeutic targets for drug development. In this contribution, we present an overview of preclinical models utilized in lymphoma translational research and provide examples of how those models are paving the road for future clinical studies. In addition, we present the limitations of each model utilized stressing the need to develop more clinically relevant laboratory models to study lymphoid malignancies.

Laboratory Models in Lymphoma

Parallel to biotechnology advances, the development and implementation of laboratory models to study lymphomas have become more complex. In general, preclinical models can be categorized depending on the material utilized (*human or murine cell lines* vs. *primary tumor cells*) and the setting tested (in vivo vs. in vitro). The use of various preclinical models to study a targeted agent is more accurate in predicting efficacy in subsequent clinical studies than preclinical evaluations conducted using only one model system. A significant number of peer-reviewed journals encourage scientists to test their therapeutic concepts in several preclinical models in order to better define the significance of their scientific findings. Each system has advantages or limitations, and for the most part, they are complementary to each other.

In Vitro Preclinical Models

Cell culture experiments are the backbone of drug discovery and development in cancer research. These experiments are usually the first step in identifying therapeutic targets and addressing the antitumor activity of a new drug. In vitro studies can be conducted in cancer cell lines or more recently from primary tumor cells derived from cancer patients.

Primary Tumor Cells

Normal and primary malignant lymphoid cells can be isolated from the peripheral blood (especially in chronic lymphocytic leukemia [CLL] patients), bone marrow aspirates, or nodal masses in patients with lymphoma. Cell suspensions can easily be generated, and malignant cells can be isolated using magnetic beads or flow cytometry cell sorting. In contrast to the majority of the B-cell lymphoma cell lines available for preclinical studies, primary tumor cells had not been coinfected with the Epstein–Barr virus (EBV) and represent a more clinically relevant source of tumor cells to test novel therapeutic agents. In addition, primary tumor cells may add more insightful information regarding the pathophysiology of a given specific subtype of lymphoma. This source of laboratory material is especially important, as the role of the tumor microenvironment and accessory cells present in the tumor bed is increasingly being recognized by the scientific community. Moreover, the development or optimization of novel agents targeting not only cancer cells but also the tumor microenvironment (i.e., lenalidomide) requires carefully designed preclinical studies utilizing primary tumor cells and stromal/accessory cells (i.e., multiple myeloma, CLL, follicular lymphoma, or Hodgkin's lymphoma [HL]).

On the other hand, the limited access to nodal masses, size of the specimen obtained, and the short-term viability of primary tumor cells once extracted from lymphoma patients are some of the limitations encountered when designing preclinical studies using tumor cells obtained from lymphoma patients.

Cell Lines and Stem Cell

The use of lymphoma cell lines has been necessary for the preclinical studies testing different agents, including monoclonal antibodies. In addition, molecular biology studies performed in cell lines have provided us with insightful information regarding the biology of human neoplasia and potential mechanisms responsible for the development of resistance to chemotherapy agents, biologics, and monoclonal antibodies. Our group of investigators believe that cell lines are excellent candidates to study mechanisms involved in the development of resistance for several reasons: (1) comparative analysis can be performed between various lymphoma cell lines and their resistant clones generated following chronic exposure of parental cells to a particular drug/biological agent (e.g., mAb), (2) availability—lymphoma cell lines can be grown in large quantities for a long period of time so that validation of initial results or clarification of conflictive data can be repeated at any time, (3) lymphoma cell lines consist of a relatively "homogeneous" population in which nonmalignant cells are absent (as opposed to tissue biopsy samples) which is important when performing sensitive assays such as gene and amino acid sequencing.

Diploid transformed (coinfected with EBV virus) or non-transformed cells can be established or are commercially available in several tissue and cell culture facilities. Transformed cells tend to proliferate faster and grow easier in vitro than non-transformed cells. EBV has been used to immortalize malignant B cells and established cell lines for several decades, and these cells harbor the EBV virus in the latent stage. The human T-cell leukemia virus-1 (HTLV-1) is a retrovirus frequently used to transform benign or malignant T cells and establish cell lines. Normal T cells isolated from peripheral blood are unable to grow spontaneously in vitro. However, they can be infected with HTLV-1 virus in order to induce growth in a liquid as well in a semisolid culture medium [2]. These transformed T cells are able to actively transcribe HTLV-1 RNA and are considered to be infectious requiring special handling by laboratory personnel.

Seeding non-transformed neoplastic cells directly into suspension cultures is the widely used procedure to establish a lymphoma cell line. The success rate is very low and often unpredictable. Examples of widely used continuous transformed or non-transformed NHL cell lines are listed in Table 1. Matsuo and Drexler [3] observed that malignant cells which were derived from the relapsed lymphoma patients or from patients with poor prognosis had an enhanced growth potential in vitro compared with cells derived from previously untreated or good prognostic features patients.

In contrast to what is observed in solid tumor malignancies, the growth in vitro of hematological malignant cells requires nonadherent culture techniques and propagates easily in cell suspensions. In addition, nonadherent cells do not require mechanical or chemical (i.e., enzymatic disruption) manipulation for harvesting, and therefore nonspecific activation or death is minimal. On the other hand, some lymphoma cell lines (i.e., natural killer- [NK] or T-cell lymphoma cell lines) require special nutrients, cytokines, or culture conditions for optimal growth.

Normal Lymphocytes

Short-term culture of peripheral lymphocytes is a standard technique in human genetics and provides an unlimited source of diagnostic material for mutational analysis, investigation of chromosomal abnormalities, and identification of hereditary

Table 1 Established transformed and non-transformed cell lines commonly utilized in lymphoma preclinical models

Human cell lines	Features
Burkitt's lymphoma (BL)	
Raji	Derived from a BL of the left maxilla of an 11-year-old black male, Epstein–Barr nuclear antigen (EBNA) positive
Daudi	Derived from a 16-year-old male with BL, cells are negative for beta-2-microglobulin and carry the translocation (t) (8;14)(q24;q32)
BL-2	BL cell line isolated from a tumor biopsy obtained from a Caucasian child. The cells carry the t(8;22)(q24;q11)
BJA-B	Epstein–Barr virus (EBV)-negative BL cell line with t(2;8)(p12;q24)
Jijoye	Lymphoblastic cell line derived from a 7-year-old boy with Burkitt's lymphoma, EBV positive
CA46	Human cell line established from the ascites fluid of a patient with Burkitt's lymphoma; the cells are EBNA-negative, carry the t(8;14), and express Bcl-2 and c-Myc proteins
Ci-1	Human B-cell lymphoma cell line with the t(2;8), t(14;22)
Diffuse large B-cell lymphoma (DLBCL)	
RL	Human germinal center B-cell (GCB) DLBCL cell line carries the translocation (t) (14;18)
SU-DHL-4	Human cell line from the peritoneal effusion of a 38-year-old man with GCB-DLBCL and carries the t(14;18)
NU-DHL-1	Human cell line established from the left inguinal lymph node of a 73-year-old Caucasian man with GCB-DLBCL and carries the t(3;8) and t(14;18)
U2932	Human cell line derived from the ascites of a 29-year-old woman with activated B-cell (ABC) DLBCL. The cells overexpress the BCL-2, BCL-6, and p53 proteins
CRO-AP/2	Human B-cell lymphoma cell line from the diagnostic pretreatment pleural effusion of a 49-year-old HIV+ homosexual male with primary effusion lymphoma (PEL) and previous history of Kaposi's sarcoma; cells were described to be EBV+ and HHV-8+ and to carry a BCL-6 point mutation
Follicular lymphoma (FL) transformed cells	
Karpas 422	Human transformed FL cell line with the t(14;18) (q32,q21)
MC116	Human cell line derived from the pleural effusion of a patient with B-cell lymphoma. Cells are EBV-negative, carried the t(8;14)(q24;q32)

(continued)

Table 1 (continued)

Human cell lines	Features
DoHH2	Human transformed FL cell line with t(14;18)(q32;q21)
Mantle cell lymphoma (MCL)	
Granta 519	Derived from a case of high-grade MCL, t(11;14)(q13;q32) is present
Mino	MCL cell line, cells expressed cyclin D1 and p53 and carried the t(11;14)
Z138	Human cell line was derived from a patient with MCL with blastoid transformation. The cells have the t(11;14)(q13;q32) abnormality and overexpress cyclin D1
Jeko	MCL cell line established from peripheral blood mononuclear cells of a patient with a blastoid variant of MCL, cells negative for Epstein–Barr virus and overexpress cyclin D1, Bcl-2, c-Myc, and Rb proteins and show Bcl-1/J(H) gene rearrangement
Rec-1	Human B-cell line established from a patient with MCL. The cells carried the t(11;14)(q13;q32) and overexpress cyclin D1
T-cell lymphoma	
SUP-T1	Human T-cell lymphoblastic lymphoma cell line
HUT 102	Human cell line was derived from the peripheral blood of a 26-year-old black male patient with mycosis fungoides
HUT 78	Human cell line derived from 50-year-old male patient with Sezary's syndrome. The cell line expresses CD52 antigen

alterations in genome structures. As with any clinical specimen, special considerations regarding biohazard safety are required to prevent infections. Isolation of peripheral lymphocytes is based on density gradient centrifugation of heparinized whole blood. Subsequently, addition of mitogens stimulates cell proliferation to obtain a large number of lymphocytes for chromosomal analysis by staining techniques, in situ hybridization or isolation, and direct sequencing of DNA.

In some circumstances, normal lymphocyte cell proliferation or "long-term" maintenance of hematological cells with differentiation properties is required; this can be accomplished using feeder cells. The usage of feeder layer cell culture was introduced by Dexter et al. [4]. Embryonic fibroblasts, macrophages, or thymocytes are examples of feeder cells that are known to provide the specific microenvironment signals required by the hematological cells. Normally, feeder cells are inactivated for cell proliferation (but not for survival) by radiation or mutagen treatment. In addition to secreting matrix proteins, growth factors, and/or other stimulating factors, feeder cells provide specific cell–cell contacts and cell adhesion.

Additional in vitro systems have been developed in order to characterize and study the process of cell differentiation in hematological cells. Terminal differentiation of hematological cells can be induced by in vitro exposure to certain chemicals (i.e., retinoid acid or lipopolysaccharides), cytokines (i.e., interleukin-2), hormones (i.e., tumor growth factor-beta, epidermal growth factor, humoral growth factor, glucagon, steroids, or thyroxine), or cell–cell/cell–matrix interactions [5–8].

Induction of cell differentiation can be achieved by homologous or heterologous cell–cell interaction. Homologous cell–cell interaction requires a high cell density to facilitate efficient cell–cell communication. However, for the investigation of hematological cell differentiation, heterologous stimulation by fibroblasts and thymocytes among other cell types is more frequently used. Earlier, Burgess and Metcalf [9, 10] and Cross and Dexter [11] developed various cloning methods for hematopoietic cells based on semisolid agar culture containing colony-stimulating growth factors. The HL-60 (lymphoblast) and the Friend erythroleukemia (MEL) cell lines are widely used examples of established progenitor cells for studying hematopoiesis [12].

Preclinical Animal Models

The development of an animal model of human lymphoma that closely resembles the biological behavior observed in lymphoma patients is difficult. Several models using subcutaneously grown xenografts in mice result in localized disease with no evidence of systemic dissemination. In 1990, Ghetie et al. described a model that injected Daudi cells intravenously in severe combined immunodeficiency (SCID) mice [13]. Inoculated animals that were left untreated developed hind leg paralysis (surrogate end point prior to death) within 3–6 weeks of tumor seeding. Following these reports, several human lymphoma cell lines have been used in similar models (Raji, Ramos, and Namalwa cells). The i.v./SCID lymphoma model is preferred to study therapeutic strategies for several reasons: (1) the inoculation of lymphoma cells via tail vein injection results in disseminated disease as opposed to localized disease (resembling disseminated lymphoma more typically seen in humans), (2) the delivery and bio-distribution of monoclonal antibodies to large subcutaneous nodules is compromised due to limited blood supply, and (3) the i.v./SCID model is highly reproducible (>90% engraftment), unlike subcutaneous lymphoma models where only 60–70% of the animals develop tumors at an even more erratic growth rate [14–17]. In addition, in vivo modeling provides essential tumor–host interactions and is a more accurate means of modeling human cancer. Murine models are used to investigate the factors involved in malignant transformation, invasion, and metastasis as well as to examine the response to therapy. Currently, existing and characterized mouse models can be divided in the following five categories: (1) syngeneic murine models, (2) syngeneic models with murine tumor cells engineered to express human antigen, (3) genetically engineered mice (GEM) predisposed to develop a specific type of cancer, (4) orthotopic xenograft of human tumors into immunodeficiency mice (SCID mice), and (5) humanized xenograft mice model:

(a) *Syngeneic models* are best used to study the interactions between cancer cells and the tumor microenvironment (Table 2). Various studies have demonstrated the importance of lymphoma in regulating the tumor microenvironment [18, 19]. Syngeneic models are also used to define the role of immune system in tumor rejection and to evaluate how specific treatments modulate the immune system (i.e., cancer vaccines). The reproducible evaluation of the immune response against cancer antigens is one of the principal applications of syngeneic mouse models. CD8+ T cells infiltrating the tumor bed or changes in cytokine production are commonly utilized surrogate markers to detect and quantify immunological responses [20]. For example, various investigators correlated CD8+ infiltration into the tumor bed following vaccination with survivin or an idiotype-binding peptide with anti-lymphoma activity [21, 22]. Alvarez and colleagues [23] studied the antitumor response of a genetically engineered vaccine in a lymphoma syngeneic mouse model. Following the administration of a FC-CD40L vaccine, they demonstrated an increased production of interleukin (IL)-17, IL-6, and interferon (IFN)-gamma compared with controls. In addition, FC-CD40L vaccination induced regression of established tumors and increased survival.
(b) *Syngeneic models with murine tumor cells engineered to express human antigens* are commonly utilized to evaluate the antitumor activity of monoclonal antibodies targeting human antigens. A classic example of this type of animal model is the murine malignant cells 38C13 expressing human CD20 antigen that has been used to evaluate the therapeutic potential of rituximab in vivo. In addition, this particular type of model has been used to define the mechanisms that affect rituximab antitumor activity. Golay et al. [24] demonstrated that complement is required for the therapeutic activity of rituximab in vivo in the 38C13 murine model of B-cell lymphoma. In addition, Dayde and colleagues [25] used the syngeneic CD20-modified EL4-mouse T-cell lymphoma model to evaluate the relationship between tumor burden and rituximab dose responses in vivo. In this model, EL4 murine T-cell lymphoma cells were transduced with human CD20 cDNA and transfected with luciferase plasmid (EL4-huCD20-Luc). Subsequently, cells were inoculated into C57BL/6J mice via tail vein injection. Using functional imaging to assess response to therapy, Dayde et al. demonstrated a linear relationship between tumor burden and rituximab efficacy. Additional examples of syngeneic lymphoma models using modified murine cancer cells are presented in Table 3.
(c) *Spontaneously developed lymphoma in genetically engineered mice (GEM) or transgenic mice models* are based on the knockout or transgenic technology and are widely used in basic and applied hematological research. GEM models are invaluable tools to study the mechanisms involved in lymphomagenesis and to characterize the relationship between disease phenotypes and underlying genetic lesions. The genetic profile of these mice is altered at the germline level in one or several genes (by mutation, deletion, or overexpression) thought to be

Table 2 Selective syngeneic models of NHL (modified from Donnou et al. [26])

Model	Injection site	Lymphoma type	Strain (haplotype)	References
Pi-BCL1 (m)	IV	DLBCL	BALB/c(H-2^d)	[55]
38C13 (m)	IV/IP	NHL	C3H/HeN(H-2^d)	[56]
FL5.12 transfected with Bcl2 (m)	IV	NHL	BALB/c(H-2^d)	[57]
A20 (m)	IV	DLBCL	BALB/c(H-2^d)	[58]
	IS			[59]
	SC			[22]
LMycSN-p53null (m)	SC	NHL	C57Bl/6(H-2^b)	[60]
S11 (m)	SC	BL	BALB/c nude(H-2^d)	[61]
BCL1 (m)	IP	DLBCL	BALB/c(H-2^d)	[56]
A20.IIA-GFP (m)	IS/IC	DLBCL/PCNSL	BALB/c(H-2^d)	[18]
Helicobacter felis	Stomach	MALT lymphoma	BALB/c(H-2^d)	[62]

IV intravenous, *IP* intraperitoneal, *IS* intrasplenic, *IC* intracerebral, *IO* intraocular, *SC* subcutaneous, *DLBCL* diffuse large B-cell lymphoma, *BL* Burkitt's lymphoma, *MALT* mucosa-associated lymphatic tissue, *PCNSL* primary central nervous system lymphoma, *PIOL* primary intraocular lymphoma, *SCID* severe combined immunodeficiency. *(m)* murine origin, *(h)* human origin

Table 3 Syngeneic lymphoma models with murine tumor cells engineered to express human antigens (modified from Donnou et al. [26])

Name	Injection site	Lymphoma model	Strain/haplotype	References
38C13 Her2/neu (m)	IV SC	NHL	C3H/HeN(H-2^K)	[63]
38C13 CD20+ (m)	IC IO	PCNSL PIOL	C3H/HeN(H-2^K)	[64]

IV intravenous, *SC* subcutaneous, *IC* intracerebral, *IO* intraocular, *NHL* non-Hodgkin's lymphoma, *PCNSL* primary central nervous system lymphoma, *PIOL* primary intraocular lymphoma

involved in the transformation process from low-grade to high-grade lymphoma or malignancy. Subsequently, the effect of altering these genes is studied over time, and therapeutic responses to these tumors may be followed in vivo. GEM or transgenic models develop malignancies whose genetic profiles and histopathology appear similar to the molecular characteristics and natural behavior of human tumors. It is also possible to assess the different stages of tumor progression including vey early manifestations of malignancy when using GEMs.

The development of "spontaneous" lymphomas in GEM/transgenic mice is considered to be more physiological than other mouse models, and lymphoma develops under no artificial selective pressure or favorable growth conditions. In general, lymphomas are allowed to develop in their physiological microenvironment. Lymphoma GEMs are immunocompetent and in contrast to lymphoma SCID mouse models, are more clinically relevant to human malignancies. Moreover, due to the presence of an intact immune system, the evaluation of cytokines and effector cell function in the biology and immunological treatment of lymphoid malignances can be more accurately studied. Recent advances in genetic engineering have facilitated the development of transgenic mouse models recapitulating major known genome modifications present in specific subtypes of lymphomas or to infect mice with oncogenic viruses capable of inducing B-cell lymphoma. In this approach, the desirable oncogenic DNA and its regulatory elements are inserted in murine cells during embryogenesis at the one cell stage (immediately after ovule fertilization). Regulatory elements specific for the oncogene of interest are indispensable in order to ensure the success in transgenesis, especially in lymphoma transgenic mouse models.

An example of GEM mouse lymphoma is the Eμ-myc mouse often used to study lymphomagenesis. The Eμ-myc model was designed based on the seminal work by Croce et al. [27]. The Eμ-myc transgenic mouse carries the c-myc oncogene coupled to the immunoglobulin heavy locus (IgH) enhancer Eu and results in the development of aggressive pre-B-cell or B-cell lymphomas accompanied by lymphoblastic leukemia but not Burkitt's lymphoma (BL). B-cell lymphoma development in the Eμ-myc model occurs in 100% of animals, but the onset of the disease is rather variable. Mori and colleagues [28] described two distinct tumor phenotypes in the Eμ-myc model: (1) the first type arises earlier in the life span of the mice and is composed mainly of immature B cells resembling BL; (2) the second type develops late in life (400 days after birth) and is composed of mature B cells simulating DLBCL [28].

Modifications of the original model had been studied with interesting findings. Kovalchuk et al. demonstrated that if the c-myc gene is placed under the enhancer region of the immunoglobulin light chain gene, the offspring of transgenic mice develop a high-grade lymphoma that resembles BL [29]. In contrast, Sheppard et al. generated a peculiar transgenic mouse model with translocation of N-myc gene under the IgH enhancer. A fraction of the transgenic mice (25%) carrying that particular gene rearrangement developed a form of indolent B-cell lymphoma late in their life span (9–12 months after birth) [30]. Infection of N-myc transgenic mice with the Moloney leukemia virus increased the incidence of lymphoma and accelerated the lymphomagenesis process [31].

Similar approaches have been utilized to establish transgenic mouse models of mantle cell lymphoma (MCL). At the molecular level, MCL is characterized by the deregulation of Bcl-2 family members (Mcl-1, BIM) altering apoptosis, as well as cell cycle (cyclin D1) regulated in part by the ubiquitin–proteasome system (UPS). Mcl-1 or cyclin D1 upregulation is the result of the chromosomal translocation t(11:14)(q13:q32), the hallmark cytogenetic abnormality of MCL [32–34]. Deregulation of cyclin D1 is considered the primary molecular event involved in the pathogenesis of MCL progression. While transgenic mice carrying the cyclin D1 gene under the IgH enhancer Eμ exhibit abnormalities in the cell cycle of B-cell lymphocytes, animals do not develop lymphoma during their life span [35]. This observation further stresses the fact that most lymphoid malignancies involve a multistep mutagenesis process.

Recent studies using comparative genomic hybridization and array-based genomic studies had demonstrated additional chromosomal changes with genomic loses of tumor suppression genes (i.e., ATM, CDKN2A, TP53) or gains of oncogenic genes (i.e., MYC, SYK, or BCL2). Such findings lead

Table 4 Lymphoma transgenic/GEM models

Model name (references)	Lymphoma type
SL/KH [65]	Pre-B lymphoma
Eμ-N-myc [30]	Indolent B-NHL
NFS.V+ [66]	Marginal zone lymphoma
B6-1-MYC [29]	Burkitt-like lymphoma
VavP-Bcl2 [67]	Follicular lymphoma
Eμ-BRD2 [31]	DLBCL
Bcl6 Knock in [68]	Germinal center, DLBCL
Bcl6/Myc transgenic [68]	Post germinal center, DLBCL
IL-14aTGxc-Myc TG (DTG) [38]	Blastoid variant of mantle cell lymphoma
Myc/BCR^{HEL}/HEL [69]	Burkitt-like lymphoma
Eμ-myc [28]	From follicular to DLBCL (time-dependent)
RzCD19Cre [70]	NHL, hepatitis C induced
UVB induced [71]	Mature B-cell lymphoma

DLBCL diffuse large B-cell lymphoma, *NHL* non-Hodgkin's lymphoma, *UVB* ultraviolet beam light

Table 5 Advantages and disadvantages of transgenic mouse models in lymphoma

Advantages	Disadvantages
1. Permits the study of the tumor and its microenvironment 2. Provides insightful information regarding tumor biology 3. Useful in validating postulated oncogenes or tumor suppression genes	1. Limited correlation between disease occurring in transgenic mice and humans (one or two genes mutated vs. hundreds of genes) 2. Cost and infrastructure needed 3. Time to develop and validate a model is long 4. Tumor development is slow and variable unless manipulated with viral infections

investigators to postulate a model of multistep genetic alterations which leads to molecular pathogenesis and progression (i.e., clonal evolution) in MCL [36]. Subsequent transgenic MCL lymphoma mouse models used a double transfection of cyclin D1, and N-myc/L-myc under the Eμ enhancer led to the development of pre-B-cell or mature B-cell murine lymphomas [37]. Another transgenic mice model developed by Ford and colleagues using the double transfection of IL-14a and c-myc genes results in a blastoid variant of MCL in vivo [38]. Additional examples of transgenic mouse models in lymphoma are summarized in Table 4.

Advances in transgenic technology continue to contribute greatly to our understanding of lymphoma development. Currently, available models assist scientists in identifying or validating new oncogenes and their role in the development, maintenance, and progression of lymphoma. On the other hand, this model has limitations (see Table 5) like other preclinical models, stressing the need to use multiple models rather than depending in only one system when conducting preclinical studies.

Table 6 Examples of severe combined immunodeficiency (SCID) mouse models in lymphoma

Name	Injection site	Lymphoma model	Strain/haplotype	References
Z138	IV	Human MCL	SCID mice(H-2^d)	[72]
BJA-B	IV/SC	Burkitt's lymphoma	SCID mice(H-2^d)	[73]
SU-DHL-4	IV	DLBCL	SCID mice(H-2^d)	[39]
	SC		C.B-17 SCID mice(H-2^d)	[47]
Ramos	SC	Burkitt's lymphoma	SCID mice(H-2^d)	[73]
SC-1	SC	Follicular lymphoma	SCID mice(H-2^d)	[73]
DoHH-2	SC	Follicular lymphoma	SCID mice(H-2^d)	[73]
Granta 519	SC	MCL	C.B-17 SCID mice(H-2^d)	[47]
HKBML	SC	Brain DLBCL	C.B-17 SCID mice(H-2^d)	[49]
Raji	IC	PCNSL	Nude mice(H-2^b)	[48]
MC116	IC	PCNSL	Nude mice(H-2^b)	[74]
CA46	IO	PIOL	SCID mice(H-2^d)	[75]

IV intravenous, *SC* subcutaneous, *IC* intracerebral, *IO* intraocular, *MCL* mantle cell lymphoma, *DLBCL* diffuse large B-cell lymphoma, *PCNSL* primary central nervous system lymphoma, *PIOL* primary intraocular lymphoma

(d) *Human tumor xenograft* is one of the most frequently used lymphoma mouse models to study human cancer. It required the implantation or injection of primary human tumor cells or cell lines subcutaneously or orthotopically (into naïve tumor site) of immunosuppressed, immune-deficient, or newborn immune naive mice. After tumor engraftment, the biological and antitumor activity of mAbs, chemotherapy drugs, or targeted agents can be determined. While results obtained from humor tumor xenograft experiments are thought to predict response to a given therapy in humans, the correlation between murine models and clinical activity observed in clinical trials is modest at best, especially when evaluating mAbs and targeted agents.

In general, there are several types of xenograft mouse models, and these are different in the degree of immunodeficiency (nude mouse vs. obese/nonobese (NOD) severe combined immunodeficiency (SCID) mouse models). It has been shown that lymphomas are the most difficult malignancies to implant and grow in nude mice. The reasons are the enhanced natural killer (NK) cell function, macrophage activity, and naturally occurring antitumor antibodies in nude mice. Failure to grow such hematological malignancies in nude mice led to the development of SCID mice (Table 6 shows some examples of SCID mice models used in NHL).

In the field of lymphoma, xenograft mouse models have been utilized to evaluate the biological activity of rituximab and to optimize its antitumor effects. Most of these studies used murine models of human tumor cell lines implanted subcutaneously or via tail vein injection in SCID mice models [15, 39].

Using xenograft mouse models, several investigators have studied the mechanisms-of-action of rituximab in B-cell lymphomas. Clynes demonstrated that FcγR receptor expression is necessary to eradicate NHL in a murine animal model, suggesting that ADCC plays a significant role in rituximab's activity

[40]. We confirmed that effector cells (both natural killer cells and neutrophils) are necessary for optimal antitumor activity of rituximab and corroborating findings have been reported by other investigators [15]. Furthermore, specific polymorphisms in the FcγRIIIa gene have been associated with differences in the clinical and molecular response to anti-CD20 mAb therapy in patients with indolent NHL [41]. Modulation of immune responses is also an attractive strategy to enhance the biological activity of mAbs. Xenograft mouse models of lymphoma had aid in evaluating the antitumor activity of rituximab in combination with agents potentiating rituximab-mediated ADCC such as cytokines (i.e., IL-2 or G-CSF) or immunomodulatory agents (i.e., lenalidomide) [16, 17, 42].

Recently, newly engineered mAbs targeting CD20 with better biological properties when compared to rituximab have been evaluated in preclinical lymphoma models or clinical trials in B-cell lymphoma. Both the EMAB-6 [43] and the humanized GA101 mAbs had been tested against the human SU-DHL4 tumor implanted in to the SCID/beige mice [44]. Our group of investigators evaluated the antitumor activity of ofatumumab in SCID and compared to rituximab in a BL in a SCID mouse model [45].

In addition to the use of disseminated lymphoma mouse models, xenograft mice studies more often used alternative routes of tumor inoculation (i.e., subcutaneous or intracerebral) to (1) evaluate the antitumor activity of biological or chemotherapy agents, (2) study the anti-angiogenic properties of certain targeted drugs, or (3) determine the degree of inhibition in a signaling pathway by a specific pharmacological inhibitor [46–50].

In contrast to GEM/transgenic mice models, human tumor xenografts develop a more homogenous cancer across animals inoculated (especially when animals are inoculated with lymphoma cell lines vs. patient-derived tumors), and the disease usually develops within weeks instead of months. These properties made human tumor xenografts an attractive model to study response to therapy. On the other hand, the major disadvantage of xenograft mouse models resides in the degree of immunodeficiency present in the host. Xenograft mouse models require a host deficient in adaptive immunity in order to engraft human cancer cells, and therefore, these models are not useful when evaluating vaccine strategies. Moreover, as the scientific community is recognizing the importance of the tumor microenvironment in cancer biology and therapeutics, it is questioning the clinical relevance of the human xenograft mouse model.

Humanized mice are immune-deficient mice reconstituted with the human immune system and then implanted with human cancer cell line cells. For the establishment of the humanized mice, the newborn mice must be irradiated and then engrafted with human CD34+ hematopoietic stem cells derived from human umbilical cord blood. However, the timing of obtaining cord blood, irradiating newborn mice, and verifying the humanized phenotype of the NOD/SCID mice after engraftment makes this procedure very complex and cumbersome [51, 52]. Recently, humanized xenograft mouse models have been developed by reconstituting SCID mice with human peripheral blood cells. This type of humanized mouse model appears to be suitable to evaluate vaccination strategies in lymphomas [53]. In response to the challenges faced when studying the biological activity of complement fixating antibodies targeting CD20 in B-cell lymphoma, Sato and colleagues developed a humanized NOD/Shi-SCID mouse model bearing lymphoma cell lines [52]. Similarly, other investigators had evaluated the biological activity of an anti-CD40 antibody (CP-870.893) [54].

Preclinical lymphoma models continue to evolve parallel to the development of newer therapeutic agents and in response to a better understanding of the biology of B-cell and T-cell neoplasm. A significant effort needs to be placed on T-cell lymphoma not only in the clinical arena but also at the bench side, where significant challenges exist in developing, using, and validating T-cell lymphoma preclinical models.

The use of well-established and characterized models is a valuable tool to identify surrogate markers of tumor response to a given treatment and to develop/optimize current or future therapeutic strategies against hematological malignancies. In addition, given the intricate biology of each subtype of lymphoma and the complex mechanism(s) of action of biological and targeted agents, adequate preclinical studies must be conducted in several types of preclinical models in order to accurately predict what may be observed in clinical practice. The constant change in the interaction between the lymphoma cells and the tumor microenvironment is challenging physicians and scientists to develop innovative preclinical models where such interactions can be studied. While cancer cell lines and novel mouse models are the backbone of preclinical modeling, the study of primary cancer cells isolated from lymphoma patients is becoming a necessary tool to study novel agents in a more clinically relevant setting. Robust and structured collaborations between clinical medicine and life sciences are needed in an attempt to obtain primary tumor cells in their microenvironment obtained from patients with de novo or relapsed/refractory lymphoid malignancies and to further develop in vitro or in vivo models using this invaluable material source.

References

1. Siegel R, Naishadham D, Jemal A (2012) Cancer statistics, 2012. CA Cancer J Clin 62:10–29
2. Miyoshi I, Kubonishi I, Yoshimoto S et al (1981) Type C virus particles in a cord T-cell line derived by co-cultivating normal human cord leukocytes and human leukaemic T cells. Nature 294:770–771
3. Matsuo Y, Drexler HG (1998) Establishment and characterization of human B cell precursor-leukemia cell lines. Leuk Res 22:567–579
4. Dexter TM, Allen TD, Lajtha LG (1977) Conditions controlling the proliferation of haemopoietic stem cells in vitro. J Cell Physiol 91:335–344
5. Osborne HB, Bakke AC, Yu J (1982) Effect of dexamethasone on hexamethylene bisacetamide-induced Friend cell erythrodifferentiation. Cancer Res 42:513–518
6. Nakamura T, Nishizawa T, Hagiya M et al (1989) Molecular cloning and expression of human hepatocyte growth factor. Nature 342:440–443

7. Massague J (1990) The transforming growth factor-beta family. Annu Rev Cell Biol 6:597–641
8. Boncinelli E, Simeone A, Acampora D, Mavilio F (1991) HOX gene activation by retinoic acid. Trends Genet 7:329–334
9. Burgess AW, Metcalf D (1980) The nature and action of granulocyte-macrophage colony stimulating factors. Blood 56:947–958
10. Metcalf D (1989) The molecular control of cell division, differentiation commitment and maturation in haemopoietic cells. Nature 339:27–30
11. Cross M, Dexter TM (1991) Growth factors in development, transformation, and tumorigenesis. Cell 64:271–280
12. Rossi GB, Friend C (1967) Erythrocytic maturation of (Friend) virus-induced leukemic cells in spleen clones. Proc Natl Acad Sci U S A 58:1373–1380
13. Ghetie MA, Richardson J, Tucker T et al (1990) Disseminated or localized growth of a human B-cell tumor (Daudi) in SCID mice. Int J Cancer 45:481–485
14. Schmid J, Moller P, Moldenhauer G et al (1993) Monoclonal antibody uptake in B-cell lymphomas: experimental studies in nude mouse xenografts. Cancer Immunol Immunother 36:274–280
15. Hernandez-Ilizaliturri FJ, Jupudy V, Ostberg J et al (2003) Neutrophils contribute to the biological antitumor activity of rituximab in a non-Hodgkin's lymphoma severe combined immunodeficiency mouse model. Clin Cancer Res 9:5866–5873
16. Hernandez-Ilizaliturri FJ, Jupudy V, Reising S et al (2005) Concurrent administration of granulocyte colony-stimulating factor or granulocyte-monocyte colony-stimulating factor enhances the biological activity of rituximab in a severe combined immunodeficiency mouse lymphoma model. Leuk Lymphoma 46:1775–1784
17. Hernandez-Ilizaliturri FJ, Reddy N, Holkova B et al (2005) Immunomodulatory drug CC-5013 or CC-4047 and rituximab enhance antitumor activity in a severe combined immunodeficient mouse lymphoma model. Clin Cancer Res 11:5984–5992
18. Donnou S, Galand C, Daussy C et al (2011) Immune adaptive microenvironment profiles in intracerebral and intrasplenic lymphomas share common characteristics. Clin Exp Immunol 165:329–337
19. Touitou V, Daussy C, Bodaghi B et al (2007) Impaired th1/tc1 cytokine production of tumor-infiltrating lymphocytes in a model of primary intraocular B-cell lymphoma. Invest Ophthalmol Vis Sci 48:3223–3229
20. Houot R, Levy R (2009) T-cell modulation combined with intratumoral CpG cures lymphoma in a mouse model without the need for chemotherapy. Blood 113:3546–3552
21. Harnack U, Eckert K, Fichtner I, Pecher G (2009) Oral administration of a soluble 1-3, 1-6 beta-glucan during prophylactic survivin peptide vaccination diminishes growth of a B cell lymphoma in mice. Int Immunopharmacol 9:1298–1303
22. Palmieri C, Falcone C, Iaccino E et al (2010) In vivo targeting and growth inhibition of the A20 murine B-cell lymphoma by an idiotype-specific peptide binder. Blood 116:226–238
23. Alvarez E, Moga E, Barquinero J et al (2010) Dendritic and tumor cell fusions transduced with adenovirus encoding CD40L eradicate B-cell lymphoma and induce a Th17-type response. Gene Ther 17:469–477
24. Golay J, Cittera E, Di Gaetano N et al (2006) The role of complement in the therapeutic activity of rituximab in a murine B lymphoma model homing in lymph nodes. Haematologica 91:176–183
25. Dayde D, Ternant D, Ohresser M et al (2009) Tumor burden influences exposure and response to rituximab: pharmacokinetic-pharmacodynamic modeling using a syngeneic bioluminescent murine model expressing human CD20. Blood 113:3765–3772
26. Donnou S, Galand C, Touitou V et al (2012) Murine models of B-cell lymphomas: promising tools for designing cancer therapies. Adv Hematol 2012:701704
27. Croce CM, Erikson J, ar-Rushdi A et al (1984) The translocated c-myc oncogene of Burkitt lymphoma is differentially regulated in lymphoblastoid vs. plasma cells. Curr Top Microbiol Immunol 113:133–145

28. Mori S, Rempel RE, Chang JT et al (2008) Utilization of pathway signatures to reveal distinct types of B lymphoma in the Emicro-myc model and human diffuse large B-cell lymphoma. Cancer Res 68:8525–8534
29. Kovalchuk AL, Qi CF, Torrey TA et al (2000) Burkitt lymphoma in the mouse. J Exp Med 192:1183–1190
30. Sheppard RD, Samant SA, Rosenberg M et al (1998) Transgenic N-myc mouse model for indolent B cell lymphoma: tumor characterization and analysis of genetic alterations in spontaneous and retrovirally accelerated tumors. Oncogene 17:2073–2085
31. Greenwald RJ, Tumang JR, Sinha A et al (2004) E mu-BRD2 transgenic mice develop B-cell lymphoma and leukemia. Blood 103:1475–1484
32. Motokura T, Arnold A (1993) Cyclins and oncogenesis. Biochim Biophys Acta 1155:63–78
33. Bertoni F, Rinaldi A, Zucca E, Cavalli F (2006) Update on the molecular biology of mantle cell lymphoma. Hematol Oncol 24:22–27
34. Dreyling M, Hoster E, Bea S et al (2010) Update on the molecular pathogenesis and clinical treatment of Mantle Cell Lymphoma (MCL): minutes of the 9th European MCL Network conference. Leuk Lymphoma 51:1612–1622
35. Lovec H, Grzeschiczek A, Kowalski MB, Moroy T (1994) Cyclin D1/bcl-1 cooperates with myc genes in the generation of B-cell lymphoma in transgenic mice. EMBO J 13: 3487–3495
36. Jares P, Colomer D, Campo E (2007) Genetic and molecular pathogenesis of mantle cell lymphoma: perspectives for new targeted therapeutics. Nat Rev Cancer 7:750–762
37. Bodrug SE, Warner BJ, Bath ML et al (1994) Cyclin D1 transgene impedes lymphocyte maturation and collaborates in lymphomagenesis with the myc gene. EMBO J 13:2124–2130
38. Ford RJ, Shen L, Lin-Lee YC et al (2007) Development of a murine model for blastoid variant mantle-cell lymphoma. Blood 109:4899–4906
39. Yan JS, Chen XY, Li WP et al (2009) Establishing SCID mouse models of B-cell non-Hodgkin's lymphoma. Ai Zheng 28:181–183
40. Clynes RA, Towers TL, Presta LG, Ravetch JV (2000) Inhibitory Fc receptors modulate in vivo cytotoxicity against tumor targets. Nat Med 6:443–446
41. Cartron G, Dacheux L, Salles G et al (2002) Therapeutic activity of humanized anti-CD20 monoclonal antibody and polymorphism in IgG Fc receptor FcgammaRIIIa gene. Blood 99:754–758
42. Munn DH, Cheung NK (1987) Interleukin-2 enhancement of monoclonal antibody-mediated cellular cytotoxicity against human melanoma. Cancer Res 47:6600–6605
43. de Romeuf C, Dutertre CA, Le Garff-Tavernier M et al (2008) Chronic lymphocytic leukaemia cells are efficiently killed by an anti-CD20 monoclonal antibody selected for improved engagement of FcgammaRIIIA/CD16. Br J Haematol 140:635–643
44. Mossner E, Brunker P, Moser S et al (2010) Increasing the efficacy of CD20 antibody therapy through the engineering of a new type II anti-CD20 antibody with enhanced direct and immune effector cell-mediated B-cell cytotoxicity. Blood 115:4393–4402
45. Barth MJ, Hernandez-Ilizaliturri FJ, Mavis C et al (2012) Ofatumumab demonstrates activity against rituximab-sensitive and -resistant cell lines, lymphoma xenografts and primary tumour cells from patients with B-cell lymphoma. Br J Haematol 156:490–498
46. Reddy N, Hernandez-Ilizaliturri FJ, Deeb G et al (2008) Immunomodulatory drugs stimulate natural killer-cell function, alter cytokine production by dendritic cells, and inhibit angiogenesis enhancing the anti-tumour activity of rituximab in vivo. Br J Haematol 140:36–45
47. Ackler S, Xiao Y, Mitten MJ et al (2008) ABT-263 and rapamycin act cooperatively to kill lymphoma cells in vitro and in vivo. Mol Cancer Ther 7:3265–3274
48. Wang W, Kardosh A, Su YS et al (2006) Efficacy of celecoxib in the treatment of CNS lymphomas: an in vivo model. Neurosurg Focus 21:E14
49. Muta D, Makino K, Nakamura H et al (2011) Inhibition of eIF4E phosphorylation reduces cell growth and proliferation in primary central nervous system lymphoma cells. J Neurooncol 101:33–39

50. Gerber HP, Kung-Sutherland M, Stone I et al (2009) Potent antitumor activity of the anti-CD19 auristatin antibody drug conjugate hBU12-vcMMAE against rituximab-sensitive and -resistant lymphomas. Blood 113:4352–4361
51. Macchiarini F, Manz MG, Palucka AK, Shultz LD (2005) Humanized mice: are we there yet? J Exp Med 202:1307–1311
52. Sato F, Ito A, Ishida T et al (2010) A complement-dependent cytotoxicity-enhancing anti-CD20 antibody mediating potent antitumor activity in the humanized NOD/Shi-scid, IL-2Rgamma(null) mouse lymphoma model. Cancer Immunol Immunother 59:1791–1800
53. Ge Y, Xi H, Zhang XG (2010) Vaccination with immature dendritic cells combined with CD40mAb induces protective immunity against B lymphoma in hu-SCID mice. Biomed Pharmacother 64:487–492
54. Gladue RP, Paradis T, Cole SH et al (2011) The CD40 agonist antibody CP-870,893 enhances dendritic cell and B-cell activity and promotes anti-tumor efficacy in SCID-hu mice. Cancer Immunol Immunother 60:1009–1017
55. Illidge T, Honeychurch J, Howatt W et al (2000) A new in vivo and in vitro B cell lymphoma model, pi-BCL1. Cancer Biother Radiopharm 15:571–580
56. Timmerman JM, Caspar CB, Lambert SL et al (2001) Idiotype-encoding recombinant adenoviruses provide protective immunity against murine B-cell lymphomas. Blood 97:1370–1377
57. Meijerink JP, Van Lieshout EM, Beverloo HB et al (2005) Novel murine B-cell lymphoma/leukemia model to study BCL2-driven oncogenesis. Int J Cancer 114:917–925
58. Chaise C, Itti E, Petegnief Y et al (2007) [F-18]-Fluoro-2-deoxy-D: -glucose positron emission tomography as a tool for early detection of immunotherapy response in a murine B cell lymphoma model. Cancer Immunol Immunother 56:1163–1171
59. Curti A, Pandolfi S, Valzasina B et al (2007) Modulation of tryptophan catabolism by human leukemic cells results in the conversion of CD25– into CD25+ T regulatory cells. Blood 109:2871–2877
60. Yu D, Thomas-Tikhonenko A (2002) A non-transgenic mouse model for B-cell lymphoma: in vivo infection of p53-null bone marrow progenitors by a Myc retrovirus is sufficient for tumorigenesis. Oncogene 21:1922–1927
61. Robertson KA, Usherwood EJ, Nash AA (2001) Regression of a murine gammaherpesvirus 68-positive b-cell lymphoma mediated by CD4 T lymphocytes. J Virol 75:3480–3482
62. Enno A, O'Rourke JL, Howlett CR et al (1995) MALToma-like lesions in the murine gastric mucosa after long-term infection with Helicobacter felis. A mouse model of Helicobacter pylori-induced gastric lymphoma. Am J Pathol 147:217–222
63. Penichet ML, Dela Cruz JS, Challita-Eid PM et al (2001) A murine B cell lymphoma expressing human HER2/neu undergoes spontaneous tumor regression and elicits antitumor immunity. Cancer Immunol Immunother 49:649–662
64. Mineo JF, Scheffer A, Karkoutly C et al (2008) Using human CD20-transfected murine lymphomatous B cells to evaluate the efficacy of intravitreal and intracerebral rituximab injections in mice. Invest Ophthalmol Vis Sci 49:4738–4745
65. Shimada MO, Yamada Y, Nakakuki Y et al (1993) SL/KH strain of mice: a model of spontaneous pre-B-lymphomas. Leuk Res 17:573–578
66. Fredrickson TN, Lennert K, Chattopadhyay SK et al (1999) Splenic marginal zone lymphomas of mice. Am J Pathol 154:805–812
67. Egle A, Harris AW, Bath ML et al (2004) VavP-Bcl2 transgenic mice develop follicular lymphoma preceded by germinal center hyperplasia. Blood 103:2276–2283
68. Cattoretti G, Pasqualucci L, Ballon G et al (2005) Deregulated BCL6 expression recapitulates the pathogenesis of human diffuse large B cell lymphomas in mice. Cancer Cell 7:445–455
69. Field KA, Charoenthongtrakul S, Bishop JM, Refaeli Y (2008) Farnesyl transferase inhibitors induce extended remissions in transgenic mice with mature B cell lymphomas. Mol Cancer 7:39
70. Kasama Y, Sekiguchi S, Saito M et al (2010) Persistent expression of the full genome of hepatitis C virus in B cells induces spontaneous development of B-cell lymphomas in vivo. Blood 116:4926–4933

71. Puebla-Osorio N, Miyahara Y, Coimbatore S et al (2011) Induction of B-cell lymphoma by UVB radiation in p53 haploinsufficient mice. BMC Cancer 11:36
72. Tefferi A, Thiele J, Orazi A et al (2007) Proposals and rationale for revision of the World Health Organization diagnostic criteria for polycythemia vera, essential thrombocythemia, and primary myelofibrosis: recommendations from an ad hoc international expert panel. Blood 110:1092–1097
73. Daniel D, Yang B, Lawrence DA et al (2007) Cooperation of the proapoptotic receptor agonist rhApo2L/TRAIL with the CD20 antibody rituximab against non-Hodgkin lymphoma xenografts. Blood 110:4037–4046
74. Muldoon LL, Lewin SJ, Dosa E et al (2011) Imaging and therapy with rituximab anti-CD20 immunotherapy in an animal model of central nervous system lymphoma. Clin Cancer Res 17:2207–2215
75. Stein R, Qu Z, Chen S et al (2006) Characterization of a humanized IgG4 anti-HLA-DR monoclonal antibody that lacks effector cell functions but retains direct antilymphoma activity and increases the potency of rituximab. Blood 108:2736–2744

Part II
Prognostic Factors

Prognostic Factors in B-Cell Lymphomas

Diana O. Treaba

Abstract The development of staging systems, especially the modified Ann Arbor staging system and of the International Prognostic Index and its type-specific lymphoma variants (i.e. FLIPI and MLIPI.) represent important steps in the therapeutic decision and prognosis. The chapter is reviewing the impact of the staging system and of the IPI on various low- and high-grade B-cell lymphomas and also is integrating various prognostic factors identified and emerged from diverse areas that characterize these lymphomas, including histologic, immunophenotypic, cytogenetic, and molecular profiles; clinical presentation; and clinical course.

Introduction

The heterogenous group of B-cell lymphomas includes low- and high-grade lymphomas, characterized by specific morphological, immunophenotypic, cytogenetic, and molecular profiles. A direct reflection of this heterogeneity is the large variety of factors evaluated for their possible association with the response to therapy, disease evolution and overall outcome. A first step in assessing prognosis was the development of the Ann Arbor lymphoma staging system, originally described in 1971 [1] for patients with Hodgkin disease (Table 1), which is now also largely used, in a slightly modified version, however (Costwolds) [2], for non-Hodgkin

D.O. Treaba, M.D. (✉)
Assistant Professor of Pathology, Brown University, Providence, RI 02903, USA

Director, Lifespan Hematopathology Laboratory, Rhode Island Hospital,
APC11, #1142, Providence, RI 02903, USA
e-mail: dtreaba@lifespan.org

P.J. Quesenberry and J.J. Castillo (eds.), *Non-Hodgkin Lymphoma: Prognostic Factors and Targets*, Cancer Drug Discovery and Development,
DOI 10.1007/978-1-4614-5851-7_7,

Table 1 Ann Arbor staging system, modified from Carbone et al. 1971 [1]

Stage	Sites of involvement
I	A single lymph node region or a single extralymphatic organ or site
II	Two or more lymph node regions on the same side of the diaphragm or involvement of a single extralymphatic organ or site and of 1 or more lymph node regions on the same side of the diaphragm
III	Lymph nodes regions on both sides of the diaphragm, may be accompanied by localized involvement of extralymphatic organ or site, or by involvement of the spleen or both
IV	Diffuse or disseminated involvement of one or more extralymphatic organs, including any involvement of the liver, bone marrow, or nodular involvement of the lungs, with or without associated lymph node enlargement

Table 2 International Prognostic Index, modified from Ship et al., 1993 [3]

Risk group	Points	5-year survival (%)
Low risk	0–1	73
Low-intermediate risk	2	51
High-intermediate risk	3	43
High risk	4–5	26

Note: one point is assigned for each of the following risk factors: age greater than 60 years; stage III or IV disease; elevated serum LDH; ECOG performance status of 2, 3, or 4; more than 1 extranodal site

lymphomas in spite of its limitations (does not take into consideration aspects such as the lymphoma grade, the presence of bulky disease, and often the bone marrow involvement in low-grade lymphomas, i.e. chronic lymphocytic leukemia/small lymphocytic lymphoma). The Ann Arbor staging system predicts a better prognosis for B-cell lymphomas with low Ann Arbor stages (I and II) than in advanced stages (III–IV) and also has an impact in the therapeutical decision. A revolutionary step in the research for assessing prognosis was the development in 1993 of the International Prognostic Index (IPI) (Table 2) [3], a clinical tool now widely used to assess survival. Five clinical prognostic factors independently associated with survival, age, stage, number of extranodal sites, performance status, and serum LDH level, are evaluated at diagnosis to assess the relative risk of death. The IPI defines four groups of patients with similar relative risk, low, low-intermediate, high-intermediate, and high associated with a predicted 5-year survival of 75%, 51%, 43%, and 26%, respectively. For patients under 60 years, the age-adjusted index was also developed, and includes only the stage of disease, performance status and LDH. The predicted 5-year survival for the age adjusted-IPI groups being 83%, 69%, 46%, and 32%, respectively [3]. The revised IPI in the Rituximab era (R-IPI) identifies three prognostic groups with a very good, good, and poor outcome and with associated 4-year overall survivals of 94%, 79%, and 55% respectively [4]. Other disease-specific variations of the IPI were later on defined: Follicular

Lymphoma International Prognostic Index—FLIPI [5], Mantle cell Lymphoma International Prognostic Index—MIPI [6], etc.

Prognostic Factors in B Lymphoblastic Lymphoma

An aggressive lymphoma of B-lymphoblasts involves nodal or extranodal sites, without or with minimal involvement of the peripheral blood and/or bone marrow. This lymphoma comprises less than 10% of the cases of lymphoblastic lymphoma, and has a better prognosis in children than in adults, with an estimated 80% cure rate in children and 50% cure rate in adults [7].

Prognostic Factors and Clinical Parameters in B Lymphoblastic Lymphoma

Amongst the poor prognosis clinical factors in children with B lymphoblastic lymphoma are considered infancy, age >10 years, slow response to initial therapy, and CNS disease at diagnosis [7]. In adults a short survival was associated with a failure to achieve complete remission, age older than 40 years, B symptoms, LDH level more than two times the upper limits of normal, and hemoglobin level of less than 10.0 g/dL [8]. In adults, a higher complete remission rate was associated with an age of less than 40 years, lactic dehydrogenase (LDH) level of less than two times the upper limits of normal, early stages of disease, and no or one extranodal site of disease [8]. The role of bone marrow involvement is controversial being not validated as a prognostic factor by Morel et al. [9] but recognized in the study of Mazza et al. [10]. Other factors with significant role in prognosis are: stage of disease [10, 11], symptoms, bulky disease, response to therapy [10].

Prognostic Factors and Cytogenetic Abnormalities in B Lymphoblastic Lymphoma

The following cytogenetic abnormalities and translocations are associated with a poor prognosis: t(9;22)(q34;q11.2); BCR-ABL1, t(v;11q23); MLL rearrangements, and hypodiploidy while the t(12;21)(p13;q22) TEL-AML1 (ETV6-RUNX1), hyperdiploidy and t(5;14)(q31;q32); IL3-IGH are associated with a good prognosis. The t(1;19)(q23;p13.3); E2A-PBX1(TCF3-PBX1) had a poor outcome when treated with conventional antimetabolite-based therapy, but has an improved prognosis with the more recently introduced intensive therapy protocols [7, 12]. In addition, mutations of the p53 gene were found to be associated with a poor overall survival, and treatment failure [13, 14].

Prognostic Factors in Chronic Lymphocytic Leukemia/Small Lymphocytic Lymphoma

Chronic lymphocytic leukemia/small lymphocytic lymphoma (CLL/SLL) is a mature B-cell neoplasm which comprises 6.7% of all non-Hodgkin lymphomas. While the chronic lymphocytic leukemia involves predominately the bone marrow and blood (>5×10^9/L circulating neoplastic lymphoid cells) the small lymphocytic lymphoma has a predominant extramedullary distribution and <5×10^9/L circulating neoplastic lymphoid cells [7]. CLL/SLL has a very heterogenous course and prognosis, with a median survival estimated at approximately 8–10 years; however, the individual survival is highly variable [15].

Prognostic Factors and Histological Features in CLL/SLL

The heterogeneity of CLL/SLL is also noticeable in its morphological presentation where not only a classical but also an atypical morphology has been described. The atypical CLL/SLL cases usually include a subset of lymphoid cells (>10% of the neoplastic cells) of medium to large size, with irregular, clefted nuclei, and conspicuous nucleoli, and include prolymphocytoid cells, more pleomorphic than the ones noted in prolymphocytic leukemia, and in some cases plasmacytoid cells. Of interest, patients with atypical CLL/SLL with Binet stage B and RAI stage I and II have a lower median survival than patients with classical CLL/SLL (5.7 vs. 8.2) [16]. Furthermore, the atypical CLL/SLL cases had a higher association of trisomy 12 than classical CLL patients [15–17], presented at a more advanced clinical stage, had a greater probability of progression to a higher stage [18], usually required immediate treatment and their survival was shorter [16].

Prognostic Factors and Immunophenotypical Markers in CLL/SLL

An atypical immunophenotype has been reported in a subset of the CLL/SLL cases CD5−, CD23−, FMC7+, CD11c+, strong sIg, or CD79b+, but does not usually associate with an atypical morphology. Criel et al. [16] identified some differences between the immunophenotype of classical CLL/SLL and the atypical CLL/SLL cases with more mature B-cell markers, strong surface Ig staining, FMC7 positivity, CD11a, and CD11c more frequently expressed in the atypical cases. In the study of Geisler et al. [19], in CD5+ CLL/SLL cases, the IgM-fluorescence intensity, CD23, and FMC7 had significant prognostic importance, with high IgM-fluorescence intensity, high FMC7, and low CD23 expression being associated with a short survival [19]. However, the expression of CD23 is debatable since other researchers, noted a higher expression of CD23 in the cases with atypical morphology than in the classical CLL control group [18]. Two independent prognostic markers, *CD38 and ZAP-70*, are associated with a poor prognosis. Damle et al. [20] suggested first the correlation between the expression of CD38, a surface adenosine diphosphate-ribosyl cyclase by the neoplastic lymphoid cells in CLL/SLL and the underlying IgVH mutational status: with positive cases, CD38+ ">" or "=" 30% correlating with unmutated IgVH genes and negative cases CD38+ "<" 30% correlating with mutated IgVH. While later studies did not support this surrogate association [20–23], with discordant results noted in up to 30% of the patients with CLL/SLL the expression of CD38+ by the CLL/SLL neoplastic lymphoid cells is documented as an important independent poor prognostic variable. Expression of ZAP-70, a cytoplasmic tyrosine kinase on neoplastic CLL/SLL cells, identifies a subtype of CLL/SLL with a distinct gene expression profile, and an inferior clinical outcome [24] and is a stronger predictor than the mutational IgVH status for the need of treatment in CLL [25]. Evaluation of the *proliferation rate* in CLL/SLL cases suggests an increased proliferation rate (increased percentage of Ki-67 positive cells) with disease progression [26]. A few studies [27, 28] showed that elevated intracellular *p27(Kip1)* level in CLL/SLL cells of early- and intermediate-stage B-CLL patients contributes to rapid progression of the disease. The expression of *p53* by immunohistochemistry (cutoff 20% positive lymphoma cells) was associated with a poor survival [13]. In the study of Masato Ito et al. [29] the expression of *MUM1/IRF4* (*multiple myeloma oncogene 1*) in CLL/SLL cases is an independent unfavorable prognostic marker, being associated with a shorter survival. Mona Leuenberger et al. [30] identified that expression of *activation-induced cytidine deaminase* (*AID*) *protein* in small lymphocytic lymphoma cells (cutoff for positivity 5%) correlates with an unfavorable clinical course and adverse biological parameters such as a higher proliferation rate (>20% MIB1 positive nuclei) and a complex genetic background.

Prognostic Factors and Clinical Features in CLL/SLL

The Ann Arbor staging system is used in the cases of strict small lymphocytic lymphoma, because of lack of significance in the classical chronic lymphocytic leukemia when the bone marrow is usually involved [7]. The 10-year freedom from relapse for stages I and II for patients treated with irradiation was 80% and 62% respectively, but decreased to 11% in stages III and IV [31]. The development of the two widely used clinical staging systems, Rai-Sawitsky (USA) and Binet (Europe) provide a separation of the CLL/SLL patients in low-, intermediate-, and high-risk patients. Originally developed in 1975, the 5-stage Rai-Sawitsky system [32] was later modified in 1987 [33] (Table 3) to include: 3-stages based on parameters such as lymphocytosis, anemia, thrombocytopenia, peripheral blood, bone marrow, lymph nodes, splenic, and liver involvement. The Binet [34] 3-staging system uses an anatomically distributed lymph node involvement and anemia/thrombocytopenia (Table 4).

Table 3 Rai-Sawitsky system, modified from [32]

Low risk (previous stage 0)	Lymphocytosis in the blood and marrow only
Intermediate risk (previous stages I and II):	Lymphocytosis with enlarged lymph nodes in any site, or splenomegaly or hepatomegaly
High risk (previous stages II and IV)	Lymphocytosis with disease-related anemia (hemoglobin <11 g/dL) or thrombocytopenia (platelets,100×10^9/L)

Table 4 Binet staging system, modified from Binet et al. 1981 [34]

Stage A	Hemoglobin greater than or equal to 10 g/dL, platelets greater than or equal to 100×10^9/L, and fewer than 3 lymph node areas involved
Stage B	Hemoglobin and platelet levels are at stage A and 3 or more lymph node areas are involved
Stage C	Hemoglobin less than 10 g/dL or platelets less than 100×10^9/L, or both

In the Binet stage the areas of involvement are defined each as one: head and neck lymph nodes (multiple sites count as one area), axillary lymph nodes (bilateral counts as one area), inguinal lymph nodes (bilateral counts as one area), splenomegaly and hepatomegaly. There are limitations within the staging systems, which do not identify amongst the patients diagnosed in early stage the ones that will have an accelerated clinical course, nor amongst the patients diagnosed in advanced stage the ones that may still retain an indolent course [15]. Furthermore the nature of cytopenias (autoimmune causes, bone marrow involvement, hypersplenism) [15], and a progressive recording of the degree of lymphocytosis are not analyzed by these clinical stages. In the study of Zent et al. [35], cytopenia in patients with CLL secondary to bone marrow failure was a predictor of poor prognosis (median survival 4.4 years), while the survival from the onset of cytopenia secondary to autoimmune disease was similar to patients with CLL but without cytopenia (median 9.3 vs. 9.7 years).

The progressive assessment of the peripheral blood lymphocytosis as an indicator of rate of disease progression was initially suggested as a potential prognostic factor by Galton in 1966 [36]. Nowadays defined as the interval required for the peripheral blood lymphocytes to double their amount, the *lymphocyte doubling time* is considered an adverse prognostic factor if rapid (<12 months), and predicts an aggressive clinical course and a short survival [37, 38]. The rate of lymphocyte proliferation assessed by the [^{3}H] thymidine uptake of the CLL lymphocytes, the percentage of the S-phase lymphocytes and also the mitogenic activity after polyclonal lymphocyte stimulation have been also reported to predict a poor prognosis [39].

Another indicator for poor prognosis is the *serum CD23* (sCD23) level. In a multivariate analysis of Binet stage A CLL patients, the sCD23 determination at study entry was the only variable predictive of disease progression with a relative risk of clinical worsening at 5.8 for patients with sCD23 value above 574 U/mL. In addition, during follow-up, sCD23 doubling time increased by 3.2 the risk of death of the entire population [40, 41]. Two other independent prognostic factors associated with a poor prognosis are the β_2 *microglobulin* and the serum *thymidine kinase*. The elevated β_2 microglobulin is an independent predictor of shortened progression free survival for both untreated and previously treated patients, and is also associated with a high tumor burden and extensive bone marrow infiltration, short duration of remission and inferior survival following treatment [41, 42]. Increased levels of serum thymidine kinase correlate with the proliferative activity in CLL/SLL and are predictive of progression-free survival in Binet stage A [43, 44].

Prognosis and Molecular, Cytogenetic, and Oncogenetic Abnormalities in CLL/SLL

The CLL/SLL has been divided in two subtypes based on the *mutational status* of the IgVH genes: unmutated (40–50% of the cases) and mutated (50–60% of the cases) [20, 45]. The unmutated subtype is characterized by a more aggressive disease, with an atypical morphology, advanced clinical stage at diagnosis, adverse cytogenetic features and resistance to therapy. The VH3-21 using CLL/SLL has a poor outcome and represents an adverse prognostic factor independent of the IgVH mutational status [46]. Cytogenetic abnormalities identify two major risk groups: low-risk: normal karyotype or isolated del(13q) (del (13q)) being noted in up to 50% of the cases; and high-risk: del(17p) (noted in up to 10% of the cases), del(11q) (noted in up to 20% of the cases), and trisomy 12 (noted in up to 18% of the cases) [7, 47, 48]. Trisomy 12 is linked to atypical morphological and immunophenotypical CLL/SLL [7, 16, 18]. The presence of high expression of *lymphocyte-activation gene 3* (LAG3) in CLL cells as well as of lipoprotein lipase (LPL) gene correlate with unmutated IGHV, a poorer prognosis and a reduced treatment-free survival [49, 50], while the expression of *metalloproteinase 29* (ADAM29), is overexpressed in mutated IGHV [49]. Furthermore, the ratio of the LPL/ADAM29 expression seems to provide a better prognostic assessment than ZAP-70 in advanced stages of the disease [49].

Prognostic Factors in Mantle Cell Lymphoma

Mantle cell lymphoma is a B-cell neoplasm, usually composed of monomorphic small to medium sized lymphoid cells with irregular nuclear contours and an underlying CCND1/IgH translocation. It comprises approximately 3–10% of the non-Hodgkin lymphomas, and has a median survival of 3–5 years [7].

Prognostic Factors and Histopathological Features in Mantle Cell Lymphoma

Argatoff et al. [51] identified that a nodular pattern of lymph node involvement by the mantle cell lymphoma is associated with an increased overall survival (47 months) than a diffuse pattern (39 months). However, this finding is not consistently reported since a study of Majilis et al. [52] concludes that both the nodular and diffuse patterns are associated with poor survival rates. Morphologically, two aggressive variants of the mantle cell lymphoma [7] have been described: blastoid and pleomorphic. In the blastoid variant the neoplastic lymphoid cells resemble lymphoblasts and have a high mitotic index of at least 20–30 mitoses/10 hpf (high power fields). The pleomorphic variant is characterized by variable in size cells, with large oval to irregular nuclei some with conspicuous nucleoli and usually a pale cytoplasm. Amongst the WHO 2008 classification's listed "other variants" [7], the small cell variant, has been associated with a better outcome [51]. The cases of "in-situ" mantle cell lymphoma may suggest a better prognosis, and an initial "wait-and-see policy" is usually considered, however if the "in-situ" mantle cell lymphoma is associated with overt lymphoma elsewhere, therapy is recommended [53]. A high mitotic score has also been identified as an adverse histopathological factor, with the high mitotic rate ranging among studies from >10/10 hpf to >20/10 hpf [7, 51, 54].

Prognostic Factors and Sites of Involvement in Mantle Cell Lymphoma

Peripheral blood involvement by mantle cell lymphoma (Fig. 1) has been usually associated with a poor prognosis [51, 55]. However, a "leukemic" presentation of mantle cell lymphoma (peripheral blood, bone marrow and splenic involvement) with minimal or without lymphadenopathy [56, 57] has been associated with a better prognosis and an improved survival, with a median survival of 156 months from diagnosis [57].

Prognostic Factors and Immunophenotypic Features in Mantle Cell Lymphoma

The mantle cell lymphoma cells classical immunophenotype is CD20, CD5, CD43, bcl2, cyclin D1 [7] and in a large number of cases SOX11 [58], positive B-lymphoid cells. Only a small subset of cases can be weakly CD23 positive, while in their large majority mantle cell lymphomas are CD23, CD10, and bcl6 negative. Aberrant immunophenotype mantle cell lymphomas have been described with CD10 and bcl6 expression in some of the blastic/pleomorphic variants, and there are also CD5 negative cases [7]. As in other lymphomas a correlation between the *index of proliferation* as highlighted by the number of Ki-67 positive cells and prognosis has been

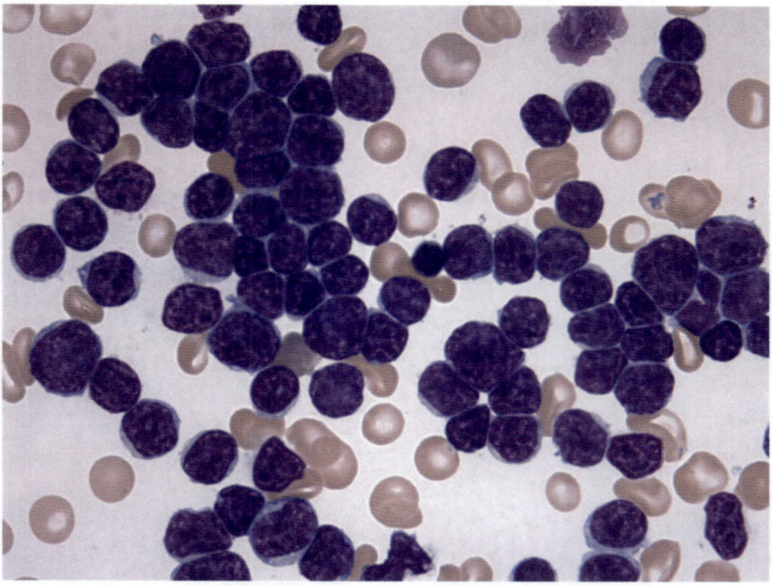

Fig. 1 Peripheral blood involvement by mantle cell lymphoma, Wright-Giemsa stain, objective 100×, oil immersion

increasingly noted, with indices of >35% being associated with a poorer prognosis [6, 59, 60]. The index of proliferation ranges from 1.2 to 91% in mantle cell lymphoma cases [6, 51], and Katzenberger et al. [59] identified median survivals of approximately 1 year for Ki-67 indices of 61–90%, and about 4 years for Ki-67 indices of 5–20% [59]. His et al. evaluating the immunohistochemical expression of *PIM1* (a cell cycle-related gene upregulated in blastoid MCL) in untreated mantle cell lymphoma patients of <70 years of age, found that the PIM1 expression was associated with shorter progression free survival and event free survival independent of clinical factors, and that the PIM1 expression is predictive of a poor outcome [60]. The rare *Cyclin D1 negative* mantle cell lymphoma, is associated with a significantly better outcome [61]. The *overexpression of p53*, (Fig. 2) by the lymphoma cells also delineates a subset of aggressive mantle cell lymphomas with a decreased overall survival [62].

Prognostic Factors and Cytogenetic and Oncogenetic Abnormalities in Mantle Cell Lymphoma

A complex karyotype and an increased number of chromosomal alterations (gains: 3q, 9q and 13q; loses: 1p, 9p, 9q, and 17p; 10p alterations) have been associated with a poorer prognosis [7, 63]. Aggressive blastoid/pleomorphic variants have a higher karyotypic complexity, a higher frequency of 1p and 17p deletions and 10p alterations,

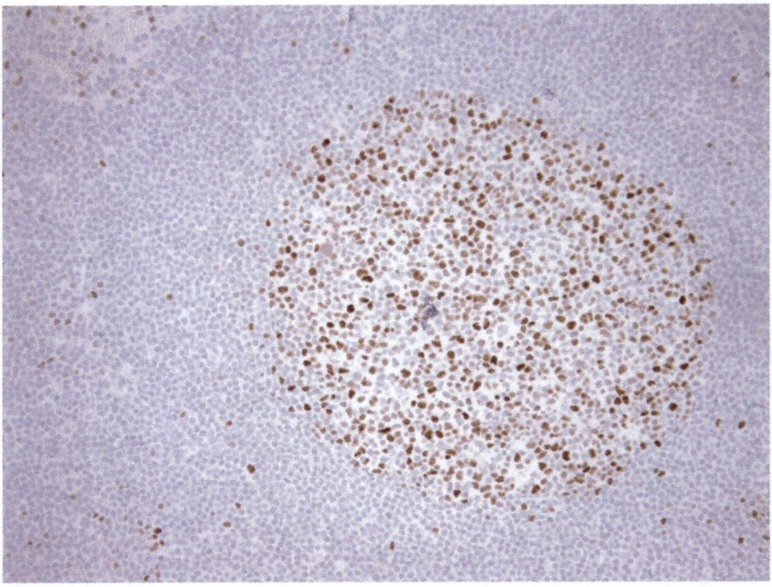

Fig. 2 p53 expression by blastoid variant of mantle cell lymphoma, objective 20×

a higher proliferation index and a poor survival. Gains of chromosomes 3q and 17p losses detected by conventional cytogenetics are prognostic markers indicating poor outcome [63] and are associated with a poorer prognosis independent of the proliferation index. Mutations in $p16^{INK4a}$ at 9p22-24, and p53 at 17p13, are associated with a worse prognosis, and often are detected in the blastoid and pleomorphic variants [7, 63–65]. Large/complex 13q losses as well as losses/copy number neutral LOH at 19p13 are reported to be associated with an improved survival [66].

Prognostic Factors and Clinical Features in Mantle Cell Lymphoma

The advanced stage disease, age >65 years, high tumor burden, the presence of B symptoms and poor performance status are all associated with a poor prognosis. In contrast, younger age (<65 years), normal LDH serum levels as well as normal beta 2-microglobulin seem to be associated with a better outcome [67]. The Mantle cell lymphoma International Prognostic Index (MIPI) [6], derived from a trial of 455 patients with advanced stage disease identifies four independent prognostic factors: age, Eastern Cooperative Oncology Group performance, lactate dehydrogenase and leukocyte count. Based on their MIPI the mantle cell lymphoma patients are separated into three risk groups: low risk (median survival was not reached after a median 32 months follow-up; the 5-year OS rate was 60%), intermediate risk (median survival 51 months) and high risk (median survival 29 months).

Prognostic Factors in Follicular Lymphoma

Follicular lymphoma is a B-cell lymphoma derived from germinal center B-lymphoid cells and consists of both centrocytes and centroblasts with usually at least a partially follicular pattern. Follicular lymphoma comprises 22% of all lymphomas, with a higher incidence (approximately 35%) in USA and Western Europe. The median age at diagnosis is 59–65 years old, and also occurs in patients less than 20 years old. The t(14;18)(q32;q21) juxtaposing the anti-apoptotic gene bcl2 to the immunoglobulin heavy chain gene locus on chromosome 14 is seen in approximately 90% of the low-grade follicular lymphomas [7].

Prognostic Factors and Histological Features in Follicular Lymphoma

In 1983 Mann and Berard [68] introduced a grading system for follicular lymphoma that remains widely used [7]. The grading is based on counting the absolute number of centroblasts in ten neoplastic lymphoid follicles, and is expressed per high-power microscopic field (hpf, 40×) of 0.159 mm^2. Grade 1 has 0–5 centroblasts per hpf, grade 2 has 6–15 centroblasts per hpf and grade 3 has >15 centroblasts per hpf. In addition, the grade 3 follicular lymphoma is subdivided in grade 3a, with >15 centroblasts per hpf, but has still admixed centrocytes, while grade 3b has solid sheets of centroblasts without centrocytes. The method of grading was maintained because of its proven capacity to predict the overall survival as well as the failure-free survival [69]. The low-grade follicular lymphomas (grade 1: 0–5 centroblasts/hpf, and grade 2: 6–15 centroblasts/hpf) are indolent lymphomas with a median survival reported as 14 years in 2004 [70]. These low-grade follicular lymphomas are often not curable with the known therapy regimens. Of interest, the more aggressive grade 3 follicular lymphomas (>15 centroblasts/hpf), are often described as a heterogenous group, with grade 3a follicular lymphoma with associated t(14;18) in 73% of the cases (and thus closer in expression to low-grade follicular lymphomas), and follicular lymphoma grade 3b with only 13% of the cases harboring the translocation and biologically, based also on the associated secondary chromosomal abnormalities, being closer to diffuse large B-cell lymphomas [71]. In their study, His et al. [72] came to the conclusion that grades 3 follicular lymphomas seem to have a similar survival rate of 44 months. While diffuse areas in low-grade follicular lymphomas do not significantly influence the overall prognosis, diffuse areas in grade 3 follicular lymphomas, now considered diffuse large B-cell lymphomas components [7] will significantly alter the overall prognosis.

Prognostic Factors and Immunophenotypical Features in Follicular Lymphoma

The neoplastic follicles are CD20 positive—B-lymphoid follicles with expression of germinal center markers (CD10 and bcl6) and also with expression of the anti-apoptotic marker bcl2. On occasions expression of MUM-1 which is generally not seen in follicular lymphomas has been described in follicular lymphomas, especially in the higher grades follicular lymphomas. Naresh et al. [73], identified that 78.9% of follicular lymphomas of grades 3a and 3b were *MUM1-positive*, while only 7.4% of the follicular lymphomas of grades 1 and 2 were MUM1-positive ($p<0.0001$). Nine of ten follicular lymphomas of grade 3b (90%) were MUM1-positive. Furthermore, MUM1 expression showed a significant inverse correlation with CD10 and Bcl-6 expression [73]. A subset of the high-grade follicular lymphomas, some with focally diffuse areas has been reported to co-express *CD43* [74]. An association between the histological grade of follicular lymphomas and the *proliferation index Ki-67* is also reported with lower grade follicular lymphomas associated with a proliferation fraction of <20% while most grade 3 follicular lymphomas have proliferation rates of >20%. In the study of Broyde et al.[75] in follicular lymphomas, the mean Ki-67 proliferation index increased with the grade, from 19.6±18% in grade 1 to 61.6±28% in grade 3. However, there was no definite association between Ki-67 proliferation index and survival. Wang et al. described [76] a subset of low-grade follicular lymphomas associated with a high proliferation rate, and this subset had a more aggressive behavior, comparable to grade 3 follicular lymphomas. Figure 3 demonstrates an example of a low-grade follicular lymphoma with a high proliferation rate. A high prevalence of *cyclin D3 IR* expression (noted in >20% of the neoplastic lymphoid cells) as well as of *p27* was reported in grade 3 follicular lymphomas [77], and was concordant with a high proliferation rate in these high-grade follicular lymphomas. This discovery raised the speculation that Cyclin D3 may have a role in driving the proliferation of the neoplastic follicular cells, and also that the association between cyclin D3 and proliferation is likely tumor-specific. A high expression of the tumor suppressor gene *p53 expression* (">" or "=" 45% of the neoplastic follicle cells) was also detected by immunostaining in neoplastic follicles and may predict histological transformation [78]. The overexpression of the suppressor of cytokine signaling 3 protein—*SOCS3* by some of de novo follicular lymphomas when evaluated immunohistochemically segregated after adjusting for FLIPI subgroups, a group of follicular lymphomas with a decreased overall survival. These findings, while reported only in a single study to date, suggest that the overexpression of SOCS3 may be an independent poor prognostic factor in patients with de novo follicular lymphomas [79].

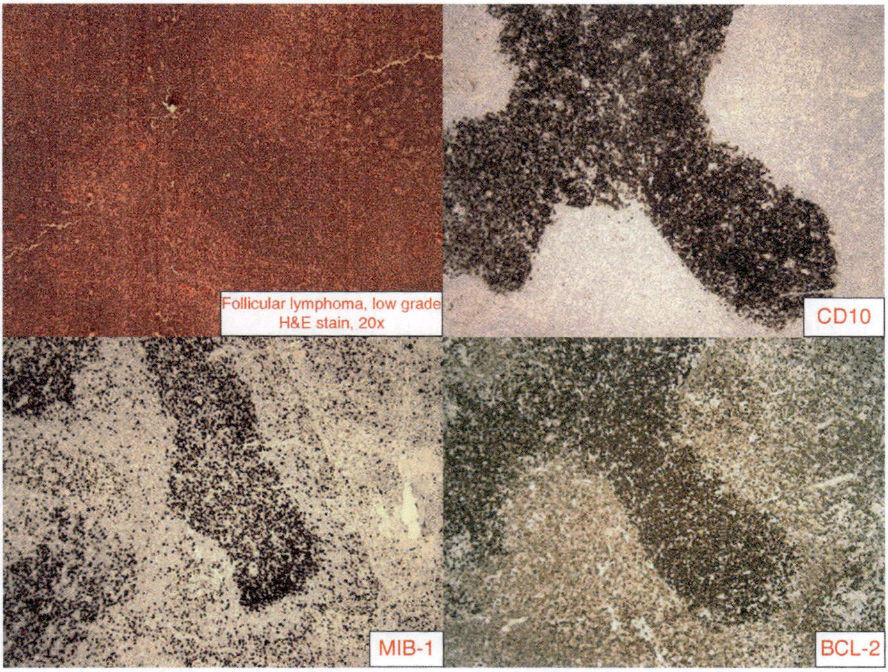

Fig. 3 Low-grade follicular lymphoma on left hematoxylin and eosin (H&E) stained slide, objective 20×; anti-CD10 antibody highlights the neoplastic follicle cells, objective 20×, anti-bcl2 antibody highlights both the neoplastic follicles and the interfollicular cells, objective 20×, and the MIB-1 antibody to the KI-67 antigen highlights the high proliferation rate (approximately 60–70%) in the neoplastic follicles, objective 20×

Prognostic Factors and Clinical Features. Follicular Lymphoma International Prognostic Index

Developed from the results of a multicentric retrospective study of 4,167 patients [5] the Follicular Lymphoma International Prognostic Index is based on five prognostic parameters: age (≥60 years vs. <60 years), Ann Arbor stage (III–IV vs. I–II), hemoglobin level (<120 g/L vs. ≥120 g/L), number of nodal areas involved (>4 vs. ≤4), serum LDH level (above normal vs. normal or below)[5]. The patients are divided in three risk groups: low, intermediate and high. Patients with a good prognosis (0–1 adverse factors) have according to this study a 10-year overall survival of 71%. Patients with intermediate risk group (2 risk factors) had a 10 years overall survival of 51% and patients in the high-risk group (= or >3 risk factors) had a 10 years overall survival of 36% [5].

In a second and prospective FLIPI study of 1,093 patients the prognostic factors were changed to age >60 years, hemoglobin 12 g/dL, serum beta 2 microglobulin higher than the upper normal limit, longest diameter of the largest lymph node >6 cm and bone marrow involvement. As a consequence, the FLIPI2 score defined three risk groups: patients in the low-risk group (number of risk factors 0) with a

3-year survival rate of 99%, patients with intermediate risk (number of risk factors 1–2) have a 3-year survival rate of 96%, while patients in a high-grade group (3–5 risk factors) have a 3-year survival rate of 77% [80].

Prognosis and Cytogenetic and Oncogenetic Abnormalities in Follicular Lymphoma

The t(14;18) has been documented in up to 90% of the low-grade follicular lymphomas, and in approximately 90% of the cases there are other genetic abnormalities [7]. The presence of a complex karyotype and also the presence of six chromosomal abnormalities are associated with a poor prognosis. Associated with a poor prognosis are chromosomal abnormalities: del6q23-26, del17p, −1p, +12, +18p, +Xp, and also mutations in TP53. Alterations of chromosomes 1p36, 9p, and 6q21 are associated with an increased risk of transformation to a higher grade lymphoma [81]. A few cases of high-grade follicular lymphomas have associated t(14;18) and MYC rearrangements. MYC rearrangements have been also described when transformation to a more aggressive lymphoma takes place [82]. Microarray studies of gene expression highlight the importance of follicular lymphoma's specific "microenvironment" signature and median overall survival. Involvement of the neoplastic tissue by T-cells and monocytes (immune response type 1) suggest a favorable prognosis, and is associated with a median overall survival of 11.2 years. The involvement by monocytes and dendritic cells (immune response type 2) suggest a poor outcome and are associated with a median overall survival of 3.9 years [83].

Transformation of Follicular Lymphomas to High-Grade Lymphomas

Transformation to high-grade lymphomas has been described in follicular lymphomas and occurs in 25–60% of the follicular lymphomas [84, 85], being associated with a poor prognosis, and disease refractory to therapy. While progression to diffuse large B-cell lymphoma, is most often encountered, progression to Burkitt lymphoma or B lymphoblastic lymphomas have also been described. In their study of 276 patients, Silvia Montoto et al. [85] described high-grade transformation of follicular lymphomas to diffuse large B-cell lymphomas in 11% (30/276) after a median follow-up of 6.5 years, with a risk of 15 and 22% at 10 years and at 15 years, respectively. In the multivariate analysis, grade 3 histology and the FLIPI retained prognostic significance. Only FLIPI predicted high-grade transformation in grade 1–2 patients. Twenty-eight patients received salvage treatment for high-grade transformation, with a CR rate of 52%. The median survival from transformation was 1.2 years.

Prognostic Factors in Marginal Zone Type Lymphomas

Prognostic Factors in Extranodal Marginal Zone Lymphoma of Mucosa-Associated Lymphoid Tissue (Malt Lymphoma)

Extranodal marginal zone lymphoma of mucosa-associated lymphoid tissue (MALT lymphoma) is an indolent B-cell lymphoma, with an incidence of 7–8% amongst the B-cell lymphomas, and comprises approximately 50% of the primary gastric lymphomas. The lymphoma cells infiltrate the marginal zone of reactive B-lymphoid follicles and also extend in the interfollicular region. In epithelial tissues the neoplastic cells infiltrate the epithelium forming lymphoepithelial lesions. Morphologically, it consists of a heterogenous lymphoid population of small centrocyte-like cells, monocytoid B-cells, immunoblasts and centroblasts like cells. Plasma cell differentiation is noted in up to 30% of the cases [7]. The median age at diagnosis is 61 years old, and the 5-year overall survival is reported between 86 and 95% and there is no significant difference between GI or non-GI lymphoma and between localized and disseminated disease [7, 86].

Prognostic Factors and Histological and Immunophenotypical Features in Extranodal Marginal Zone Lymphoma of Mucosa-Associated Lymphoid Tissue (MALT Lymphoma)

The low depth of lymphoma invasion in GI locations is associated with a better outcome [87]. In prior studies a histological separation of "low-grade" and "high-grade" MALT lymphomas was made [88, 89], based on an increased number of large transformed cells in the later, with the higher grades reported to be associated with a poorer outcome. However, this "grading" of MALT lymphomas is not recognized in the 4th edition of the WHO Classification [7]. MALT lymphoma's transformation to diffuse large B-cell lymphoma is associated with a poorer outcome [87, 89–91]. The *proliferation rate* as highlighted by the number of Ki-67 positive nuclei is usually low (ranges from 3 to 35%, average 13.2%)[75], and no significant association was found between Ki-67 and overall survival. Of interest, expression of *CD43* positive in ocular lymphomas was found to be associated with a higher rate of subsequent distant recurrence and the rate of lymphoma-related death [92]. The expression of *bcl-10* by immunohistochemistry appears to identify those MALT lymphomas with underlying genetic aberrations [93].

Prognostic Factors and Clinical Features in Extranodal Marginal Zone Lymphoma of Mucosa-Associated Lymphoid Tissue (MALT Lymphoma)

Amongst the adverse clinical prognostic factors are the poor performance status, bulky tumor, and incompletely resected tumor [93], and high levels of LDH, beta 2-microglobulin, and serum albumin [89, 93]. An early stage MALT lymphoma had the best prognosis [93] while presentation with disseminated disease was reported to carry a poorer prognosis [94].

Prognostic Factors and Cytogenetic Abnormalities Extranodal Marginal Zone Lymphoma of Mucosa-Associated Lymphoid Tissue (MALT Lymphoma)

A prognostic role has been designated by several studies to the presence of t(11;18)(q21;q21), in gastric MALT lymphomas. The translocation between API2-MALT is predictive of resistance to antibiotic therapy to H. pylori [95], and also to resistance to oral alkylating agents, with less than 10% of durable remission at long-term follow-up [96]. In addition, patients with t(11;18)-positive or aneuploidy-positive MALT lymphomas have a higher tendency for recurrence and for bone marrow involvement than the MALT lymphomas that lacked chromosomal abnormalities (recurrence rate approximately 50% vs. 20%, bone marrow involvement 25% vs. none)[97]. In addition, both *API2-MALT1* fusion and aneuploidy were disproportionately detected in the lung (90% of the primary pulmonary MALT lymphomas had either t(11;18) or trisomy 3 and/or 18) findings suggesting that primary pulmonary MALT lymphomas may have a poorer prognosis than those arising in other sites [97, 98].

Prognostic Factors in Nodal Marginal Zone Lymphoma

This B-cell lymphoma comprises less than 2% of all non Hodgkin lymphomas, and morphologically resembles lymph nodes involved by extranodal marginal zone lymphoma or splenic marginal lymphoma types without evidence of extranodal or splenic disease. The median age at diagnosis is 60 years, and the 5-year survival ranges from 60 to 80% [7, 99, 100].

About half of all patients have an International Prognostic Index (IPI) score between 1 and 2 at diagnosis. The Follicular Lymphoma International Prognostic Index can be also used to assess the risk score. In the study of Arcaini et al. on 51 patients, the univariate analysis identified a worse overall survival associated with FLIPI, age >60 years and increased lactate dehydrogenase while on the multivariate analysis, only FLIPI predicted a worse overall survival [101]. The prognosis of nodal marginal zone lymphoma appears to be less favorable than other marginal zone lymphomas [99, 102]. A pediatric form has been also described, with a male sex predominance, usually localized in the head and neck regions, and characterized by a long survival and a very low relapse rate [103, 104].

Prognostic Factors in Splenic Marginal Zone Lymphoma

A rare B-cell lymphoma, splenic marginal zone lymphoma (SMZL) comprises less than 2% of all non Hodgkin lymphomas, characterized by small lymphoid cells that surround and replace the splenic white pulp germinal centers, efface the follicle mantle and merge with a peripheral (marginal) zone of larger cells; both small and large cells infiltrate the red pulp [7]. The lymphoma involves the splenic hilar lymph nodes, the bone marrow and the peripheral blood where characteristic "villous" lymphocyte morphology has been described.

Arcaini et al. [105] described three risk adverse prognostic factors: hemoglobin <12 g/dL, albumin <3.5 g/dL, and lactate dehydrogenase (LDH) > upper limits of normal. Three risk groups were identified using this model: low risk (0 factors), intermediate risk (1 factor), and high risk (2–3 risk factors) with 5-year cause-specific survival of 88%, 73%, and 50%, respectively. A subset of cases has unmutated IgVH genes and in this group 7q31 deletions are more frequent as is a shorter overall survival [106]. A study of cDNA microarray analysis identified a shorter survival with CD38 expression, naive IgV_H genes, and the expression of a set of NF-κB pathway genes, including TRAF5, REL, and PKCA [107], while on a study of splenic a marginal zone lymphoma on mice Bahler et al. [108] suggest the existence of two different groups of splenic marginal zone lymphomas one IgD+, and carrying unmutated V_H genes consistent with a naïve B-cell origin and the other one IgD−, with mutated V_H genes consistent with a memory B-cell origin. Other adverse prognostic factors suggested are: lack of response to therapy, involvement of nonhematopoietic sites, bone marrow involvement, the presence of M component, elevated, beta 2-microglobulin level, leukocyte count >20,000/μL, lymphocyte count >9,000/μL, and the overexpression of p53 [109, 110]. Loses of 7 and 17p have been associated with a shorter survival [111], while translocations t(2;8)(p12;q24) and t(14;18)(q32;q21) seem to be associated with a more aggressive disease [110].

Prognostic Factors in Splenic B-Cell Lymphoma/Leukemia, Unclassifiable

A rare B-cell lymphoma, comprising <1% of the non-Hodgkin lymphomas, characterized by with diffuse infiltration of the splenic red pulp by a population of small monomorphous B-lymphoid cells. There is peripheral blood involvement with villous lymphocytes and also involvement of the bone marrow (sinusoids). This is an indolent lymphoma, with good response after splenectomy [7, 112]. An increased p53 expression [7] was noted in some cases, and it seemed to be associated with a more aggressive disease, and a poorer prognosis [113, 114]. A more detailed evaluation of specific prognostic factors is however still lacking, due to the rarity of this disease.

Prognostic Factors in Lymphoplasmacytic Lymphoma

This B-cell lymphoma comprises approximately 1% of the non-Hodgkin lymphomas, and is characterized by a clonal population of small lymphoid cells, plasmacytoid lymphocytes, and plasma cells, with usual involvement of the bone marrow and occasionally lymph node and splenic involvement. This lymphoma does not fulfill the criteria for other B-cell lymphomas with plasmacytic differentiation. The median survival is 5–10 years, and there is a slight male predominance. An association with hepatitis C virus infection, cryoglobulinemia type II, and rarely amyloid deposition was reported. A monoclonal paraprotein, often of IgM type is associated, but some cases can have other paraproteins or no paraproteins. Waldenstroms' macroglobulinemia is considered a lymphoplasmacytic lymphoma with bone marrow involvement and an IgM paraprotein of any concentration [7].

Prognostic Factors and Histological Features in Lymphoplasmacytic Lymphoma

Involvement of >50% of the bone marrow space by lymphoma, as well as an increased number of large transformed cells, a polymorphous variant, and the transformation to diffuse large B-cell lymphoma are indicators of a more aggressive behavior [115–117].

Prognostic Factors and Immunophenotypical Features in Lymphoplasmacytic Lymphoma

The proliferation index (percentage of Ki-67 positive cells) ranged from 5 to 20% in patients with lymphoplasmacytic lymphoma in one study [75], where an association between Ki-67 and prognosis was not identified, while in other studies [117, 118] an increased Ki-67 was indicative of a more aggressive disease.

Prognostic Factors and Clinical Features in Lymphoplasmacytic Lymphoma

In 2009, the International Prognostic Scoring System for Waldenstrom macroglobulinemia was developed based on five high-risk covariates (ISSWM): age >65 years, hemoglobin ≤11·5 g/dL, platelet count ≤100 × 109/L, beta 2-microglobulin >3 mg/L and serum monoclonal protein concentration (IgM paraproptein) >7.0 g/dL estimated by densitometry. Three risk group patients were identified: low risk: with ≤1 adverse characteristic and age ≤65 years, intermediate risk with 2 adverse characteristics or only age >65 years, and high-risk patients with >2 adverse characteristics. The 5-year survival rates were 87%, 68%, and 36% respectively [119].

Several studies indicate that some pretreatment parameters: including older age, male sex, B-symptoms, cytopenias, low albumin serum levels and high beta 2-microglobulin (41 U/L) are markers of poor prognosis in Waldenstrom macroglobulinemia [120–123]. In particular, hemoglobin and high beta 2-microglobulin levels at diagnosis are important prognostic markers in Waldenstrom macroglobulinemia [120, 123]. In early disease stages, serum beta 2-microglobulin, serum thymidine kinase, Karnofsky performance status, and platelet count independently predict progression-free survival in patients with lymphoplasmacytic lymphoma [123].

Prognosis and Molecular and Cytogenetic Abnormalities in Lymphoplasmacytic Lymphoma

Molecular and cytogenetics-based studies have been also used to identify possible prognostic factors in lymphoplasmacytic lymphoma and amongst the various cytogenetic abnormalities encountered the most frequent structural abnormality (approximately 30–50% of the cases) identified was del(6q) which involves the q13 to q25 region [124]. While the presence of the deletion of 6q does not influence the disease presentation, initiation of treatment or survival, it has been suggested as a possible marker of transformation in LPL/WM to large cell lymphoma [116, 124].

Studies of micro RNA profiling identified in Waldenstrom macroglobulinemia (WM) a characteristic microRNA signature with an increased expression of microRNA-363*/-206/-494/-155/-184/-542-3p, and a decreased expression of microRNA-9*. The increased expression of the five miRNAs is an important adverse prognostic factor and correlates with the International Prognostic Staging System. In addition, because therapeutic agents alter the levels of the major miRNAs identified, by downmodulation of five increased miRNAs and up-modulation of patient-downexpressed miRNA-9*, the microRNAs may provide the basis for the development of new microRNA-restricted therapeutic target in WM [123].

Prognostic Factors in Burkitt Lymphoma

A highly aggressive B-cell lymphoma composed of monomorphic medium-sized transformed cells, with an extremely short doubling time and with often presentation in extranodal sites or as an acute leukemia [7]. The incidence is approximately 1% of the non-Hodgkin lymphomas in USA and 2.2% in Europe. The large majority of the cases are associated with MYC rearrangements, with t(8;14)(q24q32) being most often encountered and with a lower incidence of translocations t(2;14) and t(14;22). However, in spite of a classical immunophenotype and morphology in up to 10% of cases of classical Burkitt lymphoma a myc translocation can not be demonstrated by FISH. There are three clinical variants recognized: endemic, sporadic and immunodeficiency associated. After the introduction of CODOX-M/IVAC combination chemotherapy, rituximab and dose-adjusted (DA)-EPOCH [124, 125], Burkitt lymphoma achieved a cure rate of more than 90%.

Prognostic Factors and Morphological Features in Burkitt Lymphoma

The clinical variants of Burkitt lymphoma do not have distinct morphological features. Burkitt lymphoma has an extremely high proliferation index (>95% Ki-67 positive cells) and a high fraction of apoptosis. The apoptotic Burkitt lymphoma cells attract benign monocytes and macrophages [126, 127] in the tumoral tissue and a characteristic "starry sky pattern" occurs. In a small group of reported cases a prominent granulomatous pattern was described and these cases were associated with a localized disease and a favorable response to chemotherapy [126–129].

Prognostic Parameters and Immunohistochemical Features in Burkitt Lymphoma

Several studies have indicated that a subset of the Burkitt lymphomas can express CD30 positivity, and in the study of Tumwine et al. the expression of CD30 by Burkitt lymphoma is associated with an improved survival—12.3 years than 6.8 year noted in the CD30 negative cases [130]. The expression of *c-Flip* [131] was found highly related to a poor prognosis, mostly characterized by adults with a chemoresistant disease, resulting in a high death rate within the first year of diagnosis. The 2-year overall survival with c-Flip expression was 24% compared with 93% in the absence of this marker. The study of Nomura Y et al. identified a significant difference in the overall survival between the Burkitt lymphoma cases with *high caspase* expression, bcl2 negative (76%) and low caspase-3, bcl2 negative (50%) groups. In addition, the association of low caspase-3 expression, bcl-2 positive identified a group of Burkitt lymphoma with the worst prognosis (16%) [132].

Prognostic Parameters and Clinical Aspects in Burkitt Lymphoma

The International Prognostic Index (IPI), based on five clinical parameters: age >60 years, stage III–IV, spread of lymphoma to more than one site beyond the lymph nodes, high levels of lactate dehydrogenase, and poor general health is used to predict disease free survival and overall survival. A low IPI score (0–1) is associated with an overall survival rate of 73%, while an IPI score of 5, is associated with a 5-year overall survival of 26%.

In patients with HIV and Burkitt lymphoma, several factors have been identified to associate with an adverse prognosis: a history of previous opportunistic infection (AIDS-defining diagnosis), a poor performance status, bone marrow involvement, and a CD4 count less than 100 cells/μL at diagnosis [133–136]. The British HIV Association (BHIVA) guidelines recommend the use of a HIV-related NHL prognostic index that combines the original IPI with the CD4 cell count at the time of diagnosis. HIV-BL treated with intensive chemotherapies, showing complete response rate ranging from 63 to 100%.

Prognostic Factors and Cytogenetics Abnormalities in Burkitt Lymphoma

Thirty to 40% of Burkitt lymphoma cases harbor only the t(8;14) or its variant translocations: t(8;22)(q24;q11) and t(2;8)(p12;q24). The variant translocations seem to have a poorer survival rate and the t(8;22)(q24;q11) has an increased frequency in patients with AIDS [137]. The rest of Burkitt lymphoma cases exhibit one to two additional abnormalities: preponderant abnormalities of 1q, trisomy 7, trisomy 12 or alterations at 13q [138]. The prognostic analysis has identified a subset of Burkitt lymphoma patients exhibiting loss of 13q, particularly 13q14.3, and with a significant decrease in 5-year overall survival (77% vs. 95%)[139]. These observations indicate that *del(13q)* occurs in childhood Burkitt lymphoma at frequencies higher than previously detected by classical cytogenetics and underscores the importance of molecular cytogenetics in risk stratification.

Prognostic Factors in Diffuse Large B-Cell Lymphoma, Not Otherwise Specified

An aggressive B-cell lymphoma, with a diffuse pattern of growth, the Diffuse Large B-cell Lymphoma consists of large neoplastic lymphoid cells with nuclei being more than twice the size of the nucleus of a small lymphocyte or larger than the nuclei of macrophages. This is the most common type of adult non-Hodgkin lymphomas with an incidence of approximately 25–30%. The median age at diagnosis is 64 years old, but it can occur at any age. A slight male predominance has been reported [7].

Prognostic Factors and Histological Features in Diffuse Large B-Cell Lymphoma, NOS

The most frequently identified morphological variants: centroblastic, immunoblastic, anaplastic, as well as the rare variants (pseudorosette formation, myxoid and fibrillary stroma, signet ring cells, spindle cells, microvillous projection, intracytoplasmic granules, etc.) do not appear to have a definite impact on the survival; however, some studies did associate the immunoblastic variant with a worst outcome [140, 141]. The discordant morphology noted in bone marrow involvement by a subset of diffuse large B-cell lymphomas was associated with older age, elevated lactate dehydrogenase, advanced stage, and increased number of extranodal sites and was not a negative prognostic factor independent of the IPI score. The morphologically concordant bone marrow involvement by diffuse large B-cell lymphoma is associated with a very poor prognosis, and remains an independent prognostic factor for progression-free survival [142].

Prognostic Factors and Immunophenotypical Features in Diffuse Large B-Cell Lymphoma, NOS

A more favorable prognosis has been reported for diffuse large B-cell lymphomas (DLBCL) with a germinal center (GC) immunophenotype (CD10 and bcl6 positive—Hans algorithm (Fig. 4) [143]) and also the LMO2 expression [144]. Furthermore, the *LMO2 expression* is associated with t(14;18) but not with bcl6 translocations in diffuse large B-cell lymphomas and appears to be a potential marker for the GC immunophenotype [144, 145]. The expression of *IRF4/MUM-1* (non germinal center—ABC immunophenotype in Hans algorithm (Fig. 4) [143]), *CD5* [146, 147] (which is also associated with an increased incidence of CNS involvement), *bcl2* [148], anaplastic lymphoma kinase [149, 150], cyclin D2 [151], and cyclin D3 [152], survivin, XIAP and CD95 positivity [153] were found to be unfavorable factors to therapy response and shorter survival. In addition, expression of caspase [153, 154], lung resistance protein [156] nuclear overexpression of P14 (ARF)[156], protein kinase C-beta [151], FOX-P1 [157, 158], adhesions molecules (CD44 and CD45 -ICAM1) [159], and lack of HLA-DR [160] expression are also associated with a worse outcome. In addition, the patients with EBV-positive DLBCL [162] (detected by in situ hybridization) have a worst clinical outcome than patients with EBV-negative DLBCL. Analysis of Ki-67 proliferation index [162, 163] has shown that high proliferation indices >40% and notable >90% is associated with a poorer prognosis. The study of Meyer et al. [164] identified *SPARC* (secreted protein, acidic and rich in cysteine) expression in the microenvironment of DLBCL, which can be used for prognosis, separating a subgroup of patients with ABC DLBCL who have significantly longer survival. More aggressive chemotherapy protocols should be considered for patients with ABC DLBCL without SPARC + stromal cells. The CD68 expression by cells present in the microenvironment did not predict survival [165].

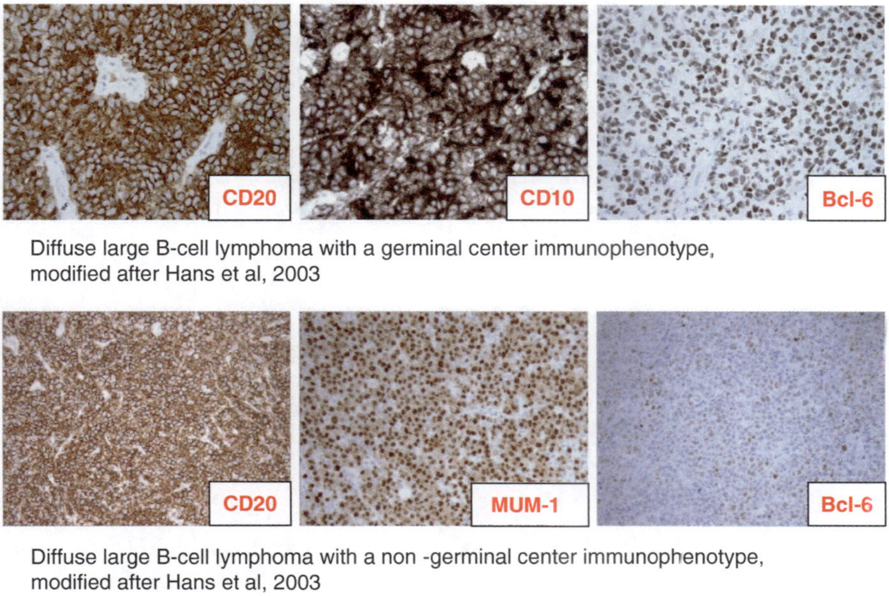

Fig. 4 Hans algorithm, modified from Hans et al., 2003 [143]

Prognostic Factors and Clinical Features in Diffuse Large B-Cell Lymphoma, NOS

The International Prognostic Index was revised in 2007 due to addition of Rituximab (R-IPI) to the therapy with CHOP [4] and identifies three prognostic groups with a very good (score 0; 4-year progression-free survival [PFS] 94%, overall survival [OS] 94%), good (score 1–2; 4-year PFS 80%, OS 79%), and poor (score 3–5; 4-year PFS 53%, OS 55%) outcome, respectively. The R-IPI does no longer identify a risk group with less than a 50% chance of survival [4].

Prognosis and Cytogenetic and Oncogenetic Abnormalities in Diffuse Large B-Cell Lymphoma, NOS

The study of Alizadeh et al. [165] identified two molecularly distinct forms of DLBCL which had gene expression patterns corresponding to different stages of B-cell differentiation: the germinal center B cells (germinal center B-like DLBCL) and genes normally induced during in vitro activation of peripheral blood B cells (activated B-like DLBC). Patients with a germinal center B-like profile DLBCL had a significantly better overall survival than those with activated B-like DLBCL. Diffuse large B-cell lymphomas with high BCL-6 gene expression have a median overall survival (OS) of 171 months, while DLBCL with low BCL-6 gene expression had a median OS of 24 months. BCL-6 gene expression was an independent survival predicting factor in multivariate analysis together with the elements of the International Prognostic Index (IPI) [166]. Adverse prognostic factors in diffuse large B-cell lymphomas are the TP53 mutations and c-myc rearrangements [167, 168].

Prognostic Factors in Diffuse Large B-Cell Lymphoma Subtypes

Prognostic Factors in T-Cell/Histiocyte-Rich Large B-Cell Lymphoma

T-cell/histiocyte-rich large B-cell lymphoma comprises approximately 1–2% of the non-Hodgkin lymphomas. The T-cell/histiocyte-rich large B-cell lymphoma has a male predominance, with a median age of 40 years [7, 169]. This is an aggressive lymphoma, usually diagnosed in an advanced disease stage. In univariate analysis, the proliferation fraction and the p53 overexpression, as well as the clinical variables incorporated in the International Prognostic Index (IPI), correlated with the response to treatment and survival. However, only the IPI score identified was relevant for prognosis in a multivariate analysis [170]. Poppe et al. identified the recurrent t(9;14)(p13;q32), PAX5/IGH gene rearrangement in cases of T-cell/histiocyte-rich large B-cell lymphomas and suggested an association between the presence of this translocation and a "de novo" diffuse large B-cell lymphoma with an adverse prognosis [171].

Prognostic Factors in Primary Large B-Cell Lymphoma of the CNS

Restricted at the time of diagnosis to primary intracerebral or intraocular locations, Primary diffuse large B-cell lymphoma of the CNS represents <1% of all non-Hodgkin lymphomas. The median age is approximately 60 years, and there is a slight male preponderance. This is an aggressive lymphoma with relapses in the CNS but also systemic [7]. The International Extranodal Lymphoma Study Group identified in a series of 378 patients with primary CNS (this study included both B and T-cell lineage lymphomas) the following adverse factors: age >60 years, performance status >1, elevated lactate dehydrogenase serum level, high CSF protein concentration, and involvement of deep regions of the brain (periventricular regions, basal ganglia, brainstem, and/or cerebellum) independently associated with a worse survival [172]. Other studies however, identified only the age and the performance status as independent prognostic factors [173, 174]. Hottinger et al., in a study of 45 patients with primary central nervous system lymphoma identified a correlation between serum markers like YKL-40 (a tissue marker of inflammation related to carcinogenesis) and MMP-9 (remodeling permeability) with the radiographic disease status, and the longitudinal increase in serum levels of YKL-40, but not the serum MMP-9 levels, can predict survival [175]. A larger subset of the primary CNS large B-cell lymphomas is of non-germinal center origin, however, a statistically significant difference in the overall survival between the germinal and non-germinal center groups was not seen [176].

Prognostic Factors in Primary Cutaneous Diffuse Large B-Cell Lymphoma, Leg Type

Primary cutaneous diffuse large B-cell lymphoma, leg type, comprises 4% of all cutaneous lymphomas. The median age at diagnosis is 76 years, has a higher incidence in women, a 5 year survival of 50% [7], and has frequent relapses and extracutaneous dissemination. Location on the leg and multiple skin lesions were predictive of death in multivariate analysis. Multiple skin lesions at diagnosis were predictive of death in a multivariate analysis [177]. FOXP1 gene gains have been identified in 82% of PCLBCL, leg type in a series [178], and the overexpression of FOXP1 is suggested to indicate an unfavorable prognosis. Inactivation of p16INK4a/CDKN2A gene might be a diagnostic feature of large B cell lymphoma leg type and is also associated with an unfavorable prognosis [179, 180].

Prognostic Factors in EBV Positive Diffuse Large B-Cell Lymphoma of the Elderly

EBV positive diffuse large B-cell lymphoma of the elderly (median age at diagnosis—71 years old) occurs in patients without a prior lymphoma or underlying immunodeficiency [7]. This is an aggressive B-cell lymphoma with a median survival of 2 years. The histological subtypes described (polymorphous and large—cell lymphoma subtype) have no association with the prognosis. The presence of B-symptoms and age >70 years are the most reliable adverse prognostic factors. The absence or the presence of one or both of these factors is associated with a median overall survival of 56, 25, and 9 months respectively [181, 182].

Prognostic Factors in Other Lymphomas of Large B-Cells

Prognostic Factors in Diffuse Large B-Cell Lymphoma with Chronic Inflammation

This Diffuse large B-cell lymphoma arises in a background of long standing chronic inflammation, is associated with Epstein Barr virus, and involves body cavities or narrow spaces (former pyothorax-associated lymphoma)[7]. It is an aggressive lymphoma with a 5-year survival of 15% in advanced clinical stages [183]. Amongst the reported adverse prognostic factors in a multivariate analysis are increased lactate dehydrogenase levels, performance status, and advanced clinical stages (III/IV)[183]. In a study of 106 patients with pyothorax-associated lymphoma, the overall prognosis was poor, with a 5-year survival of 21.6% [184]. Of interest, loss of EBV nuclear antigen-2 (EBNA-2) expression in pyothorax-associated lymphomas is correlated with a poor prognosis, with a 1 year survival [185].

Prognostic Factors in Primary Mediastinal (Thymic) Large B-Cell Lymphoma

Primary mediastinal (thymic) large B-cell lymphoma arises within the thymus from putative B-cell origin, and accounts for 2–4% of the non-Hodgkin lymphomas. The patients are young adults with a female predominance [7]. These lymphomas have usually a good prognosis. More than half of the patients usually present in Ann Arbor stage I/II [186, 187], and amongst adverse prognostic factors are considered: an elevated serum lactate dehydrogenase level, a low performance score, more than one extranodal site, and an intermediate or high International Prognostic Index score [186, 187]. The age-adjusted International Prognostic Index was not predictive of survival in the study of Savage et al. [188]. Extension into adjacent thoracic viscera and pleural or pericardial effusion [7, 189] are associated with a poor prognosis.

Prognostic Factors in Intravascular Large B-Cell Lymphoma

Intravascular large B-cell lymphoma is a rare extranodal large B-cell lymphoma, which occurs in adults (median age 67 years old) with an almost equal male to female ratio [7]. This is an aggressive lymphoma with neoplastic lymphoid cells noted within the lumina of small blood vessels from various organs, with a protean clinical presentation, and a poor response to chemotherapy [190–192]. The multivariate analysis revealed that a lack of anthracycline-based chemotherapies, age older than 60 years, and thrombocytopenia less than 100×10^9/L were independently unfavorable prognostic factors, while the CD5 positivity was not [191]. Isolated skin involvement is rare, and has been suggested to have a significantly better prognosis overall [7].

Prognostic Factors in ALK-Positive Large B-Cell Lymphoma

ALK-positive large B-cell lymphoma is a very rare lymphoma (<1% of DLBCL), which associated t(2;17)(p23;q23) clathrin (CLTC)-ALK with an overall median survival for advanced stage patients III/IV of 11 months [7, 193, 194]. A longer survival (>156 months) has been occasionally reported in children [195, 196].

Prognostic Factors in Large B-Cell Lymphoma Arising in HHV8-Associated Multicentric Castleman Disease

A rare lymphoma composed of a monoclonal proliferation of HHV-8 infected lymphoid cells expressing IgM and arising in the setting of multicentric Castleman disease. An increased association with HIV infection is also noted [7]. These are rare but very aggressive lymphomas with a very short survival [197], and the search is still in process for more detailed prognostic factors identification.

Prognosis in Borderline B-Cell Lymphomas with Features Intermediate Between Distinct Entities

Two variant B-cell lymphoma entities are recognized by the 4th Edition of the WHO Classification of Lymphomas that have emerged from the territory of "grey-zone" lymphomas: a B-cell lymphoma unclassifiable, with features intermediate between diffuse large B-cell lymphoma and Burkitt lymphoma and a B-cell lymphoma unclassifiable, with features intermediate between diffuse large B-cell lymphoma and classical Hodgkin lymphoma [7]. The B-cell lymphoma unclassifiable, with features intermediate between diffuse large B-cell lymphoma and Burkitt lymphoma, is also called "double hit lymphoma" due to the presence of dual *MYC* and *BCL2* translocations. Of interest, the incidence of dual *MYC* and *BCL2* translocations in de novo DLBCL was reported as 3–4% in separate studies [198–200]. These lymphomas have poor prognostic parameters, including elevated LDH, bone marrow and CNS involvement, and a high IPI score. This poor outcome is probably secondary to the combination of MYC and BCL2, and/or related high genomic alterations. The *BCL6+*/*MYC+* double hit lymphomas are less common, and many of these cases represent *BCL2+/BCL6+/MYC+* triple-hit lymphomas with involvement of *BCL2* as well [7, 201–203]. The B-cell lymphoma unclassifiable, with features intermediate between diffuse large B-cell lymphoma and classical Hodgkin lymphoma is more common in young men, who usually present with symptoms secondary to a large mediastinal mass. This lymphoma is usually associated with a poorer prognosis and a more aggressive course than classical Hodgkin lymphoma or primary mediastinal large B-cell lymphoma.

References

1. Carbone PP, Kaplan HS, Musshoff K, Smithers DW, Tubiana M (1971) Report of the committee on Hodgkin's disease staging classification. Cancer Res 31:1860
2. Lister TA, Crowther D, Sutcliffe SB, Glatstein E, Canellos GP, Young RC, Rosenberg SA, Coltman CA, Tubiana M (1989) Report of a committee convened to discuss the evaluation and staging of patients with Hodgkin's disease: Cotswolds meeting. J Clin Oncol 7:1630–1636
3. Shipp MA, Harrington DP, Anderson JR et al (1993) The international non-Hodgkin's lymphoma prognostic factors project: a predictive model for aggressive non-Hodgkin's lymphoma. N Engl J Med 329:987–994
4. Sehn LH, Berry B, Chhanabhai M, Fitzgerald C, Gill K, Hoskins P, Klasa R, Savage KJ, Shenkier T, Sutherland J, Gascoyne RD, Connors JM (2007) The revised International Prognostic Index (R-IPI) is a better predictor of outcome than the standard IPI for patients with diffuse large B-cell lymphoma treated with R-CHOP. Blood 109(5):1857–1861
5. Solal-Céligny P, Roy P, Colombat P, White J, Armitage JO, Arranz-Saez R, Au WY, Bellei M, Brice P, Caballero D, Coiffier B, Conde-Garcia E, Doyen C, Federico M, Fisher RI, Garcia-Conde JF, Guglielmi C, Hagenbeek A, Haïoun C, LeBlanc M, Lister AT, Lopez-Guillermo A, McLaughlin P, Milpied N, Morel P, Mounier N, Proctor SJ, Rohatiner A, Smith P, Soubeyran P, Tilly H, Vitolo U, Zinzani PL, Zucca E, Montserrat E (2004) Follicular lymphoma international prognostic index. Blood 104(5):1258–1265
6. Hoster E, Dreyling M, Klapper W, Gisselbrecht C, van Hoof A, Kluin-Nelemans HK, Pfreundschuh M, Reiser M, Metzner B, Einsele H, Peter N, Jung W, Wormann B, Ludwig WD, Duhrsen U, Eimermacher H, Wandt H, Hasford J, Hiddemann W, Unterhalt M, for the German Low Grade Lymphoma Study Group (GLSG) and the European Mantle Cell Lymphoma Network (2008) A new prognostic index (MIPI) for patients with advanced-stage mantle cell lymphoma. Blood 111:558–565
7. Swerdlow SH, Campo E, Harris NL, Jaffe ES, Pileri SA, Stein H, Thiele J, Vardiman J (2008) WHO classification of tumors of haematopoietic and lymphoid tissues, 4th edn. International Agency for Research on Cancer (IARC), Lyon, France
8. Le Gouill S, Lepretre S, Brière J, Morel P, Bouabdallah R, Raffoux E, Sebban C, Lepage E, Brice P (2003) Adult lymphoblastic lymphoma: a retrospective analysis of 92 patients under 61 years included in the LNH87/93 trials. Leukemia 17:2220–2224
9. Morel P, Lepage E, Brice P, Dupriez B, D'Agay MF, Fenaux P, Gosselin P, Bauters F, Gisselbrecht C (1992) Prognosis and treatment of lymphoblastic lymphoma in adults: a report on 80 patients. J Clin Oncol 10:1078–1085
10. Mazza P, Bertini M, Macchi S, Lauria F, Pileri S, Rivano MT, Baccarani M, Ricci P, Fiacchini M, Vitolo U, Canta M, Paolino W, Zinzani PL, Poletti G, Verlicchi F, Gherlinzoni F, Tura S (1986) Lymphoblastic lymphoma in adolescents and adults. Clinical, pathological and prognostic evaluation. Eur J Cancer Clin Oncol 22(12):1503–1510
11. Ducassou S, Ferlay C, Bergeron C, Girard S, Laureys G, Pacquement H, Plantaz D, Lutz P, Vannier JP, Uyttebroeck A, Bertrand Y (2011) Clinical presentation, evolution, and prognosis

of precursor B-cell lymphoblastic lymphoma in trials LMT96, EORTC 58881, and EORTC 58951. Br J Haematol 152(4):441–451

12. Reddy KS, Perkins SL (2004) Advances in the diagnostic approach to childhood lymphoblastic malignant neoplasms. Am J Clin Pathol 122(Suppl 1):S3–S18
13. Møller MB, Gerdes AM, Skjødt K, Mortensen LS, Pedersen NT (1999) Disrupted p53 function as predictor of treatment failure and poor prognosis in B- and T-cell non-Hodgkin's lymphoma. Clin Cancer Res 5:1085–1091
14. Ichikawa A, Kinoshita T, Watanabe T, Kato H, Nagai H, Tsushita K, Saito H, Hotta T (1997) Mutations of the p53 gene as a prognostic factor in aggressive B-cell lymphoma. N Engl J Med 337:529–534
15. Montserrat E (2004) Assessing prognosis in patients with chronic lymphocytic leukemia a quarter of a century after Rai and Binet staging systems. Ann Oncol 15:1450–1451, Editorial
16. Criel A, Verhoef G, Vlietinck R et al (1997) Further characterization of morphologically defined typical and atypical CLL: a clinical, immunophenotypic, cytogenetic, and prognostic study on 390 cases. Br J Haematol 97:383–391
17. Matutes E, Oscier D, Garcia-Marco J et al (1996) Trisomy 12 defines a group of CLL with atypical morphology: correlation between cytogenetic, clinical, and laboratory features in 544 patients. Br J Haematol 92:382–388
18. Frater JL, Hammel JP, Shapiro JL, Miller ML, Tubbs RR, Pettay J, His ED (2001) Typical and atypical chronic lymphocytic leukemia differ clinically and immunophenotypically. Am J Clin Pathol 116:655–664
19. Geisler CH et al (1991) Prognostic importance of flow cytometric immunophenotyping of 540 consecutive patients with B-cell chronic lymphocytic leukemia. Blood 79:1795–1802
20. Damle RN, Wasil T, Fais F et al (1999) IgV gene mutation status and CD38 expression as novel prognostic indicators in chronic lymphocytic leukemia. Blood 94:1840–1847
21. Del Poeta G, Maurillo L, Venditti A, Buccisano F, Epiceno AM, Capelli G, Tamburini A, Suppo G, Battaglia A, Del Principe MI, Del Moro B, Masi M, Amadori S (2001) Clinical significance of CD38 expression in chronic lymphocytic leukemia. Blood 98(9):2633–2639
22. Ibrahim S, Keating M, Do KA, O'Brien S, Huh YO, Jilani I, Lerner S, Kantarjian HM, Albitar M (2001) CD38 expression as an important prognostic factor in B-cell chronic lymphocytic leukemia. Blood 98(1):181–186
23. Hamblin TJ, Orchard JA, Ibbotson RE, Davis Z, Thomas PW, Stevenson FK et al (2002) CD38 expression and immunoglobulin variable region mutations are independent prognostic variables in chronic lymphocytic leukemia, but CD38 expression may vary during the course of the disease. Blood 99:1023–1029
24. Wiestner A et al (2003) ZAP-70 expression identifies a chronic lymphocytic leukemia subtype with unmutated immunoglobulin genes, inferior clinical outcome, and distinct gene expression profile. Blood 101(12):4944–4951
25. Rassenti LZ, Huynh L, Toy TL, Chen L, Keating MJ, Gribben JG, Neuberg DS, Flinn IW, Rai KR, Byrd JC, Kay NE, Greaves A, Weiss A, Kipps TJ (2004) ZAP-70 compared with immunoglobulin heavy-chain gene mutation status as a predictor of disease progression in chronic lymphocytic leukemia. N Engl J Med 351(9):893–901
26. Cordone I, Matutes E, Catovsky D (1992) Monoclonal antibody Ki-67 identified B and T cells in chronic lymphocytic leukemia: correlation with disease activity. Leukemia 6:902–906
27. Wolowiec D, Wojtowicz M, Ciszak L, Kosmaczewska A, Frydecka I, Potoczek S, Urbaniak-Kujda D, Kapelko-Slowik K, Kuliczkowski K (2009) High intracellular content of cyclin-dependent kinase inhibitor p27(Kip1) in early- and intermediate stage B-cell chronic lymphocytic leukemia lymphocytes predicts rapid progression of the disease. Eur J Haematol 82(4):260–266
28. Vrhovac R, Delmer A, Tabg R, Marie JP, Zittoun R, Ajchenbaum-Cymbalista F (1998) Prognostic significance of the cell cycle inhibitor p27Kip1 in chronic B-cell lymphocytic leukemia. Blood 91:4694–4700
29. Ito M, Iida S, Inagaki H, Tsuboi K, Komatsu H, Yamaguchi M, Nakamura N, Suzuki R, Seto M, Nakamura S, Morishima Y, Ueda R (2002) MUM1/IRF4 Expression is an unfavorable

prognostic factor in B-cell chronic lymphocytic leukemia (CLL)/small lymphocytic lymphoma (SLL). Jpn J Cancer Res 93:685–694
30. Leuenberger M, Frigerio S, Wild PJ, Noetzli F, Korol D, Zimmermann DR, Gengler C, Probst-Hensch NM, Moch H, Tinguely M (2010) AID protein expression in chronic lymphocytic leukemia/small lymphocytic lymphoma is associated with poor prognosis and complex genetic alterations. Mod Pathol 23:177–186
31. Morrison W, Hoppe R, Weiss L et al (1989) Small lymphocytic lymphoma. J Clin Oncol 7:598–606
32. Rai KR, Sawitsky A, Cronkite EP et al (1975) Clinical staging of chronic lymphocytic leukemia. Blood 46:219–234
33. Rai KR (1987) A critical analysis of staging in CLL. In: Gale RP, Rai KR (eds) Chronic lymphocytic leukemia: recent progress and future direction: 1987 UCLA symposia on molecular and cellular biology, vol 59, New series. Liss, New York, pp 253–264
34. Binet JL, Auquier A, Dighiero G et al (1981) A new prognostic classification of chronic lymphocytic leukemia derived from a multivariate survival analysis. Cancer 48:198–206
35. Zent CS, Ding W, Schwager SM, Reinalda MS, Hoyer JD, Jelinek DF, Tschumper RC, Bowen DA, Call TG, Shanafelt TD, Kay NE, Slager SL (2008) The Prognostic significance of cytopenia in chronic lymphocytic leukemia/small lymphocytic lymphoma (CLL). Br J Haematol 141(5):615–621
36. Galton DAG (1996) The pathogenesis of chronic lymphocytic leukemia. Can Med Assoc J 94:1005–1010
37. Molica S, Alberti A (1987) Prognostic value of lymphocyte doubling time in chronic lymphocytic leukemia. Cancer 60:2712–2716
38. Molica S, Reverter JC, Alberti A et al (1990) Timing of diagnosis and lymphocyte accumulation patterns in chronic lymphocytic leukemia: analysis of their clinical significance. Eur J Haematol 44:277–281
39. Montserrat E, Sanchez BJ, Vinolas N et al (1986) Lymphocyte doubling time in chronic lymphocytic leukaemia: analysis of its prognostic significance. Br J Haematol 62:567–575
40. Sarfati M, Chevret S, Chastang C, Biron G, Stryckmans P, Delespesse G, Binet JL, Merle-Beral H, Bron D (1996) Prognostic importance of serum soluble CD23 level in chronic lymphocytic leukemia. Blood 88:4259–4263
41. Molica S, Levato D, Cascavilla N et al (1999) Clinico-prognostic implications of simultaneous increased serum levels of soluble CD23 and beta2-microglobulin in B-cell chronic lymphocytic leukemia. Eur J Haematol 62:117–122
42. Hallek M, Wanders L, Ostwald M et al (1996) Serum beta(2)-microglobulin and serum thymidine kinase are independent predictors of progression-free survival in chronic lymphocytic leukemia and immunocytoma. Leuk Lymphoma 22:439–447
43. Hallek M, Langenmayer I, Nerl C et al (1999) Elevated serum thymidine kinase levels identify a subgroup at high risk of disease progression in early, nonsmoldering chronic lymphocytic leukemia. Blood 93:1732–1737
44. Matthews C, Catherwood MA, Morris TC et al (2006) Serum TK levels in CLL identify Binet stage A patients within biologically defined prognostic subgroups most likely to undergo disease progression. Eur J Haematol 77:309–317
45. Hamblin TJ, Davis Z, Gardiner A et al (1999) Unmutated IgV(H) genes are associated with a more aggressive form of chronic lymphocytic leukemia. Blood 94:1848–1854
46. Thorselius M, Krober A, Murray F et al (2006) Strikingly homologous immunoglobulin gene rearrangements and poor outcome in VH3-21-using chronic lymphocytic leukemia patients independent of geographic origin and mutational status. Blood 107:2889–2894
47. Dohner H, Stilgenbauer S, Benner A et al (2000) Genomic aberrations and survival in chronic lymphocytic leukemia. N Engl J Med 343:1910–1916
48. Mayr C, Speicher MR, Kofler DM et al (2006) Chromosomal translocations are associated with poor prognosis in chronic lymphocytic leukemia. Blood 107:742–751
49. Oppezzo P, Vasconcelos Y, Settegrana C et al (2005) The LPL/ADAM29 expression ratio is a novel prognosis indicator in chronic lymphocytic leukemia. Blood 106(2):650–657

50. Kotaskova J, Tichy B, Trbusek M, Francova HS, Kabathova J, Malcikova J, Doubek M, Brychtova Y, Mayer J, Pospisilova S (2010) High expression of lymphocyte-activation gene 3 (LAG3) in chronic lymphocytic leukemia cells is associated with unmutated immunoglobulin variable heavy chain region (IGHV) gene and reduced treatment-free survival. J Mol Diagn 12(3):328–334
51. Argatoff LH, Connors JM, Klasa RJ, Horsman DE, Gascoyne RD (1997) Mantle cell lymphoma: a clinicopathologic study of 80 cases. Blood 89(6):2067–2078
52. Majlis A, Pugh WC, Rodriguez MA, Benedict WF, Cabanillas F (1997) Mantle cell lymphoma: correlation of clinical outcome and biologic features with three histologic variants. J Clin Oncol 15(4):1664–1671
53. Carbone A, Santoro A (2011) How I treat: diagnosing and managing "in situ" lymphoma. Blood 117(15):3954–3960
54. Duggan MJ, Weisenburger DD, Ye YL, Bast MA, Pierson JL, Armitage JO (1990) Mantle zone lymphoma. A clinicopathologic study of 22 cases. Cancer 66:522
55. Jares P, Campo E (2008) Advances in the understanding of mantle cell lymphoma. Br J Haematol 142:149–165
56. Ondrejka SL, Lai R, Kumar N, Smith SD, Hsi ED (2011) Indolent mantle cell leukemia: clinicopathologic variant characterized by isolated lymphocytosis, interstitial bone marrow involvement, kappa light chain restriction, and good prognosis. Haematologica. doi:10.3324/haematol.2010.036277
57. Chen D, Viswanatha DS, Zent CS, Shanafelt TD, Call TG, Kay NE, Van Dyke DL, Ketterling RP, Witzig TE, Morice WG, Hanson CA (2009) Indolent mantle cell lymphoma: a distinct subgroup characterized by leukemic phase disease without lymphadenopathy. 51th ASH Annual Meeting and Exposition, New Orleans, LA, 5–8 Dec 2009
58. Mozos A, Royo C, Hartmann E, De Jong D, Baró C, Valera A, Fu K, Weisenburger DD, Delabie J, Chuang SS, Jaffe ES, Ruiz-Marcellan C, Dave S, Rimsza L, Braziel R, Gascoyne RD, Solé F, López-Guillermo A, Colomer D, Staudt LM, Rosenwald A, Ott G, Jares P, Campo S (2009) SOX11 expression is highly specific for mantle cell lymphoma and identifies the cyclin D1-negative subtype. Haematologica 94(11):1555–1562
59. Katzenberger T, Petzoldt C, Höller S, Mäder U, Kalla J, Adam P, Ott MM, Müller-Hermelink HK, Rosenwald A, Ott G (2006) The Ki67 proliferation index is a quantitative indicator of clinical risk in mantle cell lymphoma. Blood 107(8):3407
60. Hsi ED, Jung SH, Lai R, Johnson JL, Cook JR, Jones D, Devos S, Cheson BD, Damon LE, Said J (2008) Ki67 and PIM1 expression predict outcome in mantle cell lymphoma treated with high dose therapy, stem cell transplantation and rituximab: a Cancer and Leukemia Group B 59909 correlative science study. Leuk Lymphoma 11:2081–2090
61. Yatabe Y, Suzuki R, Tobinai K, Matsuno Y, Ichinohasama R, Okamoto M, Yamaguchi M, Tamaru J, Uike N, Hashimoto Y, Morishima Y, Suchi T, Seto M, Nakamura S (2000) Significance of cyclin D1 overexpression for the diagnosis of mantle cell lymphoma: a clinicopathologic comparison of cyclin D1-positive MCL and cyclin D1-negative MCL-like B-cell lymphoma. Blood 95(7):2253–2261
62. Hernandez L, Fest T, Cazorla M, Teruya-Feldstein J, Bosch F, Peinado MA, Piris MA, Montserrat E, Cardesa A, Jaffe ES, Campo E, Raffeld M (1996) p53 gene mutations and protein overexpression are associated with aggressive variants of mantle cell lymphomas. Blood 87(8):3351–3359
63. Espinet B, Salaverria I, Beà S, Ruiz-Xivillé N, Balagué O, Salido M, Costa D, Carreras J, Rodríguez-Vicente AE, Luís García J, Hernández-Rivas JM, Calasanz MJ, Siebert R, Ferrer A, Salar A, Carrió A, Polo N, García-Marco JA, Domingo A, González-Barca E, Romagosa V, Marugán I, López-Guillermo A, Millá F, Luís Mate J, Luño E, Sanzo C, Collado R, Oliver I, Monzó S, Palacín A, González T, Sant F, Salinas R, Ardanaz MT, Font L, Escoda L, Florensa L, Serrano S, Campo E, Solé F (2010) Incidence and prognostic impact of secondary cytogenetic aberrations in a series of 145 patients with mantle cell lymphoma. Genes Chromosomes Cancer 49(5):439–451

64. Beà S, Ribas M, Hernández JM et al (1999) Increased number of chromosomal imbalances and high-level DNA amplifications in mantle cell lymphoma are associated with blastoid variants. Blood 93:4365–4374
65. Ott G, Kalla J, Hanke A et al (1998) The cytomorphological spectrum of mantle cell lymphoma is reflected by distinct biological features. Leuk Lymphoma 32:55–63
66. Halldórsdóttir AM, Sander B, Göransson H, Isaksson A, Kimby E, Mansouri M, Rosenquist R, Ehrencrona H (2011) High-resolution genomic screening in mantle cell lymphoma—specific changes correlate with genomic complexity, the proliferation signature and survival. Genes Chromosomes Cancer 50(2):113–121
67. Dreyling M, Hiddemann W for The European MCL Network (2009) Current treatment standards and emerging strategies in mantle cell lymphoma. Hematology Am Soc Hematol Educ Program 542–551. Review. Erratum in: Hematology Am Soc Hematol Educ Program 2011:562
68. Mann RB, Berard CW (1983) Criteria for the cytologic classification of follicular lymphomas: a proposed alternative method. Hematol Oncol 1:187–192
69. Martin AR, Weisenburg DD et al (1995) Prognostic value of cellular proliferation and histologic grade in follicular lymphoma. Blood 85(12):3671–3678
70. Moskowitz CH (2005) Rituximab and poor-risk follicular lymphoma. Blood 105(4):1380
71. Ott G, Katzenberger T, Lohr A, Kindelberger S, Rudiger T, Wilhelm M, Kalla J, Rosenwald A, Muller JS, Ott MM, Muller-Hermelink HK (2002) Cytomorphologic, immunohistochemical, and cytogenetic profiles of follicular lymphoma: 2 types of follicular lymphoma grade 3. Blood 99:3806–3812
72. Hsi ED, Mirza I, Lozanski G, Hill J, Pohlman B, Karafa MT, Coupland R (2004) A clinicopathologic evaluation of follicular lymphoma grade 3A versus grade 3B reveals no survival differences. Arch Pathol Lab Med 128(8):863–868
73. Naresh KN (2007) MUM1 expression dichotomizes follicular lymphoma into predominantly, MUM1-negative low-grade and MUM1-positive high-grade subtypes. Haematologica 92:267–268
74. Lai R, Weiss LM, Chang KL, Arber DA (1999) Frequency of CD43 expression in non-Hodgkin lymphoma. Am J Clin Pathol 111(4):488–494
75. Broyde A, Boycov O, Strenov Y, Okon E, Shpilberg O, Bairey O (2009) Role and prognostic significance of the Ki-67 index in non-Hodgkin's lymphoma. Am J Hematol 84:338–343
76. Wang SA, Wang L, Hochberg EP, Muzikansky A, Harris NL, Hasserjian RP (2005) Low histologic grade follicular lymphoma with high proliferation index: morphologic and clinical features. Am J Surg Pathol 29(11):1490–1496
77. Pruneri G, Valentini S, Fabris S, Del Curto B, Laszlo D, Bertoloni F, Martinelli G, Leocata P, Viale G, Neri A (2004) Cyclin D3 immunoreactivity in follicular lymphoma is independent of the t(6;14)(p21.1;q32.3) translocation or Cyclin D3 gene amplification and is correlated with histologic grade and Ki-67 labeling. Int J Cancer 112:71–77
78. Symmans WF, Katz RL, Ordoñez NG, Dalton H, Romaguera JE, Cabanillas F (1995) Transformation of follicular lymphoma. Expression of p53 and bcl-2 oncoprotein, apoptosis and cell proliferation. Acta Cytol 39(4):673–682
79. Krishnadasan R, Bifulco C, Kim J, Rodo S, Zieske AW, Vanasse GJ (2006) Overexpression of SOCS3 is associated with decreased survival in a cohort of patients with de novo follicular lymphoma. Br J Haematol 135(1):72–75
80. Federico M, Bellei M, Marcheselli L et al (2009) Follicular lymphoma international prognostic index 2: a new prognostic index for follicular lymphoma developed by the international follicular lymphoma prognostic factor project. J Clin Oncol 27:4555–4562
81. Tilly BH, Rossi A, Stamatoullas A, Lenormand B, Bigorgne C, Kunlin A, Monconduit M, Bastard C (1994) Prognostic value of chromosomal abnormalities in follicular lymphoma. Blood 84(4):1043–1049
82. Lossos IS, Alizadeh AA, Diehn M, Warnke R, Thorstenson Y, Oefner PJ, Brown PO, Botstein D, Levy R (2002) Transformation of follicular lymphoma to diffuse large-cell lymphoma: alternative patterns with increased or decreased expression of c-myc and its regulated genes. Proc Natl Acad Sci U S A 99(13):8887–8891

83. Dave SS, Wright G, Tan B et al (2004) Prediction of survival in follicular lymphoma based on molecular features of tumor-infiltrating immune cells. N Engl J Med 351:2159–2169
84. Hart J, Lai R, Montoto S, Gribben JG, Lister TA, Carlotti JFE, Wrench D, Matthews J, Iqbal S, Davies A, Norton A (2009) Transformation of follicular lymphoma to diffuse large B-cell lymphoma may occur by divergent evolution from a common progenitor cell or by direct evolution from the follicular lymphoma clone. Blood 113:3553–3557
85. Montoto S, Davies AJ, Matthews J, Calaminici M, Norton AJ, Amess J, Vinnicombe S, Waters R, Rohatiner AZS, Lister TA (2007) Risk and clinical implications of transformation of follicular lymphoma to diffuse large B-cell lymphoma. J Clin Oncol 25(17):2426–2433
86. Thieblemont C (2005) Clinical presentation and management of marginal zone lymphomas. Hematology 1:307–313
87. Pinotti G, Zucca E, Roggero E et al (1997) Clinical features, treatment and outcome in a series of 93 patients with low-grade gastric MALT lymphoma. Leuk Lymphoma 26:527–537
88. Hoeve MA, Gisbertz IAM, Schouten HC, Schuuring E, Bot FG, Hermans J, Hopman A, Kluin PM, Arends J-W, van Krieken JHJM (1999) Gastric low-grade MALT lymphoma, high-grade MALT lymphoma and diffuse large B cell lymphoma show different frequencies of trisomy. Leukemia 13(5):799–807
89. Thieblemont C, Bastion Y, Berger F et al (1997) Mucosa-associated lymphoid tissue gastrointestinal and nongastrointestinal lymphoma behavior: analysis of 108 patients. J Clin Oncol 15:1624–1630
90. Zuca E, Conconi A, Pedrinis E et al (2003) Nongastric marginal zone B-cell lymphoma of mucosa-associated lymphoid tissue. Blood 101:2489–2495
91. Nola M, Lukenda A, Bollmann M, Kalauz M, Petrovecki M, Bollmann R (2004) Outcome and prognostic factors in ocular adnexal lymphoma. Croat Med J 45(3):328–332
92. Sagaert X, Laurent M, Baens M, Wlodarska I, De Wolf-Peeters C (2006) MALT1 and BCL10 aberrations in MALT lymphomas and their effect on the expression of BCL10 in the tumour cells. Mod Pathol 19:225–232
93. Radaszkiewicz T, Dragosics B, Bauer P (1992) Gastrointestinal malignant lymphomas of the mucosa-associated lymphoid tissue: factors relevant to prognosis. Gastroenterology 102:1628–1638
94. Montalban C, Castrillo J, Abraira V et al (1995) Gastric B-cell mucosa-associated lymphoid tissue (MALT) lymphoma. Clinicopathological study and evaluation of the prognostic factors in 143 patients. Ann Oncol 6:355–362
95. Liu H, Ruskon-Fourmestraux A, Lavergne-Slove A et al (2001) Resistance of t(11;18) positive gastric mucosa-associated lymphoid tissue lymphoma to Helicobacter pylori eradication therapy. Lancet 357:39–40
96. Levy M, Copie-Bergman C, Gameiro C et al (2005) Prognostic value of translocation t(11;18) in tumoral response of low-grade gastric lymphoma of mucosa-associated lymphoid tissue type to oral chemotherapy. J Clin Oncol 23:5061–5066
97. Remstein ED, Kurtin PJ, James CD, Wang XY, Meyer RG, Dewald GW (2002) Mucosa-associated lymphoid tissue lymphomas with t(11;18)(q21;q21) and mucosa-associated lymphoid tissue lymphomas with aneuploidy develop along different pathogenetic pathways. Am J Pathol 161:63–71
98. Kurtin PJ, Myers JL, Adlakha H, Strickler JG, Lohse C, Pankratz VS, Inwards DJ (2001) Pathologic and clinical features of primary pulmonary extranodal marginal zone B-cell lymphoma of MALT type. Am J Surg Pathol 25:997–1008
99. Nathwani B, Anderson J, Armitage J et al (1999) Marginal zone B-cell lymphoma: a clinical comparison of nodal and mucosa-associated lymphoid tissue types. Non-Hodgkin's Lymphoma Classification Project. J Clin Oncol 17:2486–2492
100. Berger F, Felman P, Thieblemont C et al (2000) Non-MALT marginal zone B-cell lymphomas: a description of clinical presentation and outcome in 124 patients. Blood 95:1950–1956
101. Arcaini L, Paulli M, Burcheri S, Rossi A, Spina M, Passamonti F, Lucioni M, Motta T, Canzonieri V, Montanari M, Bonoldi E, Gallamini A, Uziel L, Crugnola M, Ramponi A, Montanari F, Pascutto C, Morra E, Lazzarino M (2007) Primary nodal marginal zone B-cell

lymphoma: clinical features and prognostic assessment of a rare disease. Br J Haematol 136:301–304

102. A clinical evaluation of the International Lymphoma Study Group classification of non-Hodgkin's lymphoma. By the Non-Hodgkin's Lymphoma Classification Project (1997) Blood 89:3909–3918
103. Taddesse-Heath L, Pittaluga S, Sorbara L, Bussey M, Raffeld M, Jaffe ES (2003) Marginal zone B-cell lymphoma in children and young adults. Am J Surg Pathol 27(4):522–531
104. Rizzo KA, Streubel B, Pittaluga S, Chott A, Xi L, Raffeld M, Jaffe ES (2010) Marginal zone lymphomas in children and the young adult population; characterization of genetic aberrations by FISH and RT-PCR. Mod Pathol 23:866–873
105. Arcaini L, Lazzarino M, Colombo N et al (2006) Splenic marginal zone lymphoma: a prognostic model for clinical use. Blood 107:4643–4649
106. Algara P, Mateo MS, Sanchez-Beato M et al (2002) Analysis of the IgV(H) somatic mutations in splenic marginal zone lymphoma defines a group of unmutated cases with frequent 7q deletion and adverse clinical course. Blood 99:1299–1304
107. Ruiz-Ballesteros E, Mollejo M, Rodriguez A et al (2005) Splenic marginal zone lymphoma: proposal of new diagnostic and prognostic markers identified after tissue and cDNA microarray analysis. Blood 106:1831–1838
108. Bahler DW, Pindzola JA, Swerdlow SH (2002) Splenic marginal zone lymphomas appear to originate from different B cell types. Am J Pathol 161:81–88
109. Chacòn JI, Mollejo M, Muñoz E (2002) Splenic marginal zone lymphoma: clinical characteristics and prognostic factors in a series of 60 patients. Blood 100(5):1648–1654
110. Batanian JR, Dunphy CH, Richart JM, Petruska PJ, Perkins SL (2000) Simultaneous presence of t(2;8)(p12;q24) and t(14;18)(q32;q21) in a B-cell lymphoproliferative disorder with features suggestive of an aggressive variant of splenic marginal-zone lymphoma. Cancer Genet Cytogenet 120(2):136–140
111. Hernández JM, García JL, Gutiérrez NC, Mollejo M, Martínez-Climent JA, Flores T, González MB, Piris MA, San Miguel JF (2001) Novel genomic imbalances in B-cell splenic marginal zone lymphomas revealed by comparative genomic hybridization and cytogenetics. Am J Pathol 158(5):1843–1850
112. Traverse-Glehen A, Baseggio L, Callet-Bauchu E, Morel D, Gazzo S, Ffrench M, Verney A, Rolland D, Thieblemont C, Magaud J-P, Salles G, Coiffier B, Berger F, Felman P (2008) Splenic red pulp lymphoma with numerous basophilic villous lymphocytes: a distinct clinicopathologic and molecular entity? Blood 111(4):2253–2260
113. Bartl R, Frisch B, Mahl G, Burkhardt R, Fateh-Moghadam A, Pappenberger R, Sommerfeld W, Hoffmann-Fezer G (1983) Bone marrow histology in Waldenström's macroglobulinaemia. Clinical relevance of subtype recognition. Scand J Haematol 31(4):359–375
114. Mansoor A, Medeiros LJ, Weber AR, Hayes K, Jones D, Lai R, Glassman A, Bueso-Ramos CE (2001) Cytogenetic findings in lymphoplasmacytic lymphoma/Waldenström macroglobulinemia chromosomal abnormalities are associated with the polymorphous subtype and an aggressive clinical course. Am J Clin Pathol 116:543–549
115. Lin P, Mansoor A, Bueso-Ramos C, Hao S, Lai R, Medeiros LJ (2003) Diffuse large B-cell lymphoma occurring in patients with lymphoplasmacytic lymphoma/Waldenström macroglobulinemia. Clinicopathologic features of 12 cases. Am J Clin Pathol 120:246–253
116. Petit B, Chaury MP, Le Clorennec C, Jaccard A, Gachard N, Moalic-Judge S, Labrousse F, Cogné M, Bordessoule D, Feuillard J (2005) Indolent lymphoplasmacytic and marginal zone B-cell lymphomas: absence of both IRF4 and Ki67 expression identifies a better prognosis subgroup. Haematologica 90(2):200–206
117. Morel P, Duhamel A, Gobbi P, Dimopoulos MA, Dhodapkar MV, McCoy J, Crowley J, Ocio EM, Garcia-Sanz R, Treon SP, Leblond V, Kyle RA, Barlogie B, Merlini G (2009) International prognostic scoring system for Waldenstrom macroglobulinemia. Blood 113(18):4163–4170
118. Hallek M, Wanders L, Ostwald M, Busch R, Senekowitsch R, Stern S, Schick HD, Kuhn-Hallek I, Emmerich B (1996) Serum beta(2)-microglobulin and serum thymidine kinase are independent predictors of progression-free survival in chronic lymphocytic leukemia and immunocytoma. Leuk Lymphoma 22(5–6):439–447

119. Dimopoulos MA, Hamilos G, Zervas K et al (2003) Survival and prognostic factors after initiation of treatment in Waldenstrom's macroglobulinemia. Ann Oncol 14:1299–1305
120. Garcia-Sanz R, Montoto S, Torrequebrada A et al (2001) Waldenstrom macroglobulinaemia: presenting features and outcome in a series with 217 cases. Br J Haematol 115:575–582
121. Dhodapkar MV, Jacobson JL, Gertz MA, Crowley JJ, Barlogie B (2003) Prognostic factors and response to fludarabine therapy in Waldenstrom's macroglobulinemia: an update of a US intergroup trial (SW0G S9003). Semin Oncol 30:220–225
122. Chang H, Qi C, Trieu Y et al (2008) Prognostic relevance of 6q deletion in Waldenstrom macroglobulinemia. Proceedings of the 5th International Workshop of Waldenstrom macroglobulinemia, Stockholm, Sweden (abstract 1125)
123. Roccaro AM, Sacco A, Chen C, Runnels J, Leleu X, Azab F, Azab AK, Jia X, Ngo HT, Melhem MR, Burwick N, Varticovski L, Novina CD, Rollins BJ, Anderson KC, Ghobrial IM (2009) MicroRNA expression in the biology, prognosis, and therapy of Waldenström macroglobulinemia. Blood 113(18):4391–4402
124. Wilson WH, Dunleavy K, Pittaluga S, Hegde U, Grant N, Steinberg SM, Raffeld M, Gutierrez M, Chabner BA, Staudt L, Jaffe ES, Janik JE (2008) Phase II study of dose-adjusted EPOCH-rituximab in untreated diffuse large B-cell lymphoma with analysis of germinal center and post-germinal center biomarkers. J Clin Oncol 26(16):2717–2724
125. Truman LA, Ogden CA, Howie SE, Gregory CD (2004) Macrophage chemotaxis to apoptotic Burkitt's lymphoma cells in vitro: role of CD14 and CD36. Immunobiology 209(1–2):21–30
126. Ogden CA, Pound JD, Batth BK, Owens S, Johannessen I, Wood K, Gregory CD (2005) Enhanced apoptotic cell clearance capacity and B cell survival factor production by IL-10-activated macrophages: implications for Burkitt's lymphoma. J Immunol 74(5):3015–3023
127. Haralambieva E, Rosati S, van Noesel C et al (2004) Florid granulomatous reaction in Epstein-Barr virus-positive nonendemic Burkitt lymphomas: report of four cases. Am J Surg Pathol 28:379–383
128. Schrager JA, Pittaluga S, Raffeld M et al (2005) Granulomatous reaction in Burkitt lymphoma: correlation with EBV positivity and clinical outcome. Am J Surg Pathol 29:1115–1116
129. Janegová A, Janega P, Ilencíková D, Babál P (2011) Burkitt lymphoma with unusual granulomatous reaction. A case report. Cesk Patol 47(1):19–22
130. Tumwine LK, Agostinelli C, Campidelli C, Othieno E, Wabinga H, Righi S, Falini B, Piccaluga PP, Byarugaba W, Pileri SA (2009) Immunohistochemical and other prognostic factors in B cell non Hodgkin lymphoma patients, Kampala, Uganda. BMC Clin Pathol 9:11
131. Valnet-Rabier MB, Challier B, Thiebault S, Angonin R, Margueritte G, Mougin C, Kantelip B, Deconinck E, Cahn JY, Fest T (2005) c-Flip protein expression in Burkitt's lymphomas is associated with a poor clinical outcome. Br J Haematol 128(6):767–773
132. Nomura Y, Yoshida S, Karube K, Takeshita M, Hirose S, Nakamura S, Yoshino T, Kikuchi M, Ohshima K (2008) Estimation of the relationship between caspase-3 expression and clinical outcome of Burkitt's and Burkitt-like lymphoma. Cancer Sci 99(8):1564–1569
133. Kenkre VP, Stock W (2009) Burkitt lymphoma/leukemia: improving prognosis. Clin Lymphoma Myeloma 9(Suppl 3):S231–S238
134. Bower M, Gazzard B, Mandalia S et al (2005) A prognostic index for systemic AIDS-related non-Hodgkin lymphoma treated in the era of highly active antiretroviral therapy. Ann Intern Med 143:265–273
135. Kaplan LD, Abrams DI, Feigal E et al (1989) AIDS-associated non-Hodgkin's lymphoma in San Francisco. JAMA 261:719–724
136. Levine AM, Sullivan-Halley J et al (1991) Human immunodeficiency virus-related lymphoma. Prognostic factors predictive of survival. Cancer 68:2466–2472
137. Kornblau SM, Goodacre A, Cabanillas F (1991) Chromosomal abnormalities in adult non-endemic Burkitt's lymphoma and leukemia: 22 new reports and a review of 148 cases from the literature. Hematol Oncol 9(2):63–78
138. Kluin P, Schuuring E (2011) Molecular cytogenetics of lymphoma: where do we stand in 2010? Histopathology 58:128–144
139. Nelson M, Perkins SL, Dave BJ, Coccia PF, Bridge JA, Lyden ER, Heerema NA, Lones MA, Harrison L, Cairo MS, Sanger WG (2010) An increased frequency of 13q deletions detected

by fluorescence in situ hybridization and its impact on survival in children and adolescents with Burkitt lymphoma: results from the Children's Oncology Group study CCG-5961. Br J Haematol 148(4):600–610
140. Engelhard M, Brittinger G, Huhn D, Gerhartz HH, Meusers P, Siegert W, Thiel E, Wilmanns W, Aydemir U, Bierwolf S, Griesser H, Tiemann M, Lennert K (1997) Subclassification of diffuse large B-cell lymphomas according to the Kiel classification: distinction of centroblastic and immunoblastic lymphomas is a significant prognostic risk factor. Blood 89(7):2291–2297
141. De Paepe P, Achten R, Verhoef G, Wlodarska I, Stul M, Vanhentenrijk V, Praet M, De Wolf-Peeters C (2005) Large cleaved and immunoblastic lymphoma may represent two distinct clinicopathologic entities within the group of diffuse large B-cell lymphomas. J Clin Oncol 23:7060–7068
142. Sehn LS, Scott DW, Chhanabhai M, BerryB RA, Berkahn L, Connors JM, Gascoyne RD (2010) Impact of concordant and discordant bone marrow involvement on outcome in diffuse large B-cell lymphoma treated with R-CHOP. J Clin Oncol 29(11):1452–1457
143. Hans CP, Weisenburger DD, Greiner TC et al (2003) Confirmation of the molecular classification of diffuse large B-cell lymphoma by immunohistochemistry using a tissue microarray. Blood 103:275–282
144. Natkunam Y, Farinha P, Hsi ED, Hans CP, Tibshirani R, Sehn LH, Connors JM, Gratzinger D, Rosado M, Zhao S, Pohlman B, Wongchaowart N, Bast M, Avigdor A, Schiby G, Nagler A, Byrne GE, Levy R, Gascoyne RD, Lossos IS (2008) LMO2 protein expression predicts survival in patients with diffuse large B-cell lymphoma treated with anthracycline-based chemotherapy with and without rituximab. J Clin Oncol 26(3):447–454
145. Durnick DK, Law ME, Maurer MJ, Natkunam Y, Levy R, Lossos IS, Kurtin JP, McPhail ED (2010) Expression of LMO2 is associated with t(14;18)/IGH-BCL2 fusion but not BCL6 translocations in Diffuse Large B-Cell Lymphoma. Am J Clin Pathol 134:278–281
146. Yamaguchi M, Nakamura N, Suzuki R, Kagami Y, Okamoto M, Ichinohasama R, Yoshino T, Suzumiya J, Murase T, Miura I, Ohshima K, Nishikori M, Tamaru J, Taniwaki M, Hirano M, Morishima Y, Ueda R, Shiku H, Nakamura S (2008) De novo CD5+ diffuse large B-cell lymphoma: results of a detailed clinicopathological review in 120 patients. Haematologica 93(8):1195–1202
147. Ennishi D, Takeuchi K, Yokoyama M, Asai H, Mishima Y, Terui Y, Takahashi S, Komatsu H, Ikeda K, Yamaguchi M, Suzuki R, Tanimoto M, Hatake K (2008) CD5 Expression is potentially predictive of poor outcome among biomarkers in patients with diffuse large B-cell lymphoma receiving rituximab plus CHOP therapy. Ann Oncol 19(11):1921–1926
148. Iqbal J, Neppalli VT, Wright G, Dave BJ, Horsman DE, Rosenwald A, Lynch J, Hans CP, Weisenburger DD, Greiner TC, Gascoyne RD, Campo E, Ott G, Müller-Hermelink HK, Delabie J, Jaffe ES, Grogan TM, Connors JM, Vose JM, Armitage JO, Staudt LM, Chan WC (2006) BCL2 expression is a prognostic marker for the activated B-cell-like type of Diffuse Large B-Cell Lymphoma. J Clin Oncol 24(6):961–968
149. Laurent C, Do C, Gascoyne RD, Lamant L, Ysebaert L, Laurent G, Delsol G, Brousset P (2009) Anaplastic lymphoma kinase-positive diffuse large B-cell lymphoma: a rare clinicopathologic entity with poor prognosis. J Clin Oncol 27(25):4211–4216
150. Beltran B, Winer ES, Castillo J (2010) ALK-positive diffuse large B-cell lymphoma: an aggressive clinicopathological entity. Eur J Clin Med Oncol 2(1):1759–8966
151. Hans CP, Weisenburger DD, Greiner TC, Chan WC, Aoun P, Cochran GT, Pan Z, Smith LM, Lynch JC, Bociek RG, Bierman PJ, Vose JM, Armitage JO (2005) Expression of PKC-beta or cyclin D2 predicts for inferior survival in diffuse large B-cell lymphoma. Mod Pathol 18(10):1377–1384
152. Pileri SA, Dirnhofer S, Went P, Ascani S, Sabattini E, Marafioti T, Tzankov A, Leoncini L, Falini B, Zinzani PL (2002) Diffuse large B-cell lymphoma: one or more entities? Present controversies and possible tools for its subclassification. Histopathology 41(6):482–509
153. Xiang XJ, He YJ (2006) Clinical significance of survivin and caspase-3 expression in diffuse large B-cell lymphoma. Zhonghua Zhong Liu Za Zhi 28(4):298–301

154. Markovic O, Marisavljevic D, Cemerikic V, Perunicic M, Savic S, Filipovic B, Mihaljevic B (2011) Clinical and prognostic significance of apoptotic profile in patients with newly diagnosed nodal diffuse large B-cell lymphoma (DLBCL). Eur J Haematol 86(3):246–255
155. Ohsawa M, Ikura Y, Fukushima H, Shirai N, Sugama Y, Suekane T, Hirayama M, Hino M, Ueda M (2005) Immunohistochemical expression of multidrug resistance proteins as a predictor of poor response to chemotherapy and prognosis in patients with nodal diffuse large B-cell lymphoma. Oncology 68(4–6):422–431
156. Sánchez-Aguilera A, Sánchez-Beato M, García JF, Prieto I, Pollan M, Piris MA (2002) p14^{ARF} nuclear overexpression in aggressive B-cell lymphomas is a sensor of malfunction of the common tumor suppressor pathways. Blood 99:1411–1418
157. Korać P, Dominis M (2008) Prognostic markers and gene abnormalities in subgroups of diffuse large B-cell lymphoma: single center experience. Croat Med 49:618–624
158. Barrans SL, Fenton JAL, Banham A, Owen RG, Jack AS (2004) Strong expression of FOXP1 identifies a distinct subset of diffuse large B-cell lymphoma (DLBCL) patients with poor outcome. Blood 104:2933–2935
159. Veelken H, Dannheim SV, Schulte Moenting J, Martens UM, Finke J, Schmitt-Graeff A (2007) Immunophenotype as prognostic factor for diffuse large B-cell lymphoma in patients undergoing clinical risk-adapted therapy. Ann Oncol 18:931–939
160. Lossos IS, Morgensztern D (2006) Prognostic biomarkers in diffuse large B-cell lymphoma. J Clin Oncol 24(6):995–1007
161. Castillo JJ, Beltran BE, Miranda RN, Paydas S, Winer ES, Butera JN (2011) Epstein-Barr virus—positive Diffuse Large B-Cell Lymphoma of the elderly: what we know so far. Oncologist 16(1):87–96
162. Miller TP, Grogan TM, Dahlberg S, Spier CM, Braziel RM, Banks PM, Foucar K, Kjeldsberg CR, Levy N, Nathwani BN et al (1994) Prognostic significance of the Ki-67-associated proliferative antigen in aggressive non-Hodgkin's lymphomas: a prospective Southwest Oncology Group trial. Blood 83(6):1460–1466
163. Yoon DH, Choi DR, Ahn HJ, Kim S, Lee DH, Kim SW, Park BH, Yoon SO, Huh J, Lee SW, Suh C (2010) Ki-67 expression as a prognostic factor in diffuse large B-cell lymphoma patients treated with rituximab plus CHOP. Eur J Haematol 85(2):149–157
164. Meyer PN, Fu K, Greiner T, Smith L, Delabie J, Gascoyne R, Ott G, Rosenwald A, Braziel R, Campo E, Vose J, Lenz G, Staudt L, Chan W, Weisenburger DD (2011) The stromal cell marker SPARC predicts for survival in patients with diffuse large B-cell lymphoma treated with rituximab. Am J Clin Pathol 135(1):54–61
165. Alizadeh AA, Eisen MB, Davis RE, Ma C, Lossos IS, Rosenwald A, Boldrick JC, Sabet H, Tran T, Yu X, Powell JI, Yang L, Marti GE, Moore T, Hudson J Jr, Lu L, Lewis DB, Tibshirani R, Sherlock G, Chan WC, Greiner TC, Weisenburger DD, Armitage JO, Warnke R, Levy R, Wilson W, Grever MR, Byrd JC, Botstein D, Brown PO, Staudt LM (2000) Distinct types of diffuse large B-cell lymphoma identified by gene expression profiling. Nature 403:503–511
166. Lossos IS, Jones CD, Warnke R, Natkunam Y, Kaizer H, Zehnder JL, Tibshirani R, Levy R (2001) Expression of a single gene, BCL-6, strongly predicts survival in patients with diffuse large B-cell lymphoma. Blood 98(4):945–951
167. Chang CC, Chang Y, Cleveland RP, Perkins SP (2000) Expression of c-Myc and p53 correlates with clinical outcome in diffuse large B-cell lymphomas. Hematopathology. Am J Clin Pathol 113:512–518
168. Savage KJ, Johnson NA, Ben-Neriah S, Connors JM, Sehn LH, Farinha P, Horsman DE, Gascoyne RD (2009) MYC gene rearrangements are associated with a poor prognosis in diffuse large B-cell lymphoma patients treated with R-CHOP chemotherapy. Blood 114(17):3533–3537
169. Ramsay AD, Smith WJ, Isaacson PG (1988) T-cell-rich B-cell lymphoma. Am J Surg Pathol 12:433–443
170. Achten R, Verhoef G, Vanuytsel L, de Wolf-Peeters C (2002) T-cell/histiocyte—rich large B-cell lymphoma: a distinct clinicopathologic entity. J Clin Oncol 20(5):1269–1277
171. Poppe B, De Paepe P, Michaux L, Dastugue N, Bastard C, Herens C, Moreau E, Cavazzini F, Yigit N, Van Limbergen H, De Paepe A, Praet M, De Wolf-Peeters C, Wlodarska I, Speleman

F (2005) PAX5/IGH rearrangement is a recurrent finding in a subset of aggressive B-NHL with complex chromosomal rearrangements. Genes Chromosomes Cancer 44(2):218–223
172. Ferreri AJ, Blay JY, Reni M et al (2003) Prognostic scoring system for primary CNS lymphomas: the International Extranodal Lymphoma Study Group experience. J Clin Oncol 21:266–272
173. Corry J, Smith JG, Wirth A et al (1998) Primary central nervous system lymphoma: age and performance status are more important than treatment modality. Int J Radiat Oncol Biol Phys 41:615–620
174. Abrey L, Porat LB, Panageas KS, Yahalom J, Berkey B, Curran W, Schultz C, Leibel S, Nelson D, Mehta M, DeAngelis LM (2006) Primary central nervous system lymphoma: the memorial Sloan-Kettering cancer center prognostic model. J Clin Oncol 24(36):5711–5715
175. Hottinger AF, Iwamoto FM, Karimi S et al (2011) YKL-40 and MMP-9 as serum markers for patients with primary central nervous system lymphoma. Ann Neurol. doi:10.1002/ana.22360
176. Hattab EM, Martin SE, Al-Khatib SM, Kupsky WJ, Vance GH, Stohler RA, Czader M, Al-Abbadi MA (2010) Most primary central nervous system diffuse large B-cell lymphomas occurring in immunocompetent individuals belong to the nongerminal center subtype: a retrospective analysis of 31 cases. Mod Pathol 23:235–243
177. Grange F, Barry MB, Courville P, Maubec E, Bagot M, Vergier B, Souteyrand P, Machet L, Dalac S, Esteve E, Templier I, Delaporte E, Avril MF, Robert C, Dalle S, Laroche L, Delaunay M, Joly P, Wechsler J, Petrella T (2007) Primary cutaneous diffuse large B-cell lymphoma, leg type. Clinicopathologic features and prognostic analysis in 60 cases. Arch Dermatol 143(9):1144–1150
178. Espinet B, García-Herrera A, Gallardo F, Baró C, Salgado R, Servitje O, Estrach T, Colomo L, Romagosa V, Barranco C, Serrano S, Campo E, Pujol RM, Solé F (2011) FOXP1 molecular cytogenetics and protein expression analyses in primary cutaneous large B cell lymphoma, leg-type. Histol Histopathol 26(2):213–221
179. Belaud-Rotureau MA, Marietta V, Vergier B, Mainhaguiet G, Turmo M, Idrissi Y, Ferrer J, Beylot-Barry M, Dubus P, Merlio JP (2008) Inactivation of p16INK4a/CDKN2A gene may be a diagnostic feature of large B cell lymphoma leg type among cutaneous B cell lymphomas. Virchows Arch 452(6):607–620
180. Dijkman R, Tensen CP, Jordanova ES, Knijnenburg J, Hoefnagel JJ, Mulder AA, Rosenberg C, Raap AK, Willemze R, Szuhai K, Vermeer MH (2006) Array-based comparative genomic hybridization analysis reveals recurrent chromosomal alterations and prognostic parameters in primary cutaneous large B-cell lymphoma. J Clin Oncol 24:296–305
181. Oyama T, Yamamoto K, Asano N, Oshiro A, Suzuki R, Kagami Y, Morishima Y, Takeuchi K, Izumo T, Mori S, Ohshima K, Suzumiya J, Nakamura N, Abe IK, Sato Y, Yoshino T, Naoe T, Shimoyama Y, Kamiya Y, Kinoshita T, Nakamura S (2007) Age-related EBV-associated B-cell lymphoproliferative disorders constitute a distinct clinicopathologic group: a study of 96 patients. Clin Cancer Res 13:5124
182. Gibson SE, Hsi ED (2009) Epstein-Barr virus-positive B-cell lymphoma of the elderly at a United States tertiary medical center: an uncommon aggressive lymphoma with a nongerminal center B-cell phenotype. Hum Pathol 40(5):653–661
183. Narimatsu H, Ota Y, Kami M, Takeuchi K, Suzuki R, Matsuo K, Matsumura T, Yuji K, Kishi Y, Hamaki T, Sawada U, Miyata S, Sasaki T, Tobinai K, Kawabata M, Atsuta Y, Ueda R, Nakamura S (2007) Clinicopathological features of pyothorax-associated lymphoma; a retrospective survey involving 98 patients. Ann Oncol 18(1):122–128
184. Nakatsuka S, Yao M, Hoshida Y, Yamamoto S, Iuchi K, Aozasa K (2002) Pyothorax-associated lymphoma: a review of 106 cases. J Clin Oncol 20(20):4255–4260
185. Takakuwa T, Ham MF, Luo WJ, Nakatsuka S, Daibata M, Aozasa K (2006) Loss of expression of Epstein-Barr virus nuclear antigen-2 correlates with a poor prognosis in cases of pyothorax-associated lymphoma. Int J Cancer 118(11):2782–2789

186. Abou-Elella AA, Weisenburger DD, Vose JM et al (1999) Primary mediastinal large B-cell lymphoma: a clinicopathologic study of 43 patients from the Nebraska Lymphoma Study Group. J Clin Oncol 17:784–790
187. De Sanctis V, Finolezzi E, Osti MF, Grapulin L, Alfò M, Pescarmona E, Berardi F, Natalino F, Moleti ML, Di Rocco A, Enrici RM, Foà R, Martelli M (2008) MACOP-B and involved-field radiotherapy is an effective and safe therapy for primary mediastinal large B cell lymphoma. Int J Radiat Oncol Biol Phys 72(4):1154–1160
188. Savage KJ, Al-Rajhi N, Voss N et al (2006) Favorable outcome of primary mediastinal large B-cell lymphoma in a single institution: the British Columbia experience. Ann Oncol 17:123–130
189. Lazzarino M, Orlandi E, Paulli M et al (1997) Treatment outcome and prognostic factors for primary mediastinal (thymic) B-cell lymphoma: a multicenter study of 106 patients. J Clin Oncol 15:1646–1653
190. Nakashima MO, Roy DB, Nagamine M, Roullet MR, Gabriel CA, Sood SL, Bagg A (2011) Intravascular large B-cell lymphoma: a mimicker of many maladies and a difficult and often delayed diagnosis. J Clin Oncol 29(6):e138–e140
191. Murase T, Yamaguchi M, Suzuki R, Okamoto M, Sato Y, Tamaru J, Kojima M, Miura I, Mori N, Yoshino T, Nakamura S (2007) Intravascular large B-cell lymphoma (IVLBCL): a clinicopathologic study of 96 cases with special reference to the immunophenotypic heterogeneity of CD5. Blood 109(2):478–485
192. Ponzoni M, Ferreri AJ, Campo E, Facchetti F, Mazzucchelli L, Yoshino T et al (2007) Definition, diagnosis, and management of intravascular large B-cell lymphoma: proposals and perspectives from an international consensus meeting. J Clin Oncol 25:3168–3173
193. Gascoyne RD, Lamant L, Martin-Subero JI, Lestou VS, Harris NL, Müller-Hermelink HK, Seymour JF, Campbell LJ, Horsman DE, Auvigne I, Espinos E, Siebert R, Delsol G (2003) ALK-positive diffuse large B-cell lymphoma is associated with Clathrin-ALK rearrangements: report of 6 cases. Blood 102(7):2568–2573
194. Reichard KK, McKenna RW, Kroft SH (2007) ALK-positive diffuse large B-cell lymphoma: report of four cases and review of the literature. Mod Pathol 20:310–319
195. Delsol G, Lamant L, Mariame B et al (1997) A new subtype of large B-cell lymphoma expressing the ALK kinase and lacking the 2;5 translocation. Blood 89:1483–1490
196. Onciu M, Behm FG, Downing JR et al (2003) ALK-positive plasmablastic B-cell lymphoma with expression of the NPM-ALK fusion transcript: report of two cases. Blood 102:2642–2644
197. Dupin N, Diss TL, Kellam P, Tulliez M, Du MQ, Sicard D, Weiss RA, Isaacson PG, Boshoff C (2000) HHV-8 is associated with a plasmablastic variant of Castleman disease that is linked to HHV-8-positive plasmablastic lymphoma. Blood 95(4):1406–1412
198. Carbone A, Gloghini A, Aiello A, Testi A, Cabras A (2010) B-cell lymphomas with features intermediate between distinct pathologic entities. From pathogenesis to pathology. Hum Pathol 41(5):621–631
199. Savage KJ, Ben-neriah S, Connors JM, Horsman D, Gascoyne RD (2008) The prognostic significance of a MYC gene rearrangement in diffuse large B cell lymphoma (DLBCL). Ann Oncol 19(Suppl 4):186
200. Aukema SM, Siebert R, Schuuring E, Imhoff GW, Kluin-Nelemans HC, Boerma EJ, Kluin PM (2011) Double-hit B-cell lymphomas. Blood 117(8):2319–2331
201. de Jong D (2009) Novel lymphoid neoplasms—the borderland between diffuse large B-cell lymphoma and Burkitt's lymphoma. Haematologica 94(7):894–896
202. Tomita N, Tokunaka M, Nakamura N, Takeuchi K, Koike J, Motomura S et al (2009) Clinicopathological features of lymphoma/leukemia patients carrying both BCL2 and MYC translocations. Haematologica 94:935–943
203. Niitsu N, Okamoto M, Miura I, Hirano M (2009) Clinical significance of 8q24/c-MYC translocation in diffuse large B-cell lymphoma. Cancer Sci 100:233–237

Prognostic Factors in Peripheral T-Cell Lymphomas

Brady E. Beltran and Jorge J. Castillo

Abstract Peripheral T-cell lymphoma (PTCL) is a heterogeneous group of diseases characterized by an aggressive clinical course and resistance to standard chemotherapy regimens. PTCL comprises approximately 10–15% of all lymphomas in the Western world, although it could be found as high as 30–40% in Asian countries. Several clinical, pathological, genetic, and molecular prognostic factors have been described in order to risk stratify and treat our patients more appropriately. However, due to the rarity of these conditions, most studies are small in size and retrospective in nature. The present chapter goes in depth into the multiplicity of prognostic factors described in patients with PTCL, according to the most common subtypes, such as PTCL, not otherwise specified, anaplastic large cell lymphoma, angioimmunoblastic lymphoma, and adult T-cell f/lymphoma, among others. Our hope is that larger, prospective studies will be done to clarify the role of prognostication and modeling of therapy for patients with these hard-to-treat lymphomas.

Introduction

Peripheral T-cell lymphomas (PTCLs) are a group of rare aggressive non-Hodgkin lymphomas [1], which constitute approximately 12% of all lymphomas in the United States and Europe [1, 2]. There is, however, a different incidence rate of

B.E. Beltran, M.D. (✉)
Department of Oncology and Radiotherapy, Hospital Nacional Edgardo Rebagliati Martins, 150 Ave. Edgardo Rebagliati, Jesus Maria, Lima, Peru
e-mail: bgbrady@hotmail.com

J.J. Castillo
Division of Hematology and Oncology, Rhode Island Hospital, The Miriam Hospital, Providence, RI, USA

P.J. Quesenberry and J.J. Castillo (eds.), *Non-Hodgkin Lymphoma: Prognostic Factors and Targets*, Cancer Drug Discovery and Development, DOI 10.1007/978-1-4614-5851-7_8,

PTCLs in different parts of the world; for example, in Asia and South America, the incidence of PTCL approximates 25–30% [1, 2]. PTCLs are a heterogeneous group of tumors and can be subdivided into specified and not otherwise specified (NOS) forms [2, 3]. PTCL-NOS represents about 60–70% of all PTCLs [1]. In general, PTCL had a bad prognosis, stage by stage, when compared to aggressive B-cell lymphomas [4].

Several prognostic systems have been developed for PTCL. Probably the most widely used tool is the International Prognostic Index (IPI), a prognostic model designed for aggressive NHL subtypes. The IPI, when applied to aggressive T-cell lymphomas, is able to identify a group of patients who had a poor outcome (correlating with high IPI scores) and a group of patients with an improved outcome (correlating with low IPI scores). These findings were similar to diffuse large B-cell lymphoma [5].

Peripheral T-Cell Lymphoma Not Otherwise Specified

PTCL-NOS is the most common subtype of systemic PTCL seen worldwide [4]. PTCL-NOS is an aggressive disease. The overall survival (OS) for this entity at 10–15 years was only 10% [5]. PTCL-NOS is a diagnosis of pathological exclusion; if a PTCL cannot be classified according to WHO criteria, then it belongs to the group of PTCL-NOS. This is probably the reason this entity is the most common subtype of PTCL and also explains the clinical and molecular heterogeneity seen in such patients. PTCL-NOS appears in the fifth or sixth decade of life and does not show a sex predilection [6–9]. PTCL-NOS presents often as advanced disease (i.e., stage III–IV) with lymph node, skin, liver, spleen, bone marrow, and peripheral blood involvement [6–9]. B symptoms are reported in about 45% of cases at diagnosis.

Several clinical prognostic factors for survival have seen described in patients with PTCL-NOS. In an early study, bulky disease and thrombocytopenia were independent predictors of survival [5]. More recently, Castillo et al. showed that lymphopenia, defined as an absolute lymphocyte count of 1,000/μL or less, was an important prognostic factor for OS in patients with a diagnosis of PTCL-NOS independent from the PIT score [10]. In a large study of 340 cases of PTCL-NOS by the International T Cell Lymphoma Project, Weisenburger et al. showed that the prognostic factors in the original IPI score were highly significant predictors of OS in patients with PTCL-NOS. However, only patients with an IPI score of 0 or 1 (low risk) had a favorable FFS [11], likely a reflection of the poor prognosis a diagnosis of PTCL-NOS carries per each IPI category when compared to DLBCL.

In 2004, Gallamini et al. developed a new prognostic model called Prognostic Index for PTCL-NOS or PIT, which includes few similar clinical parameters than the IPI score such as age, lactate dehydrogenase (LDH) levels, and performance status. However, a new criterion was introduced, bone marrow involvement [12]. The PIT score reportedly separated patients into more specific prognostic groups than the IPI score. From the 322 PTCL-NOS patients who were evaluated, 20% had no adverse features, 34% had one adverse feature, 26% had two, and 20% had three or more. The 5-year OS for the group with no adverse prognostic features was 62% compared to 18% for patients with 3–4 adverse prognostic factors. However, in the above mentioned analysis by Weisenburger et al., the PIT score did not appear to be superior to the IPI score [11].

To refine the prognosis of patients with PTCL-NOS, new models have been proposed. Went et al. developed a clinicopathological index that has also shown prognostic value, with the addition of the immunohistochemical expression of Ki-67 (a proliferation marker) to other clinical factors (i.e., age, performance status, and LDH levels) [13, 14]. More recently, the International PTCL Clinical and Pathology Review Project established the IPTCLP score; three variables were used to construct this score: age, performance status, and platelet counts. Depending on the number of adverse prognostic factors (0, 1, 2, or 3), patients were classified into low-risk, low-intermediate risk, high-intermediate risk, or high-risk groups, respectively. Gutierrez-Garcia et al. demonstrated that the IPTCLP score as reported above was the most significant to predict OS in comparison with other PTCL scores [15].

Moving into pathological and molecular prognostic factors, a study demonstrated p53 was the most important prognostic factor and was correlated with expression of p-glycoprotein [16]. Also, anti-apoptotic genes like BCL2 and BCLXL are considered as bad prognostic markers [17]. Molecules involved with chemotaxis such as CXCR3 and CCR4 were expressed in PTCL-NOS [13], and the phenotype CXCR3-positive/CCR4-negative showed to be an adverse independent prognostic factor for survival in PTCL-NOS [13]. In a separate study, EBV expression by the malignant cells was an adverse predictor of survival in older patients with PTCL-NOS [18]. Furthermore, in a recent large study, EBV infection defined by expression of EBV-encoded RNA detected by an in situ hybridization technique was also predictive of poor survival in younger patients [11].

The T helper cell phenotype (CD4 positive, CD8 negative) was identified as a favorable prognostic factor when compared to a cytotoxic phenotype (CD4 negative, CD8 positive) [11, 13, 14]. In fact, Asano et al. have reported that a cytotoxic phenotype is predictive of poor survival in PTCL-NOS [19], but other investigators did not find similar association [11, 20, 21]. However, a study using gene expression profiling (GEP) identified a molecular subgroup of PTCL-NOS with features of cytotoxic lymphocytes and a poor survival [22]. Additionally, by using GEP methods, evidence of nuclear factor-kappa B (NF-κB) inactivity showed a better survival in patients with PTCL-NOS with a median OS of 25 months versus a median OS of 12 months in patients with increased NF-κB activity [23, 24]. In a separate GEP-based study, PTCL-NOS was characterized by an overexpression of genes involved in a "proliferation signature," and it was associated with a shorter survival [25].

Angioimmunoblastic Lymphoma

Angioimmunoblastic T-cell lymphoma (AITL) represents a particular clinicopathological entity, among predominantly nodal peripheral T-cell lymphomas. It generally occurs in elderly patients presenting with skin rash, arthralgias, generalized lymphadenopathy, hepatosplenomegaly, anemia, hypergammaglobulinemia, and autoimmune phenomena. The histologic features of AITL are a partial or complete effacement of the lymph node architecture by a polymorphous infiltrate that is typically associated with a proliferation of follicular dendritic cells (FDCs) and a prominent arborization of high endothelial venules. The neoplastic cells are small- to medium-sized cells typically with a clear cytoplasm, usually aggregate in small clusters and display minimal cytologic atypia. An increase in background EBV-infected B cells may also occur, and, in rare cases, an overt diffuse large B-cell lymphoma could develop concurrently or after therapy for AITL [26–29]. It is though that the cell of origin of AITL derives from a follicular helper T-cell (TFH) subset [30–36], as AITL tumor cells usually express CD4, CD10, BCL6, and CXCL13 [33–36].

AITL is rare accounting for approximately 2% of all non-Hodgkin lymphomas (15G). In previous studies, the 7-year overall survival was reported at 30% [37]. Results from a retrospective study from an Italian group described male sex, mediastinal lymphadenopathy, and anemia as adverse prognostic factors [37], and interestingly, the International Prognostic Index (IPI) and the Prognostic Index for PTCL (PIT) were of limited value to stratify risk groups in this entity [37]. Finally, specific chromosomal abnormalities do not seem to be associated with survival, but complex karyotypes adversely impact the outcome [38].

Adult T-Cell Leukemia/Lymphoma

Adult T-cell leukemia/lymphoma (ATLL) is a distinct peripheral T-cell malignancy associated with a retrovirus as HTLV 1 [39–41]. HTLV-1 is an RNA retrovirus, endemic in southwestern Japan, the Middle East, North Africa, the Caribbean, and South America. The Shimoyama classification defined four clinical subtypes: acute, lymphomatous, chronic, and smoldering [42]. The acute and the lymphomatous forms are considered aggressive entities with very short survival, and the remaining variants are considered indolent with survival times between 2 and 5 years. More recently, a cutaneous form has also been described [43].

A Japanese study analyzed clinical data of 854 ATLL patients to find relevant prognostic factors. It demonstrated that advanced performance status (PS), high lactic dehydrogenase (LDH) level, age >40 years, more than three lesions, and hypercalcemia are prognostic factors defined in multivariate analysis [44]. However, other clinical factors were related to poor prognosis, such as thrombocytopenia, eosinophilia, and bone marrow involvement [45–47]. Takasaki et al. [48]

Table 1 Clinical and molecular prognostic factors in ATLL

Clinical	Molecular
Eosinophilia	p53
Hypercalcemia	p16
Bone marrow involvement	IL-5
LDH	CCR-4
ECOG	Lung resistance-related protein
>40 years old	–
Thrombocytopenia	–
>3 involved lesions	–
International prognostic index	–
Prognostic index for peripheral Lymphopenia T-cell lymphoma, NOS	–

reported that visceral organ involvement, including the bone marrow, was an adverse prognostic factor in ATLL. Thrombocytopenia ($<100\times10^9$/l) and monocytosis ($\geq0.8\times10^9$/l) were also found to be significant adverse prognostic factors by multivariate analysis (Table 1).

Beltran et al. described different clinical factors in acute and lymphomatous subtypes. Low albumin level and presence of B symptoms were independent factors for worse survival in lymphomatous ATLL, and high β2-microglobulin level was independent factor for worse survival in acute ATLL [49]. Aggressive ATLL variants have a distinct, almost mutually exclusive profile of prognostic factors. Recently, IPI was described as a good model prognostic only in lymphomatous form of ATLL [50]. Beltran et al. confirmed this founding and suggested PIT score could be useful as prognostic model in aggressive ATLL [51]. Phillips et al. published a new prognostic model obtained from 89 ATLL patients from a multicenter US study. The study identified 3 prognostic categories based on Eastern Cooperative Oncology Group performance status, stage, age, and calcium level at diagnosis [52].

Immune and molecular factors are seen to be associated with a unfavorable survival in ATLL like high interleukin-5 (IL-5) serum level, CCR-4 expression, lung resistance-related protein, p53 mutation, and p16 deletion [45, 53–56].

Anaplastic Large Cell Lymphoma

Anaplastic large cell lymphoma (ALCL) is a CD30-positive neoplasm of T-cell or null-cell lineage with characteristic clinicopathologic features and accounts for 28% of all lymphomas [57]. Two subtypes of systemic ALCL are in the World Health Organization (WHO) classification scheme [58], depending of the expression of anaplastic lymphoma kinase (ALK). ALK-positive ALCL is a group with an excellent prognosis when treated with standard chemotherapy [59–62]. ALK-positive ALCL usually affects young patients and has a better prognosis compared with patients with ALK-negative ALCL. However, ALK-negative ALCL may have a more favorable prognosis than those with PTCL-NOS [63].

With gene profile and comparative genomic hybridization (CGH) studies, it was confirmed that ALK-positive and ALK-negative ALCL have unique gene expression signatures and genomic imbalances and was defined that there are different diseases at a molecular and genetic levels [64–66].

Despite this biological difference, the IPI score is a good prognostic tool for this entity, although with expected survival differences. The 5-year survival for IPI score 0–1 patients was 90% and 74% for ALK-positive and ALK-negative patients, respectively; however, patients with IPI score of 4–5 had a poor outcome with 5-year survivals of 33% and 13%, respectively [63]. The presence of stage IV and anemia is an important unfavorable prognostic factor in patients with ALK-positive ALCL [67]. Similarly, the PIT score identified different risk categories within ALCL. However, given the relative low frequency of bone marrow involvement, it essentially gives the same information already provided by the IPI score [68].

The dominant chemokine expression found CXCR3-positive/CCR4-negative to be an independent prognostic factor and significantly prognostic of a poor prognosis in ALK-negative ALCL [13].

Extranodal T/NK Lymphoma Nasal Type

Extranodal natural killer/T-cell lymphoma (NKTCL), nasal type is a distinct entity in the WHO classification of lymphoid tumors. NKTCL has a specific geographical distribution and is more prevalent in Asia and in Central and South America [68–73]. EBV is present in the genome of neoplastic cells in virtually all cases [72]. The NKTCL cell of origin has a typical NK phenotype, but in some cases, a cytotoxic T-lymphocyte phenotype could be found [72]. The nasal cavity and the upper aerodigestive tract are the most commonly involved sites, but skin, the gastrointestinal tract, lung, testis, and soft tissues can be also affected [68, 69, 72, 74]. The prognosis of extranodal NK/T-cell lymphoma is very poor [73]. The survival rate is 30% to 40%. Nonnasal disease is more aggressive than nasal disease [72, 73, 75]. Radiotherapy is an excellent treatment in early-stage NKTCL with nasal disease and has been associated with a good outcome [71–73, 76, 77].

Adverse prognostic factors for nasal disease are unfavorable IPI score, advanced-stage disease (stage III or IV), high circulating EBV DNA levels, and detection of EBV in bone marrow cells by in situ hybridization [72, 73, 76, 78–82]. In a separate study, lymphopenia, B symptoms, and advanced stage were independent predictors for OS and PFS in this entity [83], and a high proportion of large/transformed cells in the tumoral population have a negative impact on survival [71–75]. As mentioned previously, extranasal cases are very aggressive and have poor response to chemotherapy [72, 73].

Two models prognostic were published in this entity. One of them is from a Korean group. They proposed a new prognostic model based using four parameters: B symptoms, LDH levels, stage, and regional lymph node involvement. In a comparative study, this model demonstrated to be better than the IPI score [70].

The second prognostic index showed that four factors, nonnasal type, stage, performance status, and extranodal involvement, were significant prognostic factors. This model demonstrated the 4-year OS was 55% for patients with no adverse factors, 33% with one adverse factor, 15% with three factors, and 6% with four factors [84].

Prognosis of Uncommon PTCL Subtypes

Subcutaneous panniculitis T-cell lymphoma (SPTCL) was seen in 1% of cases evaluated in the International PTCL project [63]. Prognosis is good, 82% to 5-year OS. It is rarely associated with hemophagocytic syndrome (17%), which is associated with a worse prognosis (5-year OS 91% vs. 46%) [85].

EATL occurs in patients with an established history of gluten-sensitive enteropathy but most often occurs following a short history of celiac disease and/or dermatitis herpetiformis. Most patients are older males presenting with refractory celiac disease or abdominal pain. It affects jejunum, often in association with intestinal perforation or obstruction. Survival is extremely short with 5-year OS of 20% [86]. A recent study found a median OS of ten months, and the median FFS was only six months. The IPI score was not a good predictor of survival in contrast with the PIT score. The presence of clinical sprue predicted for adverse survival independently of the PIT [86].

Hepatosplenic T-cell lymphoma (HSTCL) is related with immunosuppression states such as transplant immunosuppressive treatment or treatment with tumor necrosis factor inhibitors [87]. This entity has recurrent cytogenetic abnormalities, like isochromosome 7q, which are associated with trisomy 8 [88, 89]. These cytogenetic abnormalities, however, do not appear to have prognostic significance [88]. HSTCL has a distinct gene expression-profiling signature in comparison with other PTCLs. KIR and killer lectin-like receptors, both NK molecules, are frequently overexpressed [89]. The clinical course aggressive with median survival is <2 years, and standard chemotherapy does not appear to be curative; however, long-term survivors have been reported following allogeneic transplant.

T-cell large granular lymphocytic (LGL) leukemia is an entity with persistent (>6 months) increase in peripheral blood LGLs and affects adults with a median age of 55 years and equal gender distribution. It arises more commonly in patients with autoimmune disorders [90]. LGL leukemia has an indolent clinical behavior with a median survival of >10 years. In contrast to the other mature T-cell leukemias, median survival is good [91]. Aggressive LGL leukemia and high-grade transformation, however, have a much poorer prognosis. A retrospective review of 286 patients with T-LGL leukemia identified anemia, severe neutropenia, and lymphopenia as poor prognostic factors [92].

References

1. Pileri S, Ralfkiaer E, Weisenburger D et al (2008) Peripheral T-cell lymphoma, not otherwise specified. In: Swerdlow S, Campo E, Harris NL et al (eds) WHO classification of tumors of hematopoietic and lymphoid tissues, 4th edn. IARC, Lyon, p 429
2. Vose J, Armitage J, Weisenburger D (2008) International peripheral T-cell and natural killer/T-cell lymphoma study: pathology findings and clinical outcomes. J Clin Oncol 26(25):4124–4130
3. Savage KJ, Harris NL, Vose JM et al (2008) ALK – anaplastic large cell lymphoma is clinically and immunophenotypically different from both ALK + ALCL and peripheral T-cell lymphoma, not otherwise specified: report from the International Peripheral TCell Lymphoma Project. Blood 111(12):5496–5504
4. Vose J, Armitage J, Weisenburger D (2008) International peripheral T-cell and natural killer/ Tcell lymphoma study: pathology findings and clinical outcomes. J Clin Oncol 26(25): 4124–4130
5. Suzumiya J, Ohshima K, Tamura K et al (2009) The International Prognostic Index predicts outcome in aggressive adult T-cell leukemia/lymphoma: analysis of 126 patients from the International Peripheral T-cell Lymphoma Project. Ann Oncol 20(4):715–721
6. Evens AM, Gartenhaus RB (2004) Treatment of T-cell non-Hodgkin's lymphoma. Curr Treat Options Oncol 5(4):289–303
7. Lopez-Guillermo A, Cid J, Salar A et al (1998) Peripheral T-cell lymphomas: initial features, natural history, and prognostic factors in a series of 174 patients diagnosed according to the R.E.A.L. Classification. Ann Oncol 9(8):849–855
8. Gisselbrecht C, Gaulard P, Lepage E et al (1998) Prognostic significance of T-cell phenotype in aggressive non-Hodgkin's lymphomas. Groupe d'Etudes des Lymphomes de l'Adulte (GELA). Blood 92(1):76–82
9. The Non-Hodgkin's Lymphoma Classification Project (1997) Effect of age on the characteristics and clinical behavior of non-Hodgkin's lymphoma patients. Ann Oncol 8(10):973–978
10. Castillo JJ, Morales D, Quinones P, Cotrina E, Desposorio C, Beltran B (2010) Lymphopenia as a prognostic factor in patients with peripheral T-cell lymphoma, unspecified. Leuk Lymphoma 51(10):1822–8
11. Weisenburger DD, Savage KJ, Harris NL et al (2011) Peripheral T-cell lymphoma, not otherwise specified: a report of 340 cases from the International Peripheral T-cell Lymphoma Project. Blood 117(12):3402–8
12. Gallamini A, Stelitano C, Calvi R et al (2004) Peripheral T-cell lymphoma unspecified (PTCL-U): a new prognostic model from a retrospective multicentric clinical study. Blood 103(7):2474–2479
13. Kojima H, Hasegawa Y, Suzukawa K et al (2004) Clinicopathological features and prognostic factors of Japanese patients with "peripheral T-cell lymphoma, unspecified" diagnosed according to the WHO classification. Leuk Res 28(12):1287–1292
14. Went P, Agostinelli C, Gallamini A et al (2006) Marker expression in peripheral T-cell lymphoma: a proposed clinical-pathologic prognostic score. J Clin Oncol 24(16):2472–2479
15. Gutiérrez-García G, García-Herrera A, Cardesa T et al (2011) Comparison of four prognostic scores in peripheral T-cell lymphoma. Ann Oncol 22(2):397–404
16. Pescarmona E, Pignoloni P, Puopolo M et al (2001) p53 over-expression identifies a subset of nodal peripheral T-cell lymphomas with a distinctive biological profile and poor clinical outcome. J Pathol 195(3):361–366
17. Rassidakis GZ, Jones D, Lai R et al (2003) BCL-2 family proteins in peripheral T-cell lymphomas: correlation with tumour apoptosis and proliferation. J Pathol 200(2):240–248
18. Dupuis J, Emile JF, Mounier N et al (2006) Prognostic significance of Epstein-Barr virus in nodal peripheral T-cell lymphoma, unspecified: a Group d'Etude des Lymphomes de l'Adulte (GELA) study. Blood 108(13):4163–4169

19. Asano N, Suzuki R, Kagami Y et al (2005) Clinicopathologic and prognostic significance of cytotoxic molecule expression in nodal peripheral T-cell lymphoma, unspecified. Am J Surg Pathol 29(10):1284–1293
20. Geissinger E, Odenwald T, Lee SS et al (2004) Nodal peripheral T-cell lymphomas and, in particular, their lymphoepithelioid (Lennert's) variant are often derived from CD8 cytotoxic T cells. Virchows Arch 445(4):334–343
21. Prochazka V, Trneny M, Pytlik R et al (2007) Peripheral T-cell lymphoma, unspecified: the analysis of the data from the Czech Lymphoma Study Group (CLSG) registry. Biomed Pap Med Fac Univ Palacky Olomouc Czech Repub 151(1):103–107
22. Iqbal J, Weisenburger DD, Greiner TC et al (2010) Molecular signatures to improve diagnosis in peripheral T-cell lymphoma and prognostication in angioimmunoblastic T-cell lymphoma. Blood 115(5):1026–1036
23. Martinez-Delgado B, Cuadros M, Honrado E et al (2005) Differential expression of NF-kappaB pathway genes among peripheral T-cell lymphomas. Leukemia 19(12):2254–2263
24. Ballester B, Ramuz O, Gisselbrecht C et al (2006) Gene expression profiling identifies molecular subgroups among nodal peripheral T-cell lymphomas. Oncogene 25(10):1560–1570
25. Cuadros M, Dave SS, Jaffe ES et al (2007) Identification of a proliferation signature related to survival in nodal peripheral T-cell lymphomas. J Clin Oncol 25(22):3321–3329
26. Matsue K, Itoh M, Tsukuda K, Kokubo T, Hirose Y (1998) Development of Epstein-Barr virus-associated B cell lymphoma after intensive treatment of patients with angioimmunoblastic lymphadenopathy with dysproteinemia. Int J Hematol 67:319–329
27. Lome-Maldonado C, Canioni D, Hermine O et al (2002) Angio-immunoblastic T cell lymphoma (AILD-TL) rich in large B cells and associated with Epstein-Barr virus infection: a different subtype of AILDTL? Leukemia 16:2134–2141
28. Attygalle AD, Kyriakou C, Dupuis J et al (2007) Histologic evolution of angioimmunoblastic T-cell lymphoma in consecutive biopsies: clinical correlation and insights into natural history and disease progression. Am J Surg Pathol 31:1077–1088
29. Abruzzo LV, Schmidt K, Weiss LM et al (1993) B-cell lymphoma after angioimmunoblastic lymphadenopathy: a case with oligoclonal gene rearrangements associated with Epstein-Barr virus. Blood 82:241–246
30. Krenacs L, Schaerli P, Kis G, Bagdi E (2006) Phenotype of neoplastic cells in angioimmunoblastic T-cell lymphoma is consistent with activated follicular B helper T cells. Blood 108:1110–1111
31. de Leval L, Rickman DS, Thielen C et al (2007) The gene expression profile of nodal peripheral T-cell lymphoma demonstrates a molecular link between angioimmunoblastic T-cell lymphoma (AITL) and follicular helper T cells (TFH). Blood 109:4952–4963
32. Vinuesa CG, Tangye SG, Moser B, Mackay CR (2005) Follicular B helper T cells in antibody response and autoimmunity. Nat Rev Immunol 5:853–865
33. Attygalle A, Al Jehani R, Diss TC et al (2002) Neoplastic T cells in angioimmunoblastic T-cell lymphoma express CD10. Blood 99:627–633
34. Dogan A, Attygalle AD, Kyriakou C (2003) Angioimunoblastic T-cell lymphoma. Br J Haematol 121:681–691
35. Dupuis J, Boye K, Martin N et al (2006) Expression of CXCL13 by neoplastic cells in angioimmunoblastic T cell-lymphoma (AITL): a new diagnostic marker providing evidence that AITL derives from follicular helper T cells. Am J Surg Pathol 30:490–494
36. Grogg KL, Attygalle AD, Macon WR, Remstein ED, Kurtin PJ, Dogan A (2005) Angioimmunoblastic T-cell lymphoma: a neoplasm of germinal-center T-helper cells? Blood 106:1501–1502
37. Mourad N, Mounier N, Brière J et al (2008) Clinical, biologic, and pathologic features in 157 patients with angioimmunoblastic T-cell lymphoma treated within the Groupe d'Etude des Lymphomes de l'Adulte (GELA) trials. Blood 111(9):4463–70
38. Nelson M, Horsman DE, Weisenburger DD et al (2008) Cytogenetic abnormalities and clinical correlations in peripheral T-cell lymphoma. Br J Haematol 141:461–469

39. Poiesz BJ, Ruscetti FW, Gazdar AF et al (1980) Detection and isolation of type C retro virus particles from fresh and cultured lymphocytes of a patient with cutaneous T-cell lymphoma. Proc Natl Acad Sci U S A 77(12):7415–9
40. Uchiyama T, Yodoi J, Sagawa K et al (1977) Adult T-cell leukemia: clinical and hematologic features of 16 cases. Blood 50(3):481–92
41. Yoshida M, Miyoshi I, Hinuma Y (1982) Isolation and characterization of retrovirus from cell lines of human adult T-cell leukemia and its implication in the disease. Proc Natl Acad Sci U S A 79(6):2031–5
42. Shimoyama M (1991) Diagnostic criteria and classification of clinical subtypes of adult T-cell leukaemia-lymphoma. A report from the Lymphoma Study Group (1984–1987). Br J Haematol 79(3):428–37
43. Bittencourt AL, Barbosa HS, Vieira MD et al (2009) Adult T-cell leukemia/lymphoma (ATL) presenting in the skin: clinical, histological and immunohistochemical features of 52 cases. Acta Oncol 48(4):598–604
44. (1991) Major prognostic factors of patients with adult T-cell leukemia-lymphoma: a cooperative study—Lymphoma Study Group (1984–1987). Leuk Res 15:81–90
45. Yamada Y, Hatta Y, Murata K et al (1997) Deletions of p15 and/or p16 genes as a poor-prognosis factor in adult T-cell leukemia. J Clin Oncol 15:1778–1785
46. Utsunomiya A, Ishida T, Inagaki A et al (2007) Clinical significance of a blood eosinophilia in adult T-cell leukemia/lymphoma: a blood eosinophilia is a significant unfavorable prognostic factor. Leuk Res 31:915–920
47. Takasaki Y, Iwanaga M, Tsukasaki K et al (2007) Impact of visceral involvements and blood cell count abnormalities on survival in adult T-cell leukemia/lymphoma (ATLL). Leuk Res 31:751–757
48. Takasaki Y, Iwanaga M, Tsukasaki K et al (2007) Impact of visceral involvements and blood cell count abnormalities on survival in adult T-cell leukemia/lymphoma (ATLL). Leuk Res 31:751–757
49. Beltran B, Quiñones P, Morales D, Cotrina E, Castillo JJ (2011) Different prognostic factors for survival in acute and lymphomatous adult T-cell leukemia/lymphoma. Leuk Res 35:334–339
50. Suzumiya J, Ohshima K, Tamura K, Karube K, Uike N, Tobinai K, Gascoyne RD, Vose JM, Armitage JO, Weisenburger DD (2009) International Peripheral T-Cell Lymphoma Project. The International Prognostic Index predicts outcome in aggressive adult T-cell leukemia/lymphoma: analysis of 126 patients from the International Peripheral T-Cell Lymphoma Project. Annal Oncol 20(4):715–21
51. Beltran B, Morales D, Quiñones P, Salas R, Castillo J (2009) Analysis of prognostic factors in patients with adult T-cell leukemia/lymphoma. J Clin Oncol 27:15s (suppl; abstr 8575)
52. Phillips AA, Shapira I, Willim RD, Sanmugarajah J, Solomon WB, Horwitz SM, Savage DG, Bhagat G, Soff G, Zain JM, Alobeid B, Seshan VE, O'Connor OA (2010) A critical analysis of prognostic factors in North American patients with human T-cell lymphotropic virus type-1-associated adult T-cell leukemia/lymphoma: a multicenter clinicopathologic experience and new prognostic score. Cancer 116(14):3438–46
53. Inagaki A, Ishida T, Ishii T et al (2006) Clinical significance of serum Th1-, Th2 and regulatory T cells-associated cytokines in adult T-cell leukemia/lymphoma: High interleukin-5 and -10 levels are significant unfavorable prognostic factors. Int J Cancer 118:3054–3061
54. Ishida T, Utsunomiya A, Iida S et al (2003) Clinical significance of CCR4 expression in adult T-cell leukemia/lymphoma: its close association with skin involvement and unfavorable outcome. Clin Cancer Res 9:3625–3634
55. Tawara M, Hogerzeil SJ, Yamada Y et al (2006) Impact of p53 aberration on the progression of adult T-cell leukemia/lymphoma. Cancer Lett 234:249–255
56. Ohno N, Tani A, Uozumi K et al (2001) Expression of functional lung resistance-related protein predicts poor outcome in adult T-cell leukemia. Blood 98:1160–1165

57. Tilly H, Gaulard P, Lepage E, Dumontet C, Diebold J, Plantier I et al (1997) Primary anaplastic large-cell lymphoma in adults: clinical presentation, immunophenotype, and outcome. Blood 90:3727–34
58. Chan JK (2001) The new World Health Organization classification of lymphomas: the past, the present and the future. Hematol Oncol 19:129–50
59. Falini B, Pileri S, Zinzani PL et al (1999) ALK+ lymphoma: clinico-pathological findings and outcome. Blood 93:2697–2706
60. Gascoyne RD, Aoun P, Wu D et al (1999) Prognostic significance of anaplastic lymphoma kinase (ALK) protein expression in adults with anaplastic large cell lymphoma. Blood 93:3913–3921
61. Berge RL, Oudejans JJ, Ossenkoppele GJ et al (2000) ALK expression in extranodal anaplastic large cell lymphoma favours systemic disease with (primary) nodal involvement and a good prognosis and occurs before dissemination. J Clin Pathol 53:445–450
62. Shiota M, Nakamura S, Ichinohasama R et al (1995) Anaplastic large cell lymphomas expressing the novel chimeric protein p80NPM/ALK: a distinct clinicopathologic entity. Blood 86:1954–1960
63. Savage KJ, Harris NL, Vose JM et al (2008) ALK anaplastic large-cell lymphoma is clinically and immunophenotypically different from both ALK+ALCL and peripheral T-cell lymphoma, not otherwise specified: report from the International Peripheral T-Cell Lymphoma Project. Blood 111(12):5496–504
64. Salaverria I, Bea S, Lopez-Guillermo A et al (2008) Genomic profiling reveals different genetic aberrations in systemic ALK-positive and ALK-negative anaplastic large cell lymphomas. Br J Haematol 140:516–526
65. Lamant L, de Reynies A, Duplantier MM et al (2007) Gene expression profiling of systemic anaplastic large-cell lymphoma reveals differences based on ALK status and two distinct morphologic ALK+subtypes. Blood 109:2156–2164
66. Zettl A, Rudiger T, Konrad MA et al (2004) Genomic profiling of peripheral T-cell lymphoma, unspecified, and anaplastic large T-cell lymphoma delineates novel recurrent chromosomal alterations. Am J Pathol 164:1837–1848
67. Hasenclever D, Diehl V (1998) A prognostic score for advanced Hodgkin's disease: International Prognostic Factors Project on Advanced Hodgkin's Disease. N Engl J Med 339:1506–1514
68. Quintanilla-Martinez L, Franklin JL, Guerrero I et al (1999) Histological and immunophenotypic profile of nasal NK/T cell lymphomas from Peru: high prevalence of p53 overexpression. Hum Pathol 30(7):849–855
69. Oshimi K, Kawa K, Nakamura S et al (2005) NK-cell neoplasms in Japan. Hematology 10(3):237–245
70. Lee J, Suh C, Park YH et al (2006) Extranodal natural killer T-cell lymphoma, nasal-type: a prognostic model from a retrospective multicenter study. J Clin Oncol 24(4):612–618
71. Barrionuevo C, Zaharia M, Martinez MT et al (2007) Extranodal NK/Tcell lymphoma, nasal type: study of clinicopathologic and prognosis factors in a series of 78 cases from Peru. Appl Immunohistochem Mol Morphol 15(1):38–44
72. Chan J, Quintanilla-Martinez L, Ferry J, Peh SC (2008) Extranodal NK/T-cell lymphoma, nasal-type. In: Swerdlow S, Campo E, Harris NL et al (eds) WHO Classification of tumors of hematopoietic and lymphoid tissues, 4th edn. IARC, Lyon, p 285
73. Au WY, Weisenburger DD, Intragumtornchai T et al (2009) Clinical differences between nasal and extranasal natural killer/T-cell lymphoma: a study of 136 cases from the International Peripheral T-Cell Lymphoma Project. Blood 113(17):3931–3937
74. Kwong YL, Chan AC, Liang R et al (1997) CD56+ NK lymphomas: clinicopathological features and prognosis. Br J Haematol 97(4):821–829
75. Chan JK (1998) Natural killer cell neoplasms. Anat Pathol 3:77–145
76. Cheung MM, Chan JK, Lau WH et al (2002) Early stage nasal NK/Tcell lymphoma: clinical outcome, prognostic factors, and the effect of treatment modality. Int J Radiat Oncol Biol Phys 54(1):182–190

77. Kuo TT, Shih LY, Tsang NM (2004) Nasal NK/T cell lymphoma in Taiwan: a clinicopathologic study of 22 cases, with analysis of histologic subtypes, Epstein-Barr virus LMP-1 gene association, and treatment modalities. Int J Surg Pathol 12(4):375–387
78. Au WY, Pang A, Choy C et al (2004) Quantification of circulating Epstein-Barr virus (EBV) DNA in the diagnosis and monitoring of natural killer cell and EBV-positive lymphomas in immunocompetent patients. Blood 104(1):243–249
79. Ng SB, Lai KW, Murugaya S et al (2004) Nasal-type extranodal natural killer/T-cell lymphomas: a clinicopathologic and genotypic study of 42 cases in Singapore. Mod Pathol 17(9):1097–1107
80. Chim CS, Ma SY, Au WY et al (2004) Primary nasal natural killer cell lymphoma: long-term treatment outcome and relationship with the International Prognostic Index. Blood 103(1):216–221
81. Huang WT, Chang KC, Huang GC et al (2005) Bone marrow that is positive for Epstein-Barr virus encoded RNA-1 by in situ hybridization is related with a poor prognosis in patients with extranodal natural killer/T-cell lymphoma, nasal type. Haematologica 90(8):1063–1069
82. Lee J, Suh C, Huh J et al (2007) Effect of positive bone marrow EBV in situ hybridization in staging and survival of localized extranodal natural killer/T-cell lymphoma, nasal-type. Clin Cancer Res 13(11):3250–3254
83. Huang JJ, Jiang WQ, Lin TY, Huang Y, Xu RH, Huang HQ, Li ZM (2011) Absolute lymphocyte count is a novel prognostic indicator in extranodal natural killer/T-cell lymphoma, nasal type. Annal Oncol 22(1):149–55
84. Suzuki R, Suzumiya J, Yamaguchi M et al (2010) Prognostic factors for mature natural killer (NK) cell neoplasms: aggressive NK cell leukemia and extranodal NK cell lymphoma, nasal type. Ann Oncol 21(5):1032–1040
85. Vose J, Armitage J, Weisenburger D (2008) International T-Cell Lymphoma Project. International Peripheral T-Cell and Natural Killer/T-Cell Lymphoma Study: pathology findings and clinical outcomes. J Clin Oncol. 26:4124–4130
86. Delabie J, Holte H, Vose JM et al. (2011) Enteropathy-associated T-cell lymphoma: clinical and histological findings from the International Peripheral T-Cell Lymphoma Project. Blood 118(1):149–155
87. Belhadj K, Reyes F, Farcet JP et al (2003) Hepatosplenic gammadelta T-cell lymphoma is a rare clinicopathologic entity with poor outcome: report on a series of 21 patients. Blood 102:4261–4269
88. Weidmann E (2000) Hepatosplenic T cell lymphoma: a review on 45 cases since the first report describing the disease as a distinct lymphoma entity in 1990. Leukemia 14:991–997
89. Miyazaki K, Yamaguchi M, Imai H et al (2009) Gene expression profiling of peripheral T-cell lymphoma including gammadelta T-cell lymphoma. Blood 113:1071–1074
90. Dearden CE, Johnson R, Pettengell R, Devereux S, Cwynarski K, Whittaker S, McMillan A (2011) British Committee for Standards in Haematology. Guidelines for the management of mature T-cell and NK-cell neoplasms (excluding cutaneous T-cell lymphoma). Br J Haematol 153(4):451–85
91. Osuji N, Matutes E, Tjonnfjord G, Grech H, Del Giudice I, Wotherspoon A, Swansbury JG, Catovsky D (2006) T-cell large granular lymphocyte leukemia: a report on the treatment of 29 patients and a review of the literature. Cancer 107:570–578
92. Nowakowski GS, Morice WG, Zent CS, Schwager SM, Li C, Markovic SN, Porrata L, Tefferi A, Phyliky RL (2006) Initial presentation and prognostic factors in 286 patients with T-cell large granular lymphocyte leukemia. Blood (ASH Ann Meeting Abstr) 108:300

Prognostic Factors in HIV-Associated Lymphoma

Jodi L. Layton and Jorge J. Castillo

Abstract In recent years, since the advent of highly active antiretroviral therapy (HAART), the incidence and prognosis of lymphoma in patients with HIV infection have changed dramatically. Although lymphoma is now not only the most common malignancy but also the most common cause of death, the prognosis in HIV-infected patients has improved, in big part due to the introduction of HAART but also due to better supportive therapy, such as antibiotic prophylaxis and growth factors. Overall, the immunological status of HIV-positive patients nowadays is not as deteriorated as it was in the past, allowing for HIV-positive patients with lymphoma to be treated with standard therapies. The identification of reliable and easy-to-use prognostic factors in this population is warranted, not only to lead discussions about goals of therapy but also to direct our therapies according to risk. In this chapter, we will review the classification and provide an overview of the therapy of HIV-associated lymphomas. We will then discuss the variety of clinical, pathological, and molecular prognostic factors associated with survival for patients with HIV and diffuse large B-cell, Burkitt, primary CNS, plasmablastic, primary effusion, and peripheral T-cell lymphoma.

Early in the AIDS epidemic, a higher incidence of several malignancies was identified. In addition to Kaposi sarcoma and invasive cervical cancer, an increased incidence of aggressive high-grade B-cell lymphomas became recognized as AIDS-defining malignancies due to their striking association with immunosuppression. In the post-HAART era, lymphoma has become the most common malignancy seen in patients with HIV/AIDS, and it is also the most common cause of mortality in these patients.

J.L. Layton • J.J. Castillo, M.D. (✉)
Division of Hematology and Oncology, The Warren Alpert Medical School of Brown University, The Miriam Hospital, 164 Summit Ave, Providence, RI 02906, USA
e-mail: jcastillo@lifespan.org

P.J. Quesenberry and J.J. Castillo (eds.), *Non-Hodgkin Lymphoma: Prognostic Factors and Targets*, Cancer Drug Discovery and Development, DOI 10.1007/978-1-4614-5851-7_9,

Classification of HIV-Associated Lymphomas

In the most recent version of the WHO classification of hematologic malignancies [1], AIDS-related lymphomas (ARL) have been classified as follows: (1) lymphomas also occurring in immunocompetent patients, which include diffuse large B-cell lymphoma (DLBCL), primary central nervous system lymphoma (PCNSL), Burkitt/Burkitt-like lymphoma (BL/BLL), and Hodgkin lymphoma, among others; (2) lymphomas occurring more specifically on HIV/AIDS patients, which include plasmablastic lymphoma (PBL) and primary effusion lymphoma (PEL); and (3) lymphomas occurring in other immunodeficient states, such as polymorphic lymphoma, which is also seen in post-transplanted patients. Of note, PCNSL, PBL, and PEL are considered variants of DLBCL but, given their distinct presentation and therapy, will be discussed separately.

General Considerations

Patients with HIV/AIDS often present with advanced lymphoma stage and a more aggressive clinical presentation. Prior to highly active antiretroviral therapy (HAART), these patients often already had history of opportunistic infections (OI) and carried a diagnosis of AIDS. Not surprisingly, response and overall survival (OS) rates were abysmal. Patients suffered increased toxicity and frequent infections during treatment of their lymphoma, requiring dose reductions and treatment delays. Trials were conducted to identify more tolerable treatment regimens and prognostic factors that could be utilized to tailor treatment based on AIDS-related clinical characteristics and tumor factors. Multiple studies attempted to improve treatment outcomes by employing several strategies: attempting low-dose chemotherapeutic regimens, supplementing with colony-stimulating factors with standard-dose regimens, and administering single-agent antiviral regimens as they became available.

Large registries following the epidemiology of the HIV population include patients from both the pre- and post-HAART eras. Analysis from the Swiss HIV Cohort Study demonstrates an overall decline of ARLs in the post-HAART era. The incidence of lymphoma in the pre-HAART era peaked at 13.6 cases per 100,000 person/years, declining to 1.8 cases per 100,000 person/years in the post-HAART era [2]. Currently, the risk of ARL is approximately 1.2% per year with a standard incidence ratio (SIR) for DLBCL of 31 and BL/BLL of 25, respectively [3]. In contrast, BL appears to be increasing in incidence in the post-HAART era as it tends to occur at relatively higher $CD4^+$ counts [4].

While the use of HAART has somewhat leveled the playing field, appropriate treatment for ARLs remains somewhat controversial. Experts emphasize utilizing clinical and histological characteristics to guide treatment choices. In general, patients with ARL should be treated with standard regimens, similar to the treatment of immunocompetent patients. For example, the combination of rituximab, cyclophosphamide, doxorubicin, vincristine, and prednisone (R-CHOP), which is considered the standard of care for immunocompetent patients with DLBCL [5], can be used at standard doses in patients with HIV-associated DLBCL [6]. Similarly, more intensive regimes such as CODOX-M/IVAC, a commonly used regimen in immunocompetent patients with BL/BLL [7], can be used in patients with HIV-associated BL/BLL [8, 9]. However, patients with ARL and CD4 count <50 cells mm^3 should not receive rituximab, given a high risk of infectious complications [10]. Any patient with a new diagnosis of ARL who is not receiving antivirals should be started on HAART, and if the patient is already on HAART and there is evidence of HIV progression, HAART should be optimized, since a response to HAART during treatment of ARL has been associated with better response and survival rates [11–13]. Zidovudine should not be used concurrently with chemotherapy, given its bone marrow suppressive properties. Finally, all patients with ARL should receive growth factor support and antibiotic prophylaxis to minimize neutropenia and potential life-threatening infections.

As therapy and survival for ARLs improve, there is an increased interest on identifying relevant prognostic factors, which should be validated prospectively, if possible and easy to use in clinical settings. Ideally, these prognostic factors will be also helpful on identifying appropriate therapeutic approaches depending on the risk stratification of our patients. Risk-stratified therapy is the current object of investigation by the AIDS Malignancy Consortium, a clinical trials unit sponsored by the National Cancer Institute to investigate novel therapeutic approaches in patients with HIV infection and cancer.

Diffuse Large B-Cell Lymphoma

The reported incidence of DLBCL is approximately 75% of all ARLs. The relative risk for ARL was estimated at 60- to 200-fold than that of immunocompetent patients [1], but appears to be declining in the post-HAART era [14]. Despite overall improved health of HIV-positive patients, they still typically present with more advanced stage disease and aggressive tumor biology with higher proliferation index, B symptoms, and extranodal involvement as compared to HIV-negative counterparts [15, 16]. Many early studies grouped all ARL patients together to determine the most effective chemotherapeutic regimens and supportive medications (i.e., growth colony-stimulating factors) in addition to defining significant prognostic indicators to better predict response and outcomes based on multiple variables. The introduction and widespread use of HAART caused a paradigm shift not just on clinical outcomes of HIV patients but also on the efficacy of treatments for ARL. As HIV became better treated, previously defined prognostic indicators became irrelevant.

Pre-HAART Era

Early studies that evaluated varying chemotherapy regimens often characterized patients via anticipated pertinent clinical characteristics including a previous AIDS diagnosis, $CD4^+$ count <50 or <100 cells/mm^3, performance status ECOG ≥2 or Karnofsky performance status (KPS) <60–70%, nodal involvement, presence of extranodal disease and number of sites, lactate dehydrogenase (LDH) levels, sexual behavior, and race [17–19] (Table 1).

During the early development of antiviral therapy for HIV (early 1990s), single-agent antivirals were utilized to help establish the safety of concurrent ARL treatment with antiviral therapy. A phase I/II dose escalation of CEOP (cyclophosphamide, epirubicin, vincristine, and prednisone) with or without single-agent didanosine (ddI) or zidovudine demonstrated that the use of a single-agent antiviral did not adversely affect overall survival. They cited $CD4^+$ count <100 cells/mm^3, previous diagnosis of AIDS, and KPS <70% as poor prognostic indicators [20]. Patarca and colleagues studied the use of modified VACOP-B (vincristine and mitoxantrone vs. doxorubicin, cyclophosphamide, etoposide, methylprednisolone, and bleomycin) with or without ddI, demonstrating $CD4^+$ count as a prognostic factor. Interestingly, the use of ddI did not affect OS, and β-2-microglobulin and HIV p24 antigen levels were of no prognostic significance [21].

Given the concern for possible safety risks with the use of growth colony-stimulating factors (early studies suggesting increasing HIV p24 antigen levels in in vitro models), multiple centers developed strategies to define the safety and efficacy of granulocyte-colony-stimulating factor (G-CSF) administration. These studies showed that G-CSF could be administered safely with an improvement in the total dose and cycle administration of chemotherapy regimens but did not improve OS [20, 22, 23].

Several studies employed a "risk-adapted" strategy by assigning patients to regimens based on factors thought to alter clinical outcomes. These studies aimed to balance higher toxicity of chemotherapeutic regimens with effective treatment of aggressive ARLs. Weiss and colleagues stratified "normal risk" patients to receive CHOP (cyclophosphamide, doxorubicin, vincristine, prednisone) for 4–6 cycles, followed by zidovudine and interferon alpha. "High-risk" patients received low-dose CHOP or vincristine plus prednisone [19]. The AIDS Clinical Trials Group (ACTG) evaluated low-dose vs. standard-dose M-BACOD (methotrexate, bleomycin, doxorubicin, cyclophosphamide, vincristine, and dexamethasone) with or without granulocyte/macrophage-colony-stimulating factor (GM-CSF). This trial demonstrated equal efficacy of both regimens with less hematologic toxicity in the low-dose group. Risk was defined by prognostic indicators previously used such as a previous diagnosis of AIDS and KPS score ≥70. While low-dose treatment was effective, this study also indicated that an absolute $CD4^+$ count >200 cells/mm^3 was a more important predictor of outcome than the dose intensity of the chemotherapy regimen administered [22]. Further analysis of the ACTG data defined further the prognostic significance of age, stage, and KPS. They found that age, $CD4^+$ count >100 cells/mm^3, early stage, and no history of intravenous drug use had more favorable outcomes regardless of treatment [18].

Table 1 Pre-HAART era regimens and prognostic indicators in HIV-associated diffuse large B-cell lymphoma

Study	Regimen(s)	Prognostic factors	Antiviral	GCSF
Patarca et al. 1996 [21]	Modified VACOP-B	Peripheral T-cell subsets KPS	Didanosine	No
Newell et al. 1996 [20]	CEOP	$CD4^+$ count <100 cells/mm^3 Previous AIDS diagnosis KPS	Zidovudine, didanosine, or zalcitabine	Yes
Straus et al. 1998 [18]	Low-dose vs. standard-dose m-BACOD	Age IVDU Sexual risk factors Prior AIDS diagnosis $CD4^+$ count LDH levels KPS Clinical stage B symptoms Nodal involvement	None	Yes
Weiss et al. 1998 [19]	Low-dose CHOP vs. CHOP + Interferon-α-2b + antiviral	$CD4^+$ count <50 cells/mm^3 Prior AIDS diagnosis WHO activity index	Zidovudine	No
Rossi et al. 1998 [23]	ProMACE-CytaBOM	$CD4^+$ count <100 cells/mm^3	None	Yes

Post-HAART Era

After 1996, treatment of HIV with HAART became widely accepted as standard of care with a substantial reduction in the morbidity and mortality from HIV infection. Earlier studies using single-agent antivirals had already established the safety of concurrent administration of HAART and chemotherapy regimens for the treatment of ARLs. As HIV/AIDs became better controlled, the overall health of patients improved, and higher rates of newly diagnosed lymphoma were seen. As such, previously utilized prognostic factors became less relevant. Additionally, risk stratification factors were developed into prognostic tools (International Prognostic Index, IPI) and were being widely used in non-HIV-associated lymphomas [24]. A retrospective analysis of immunocompetent NHL patients determined that age >60, stage III or IV disease, elevated serum LDH, ECOG performance status ≥2, and >1 extranodal site involved are the most significant patient characteristics influencing prognosis. While the IPI score was developed in non-HIV-associated lymphomas, its applicability became apparent particularly in the post-HAART era, although few studies have shown prognostic value of the IPI score in the pre-HAART era as well [25]. In the post-HAART era, many studies demonstrated the usefulness of the IPI score on risk-stratifying patients with ARLs, as well as defining further prognostic value of histological diagnosis [26] (Table 2).

During the post-HAART era, further distinction has been made among the various pathological variants of ARL with possible treatment and prognostic significance. Most notably, the distinction of the pathophysiology and natural history between DLBCL and BL was further elucidated [27]. This prompted the design of prospective studies evaluating different therapies for these conditions, which were "lumped together" in prior studies. In general, patients with BL are treated with more intensive regimens universally including CNS prophylaxis [28], while DLBCL patients are treated with less-intensive regimens and CNS prophylaxis is given in a case-by-case basis [29].

Many studies have demonstrated that prognostic factors can now be mostly attributed to tumor-related factors and histology. While $CD4^+$ count, viral load, and risk of opportunistic infections had clinical significance in the overall health of HIV/AIDS patients, these factors no longer infer prognostic significance in the outcomes of ARLs. Specifically, factors independently associated with complete response (CR) were histology and IPI score; improved overall survival (OS) was associated with achievement of CR, low IPI score, and histology [30–33]. Virological response to HAART is an independent prognostic factor regardless of treatment [34–36]. More recent studies emphasize even further that tumor biology such as germinal center (GC) vs. non-germinal center (NGC) phenotype and Ki67 expression, as a marker of proliferation rate, may be of prognostic significance [37, 38].

With the introduction of anti-CD20 therapy and its efficacy in non-AIDS-related lymphomas, several studies evaluated the safety and efficacy of rituximab (Rituxan®, Genentech, South San Francisco, CA) in ARLs [10, 34, 37, 39, 40]. In the last decade, the use of rituximab in non-AIDS-related lymphomas has increased

Table 2 Post-HAART era regimens and prognostic factors in HIV-associated diffuse large B-cell lymphoma

Study	Regimen(s)	Prognostic factors	Antiviral	GCSF
Tirelli et al. 2002 [40]	R-CDE	Clinical stage IPI score CD4+ count	HAART	Yes
Sawka et al. 2005 [74]	VACOP-B	IPI score	HAART	Yes
Mounier et al. 2006 [32]	ACVBP vs. standard CHOP vs. low-dose CHOP	Age-adjusted IPI score CD4+ count	HAART	Yes
Spina et al. 2005 [39]	R-CHOP	CD4+ count ECOG performance status History of OIs	HAART	No
Navarro et al. 2007 [34]	CHOP	IPI score ECOG performance status Clinical stage	HAART	Yes
Ribera et al. 2007 [75]	R-CHOP	IPI score Virological response to HAART	HAART	Yes
Sparano et al. 2010 [37]	R-EPOCH	Age-adjusted IPI score CD4+ count Ki67%	HAART	

significantly. Given the improved CR and OS with rituximab-containing regimens, several studies were developed to assess its efficacy in ARLs. Kaplan and colleagues demonstrated no statistical improvement in CR or OS in ARLs treated with CHOP and R-CHOP despite a trend toward tumor response [10]. This and other studies also demonstrated a significant increase in the incidence of infection-related deaths with the use of rituximab in patients with CD4 ≤50 cells/mm^3 [37, 39, 41]. More recent data suggests safe use of rituximab-containing regimens if CD4$^+$ >200 cells/mm^3 at initiation of therapy with concurrent administration of antibiotic prophylaxis for opportunistic infections [6, 37]. Further studies are necessary to better define the safety and efficacy of rituximab-containing treatments. Current NCCN guidelines do *not* recommend the use of rituximab in patients with ARL and CD4$^+$ counts <100 cells/mm^3 [42].

Burkitt/Burkitt-Like Lymphoma

BL was the first lymphoma to be associated with HIV infection and became recognized early on as an AIDS-defining malignancy. BL accounts for approximately 30% of all the ARLs [1]. During the early years of the HIV/AIDS epidemic, all lymphomas were treated with similar regimens, regardless of their histological subtype. BL was described and classified typically as small, non-cleaved lymphoma during the pre-HAART era. The natural history and clinical presentation of BL are that of a more aggressive lymphoma. As HIV has been more effectively treated with HAART, there has been more focus on aggressive treatments for BL as compared to DLBCL. Lim et al. demonstrated poorer outcomes for BL treated with the same regimens as DLBCL in the pre- vs. post-HAART eras [27]. More aggressive regimens have since been studied, leading to more aggressive treatment regimens. Current published recommendations by the National Comprehensive Cancer Network (NCCN) for the treatment of HIV-associated BL include CODOX-M (cyclophosphamide, vincristine, doxorubicin, high-dose methotrexate) alternating with IVAC (ifosfamide, etoposide, high-dose cytarabine), dose-adjusted EPOCH (etoposide, prednisone, vincristine, cyclophosphamide, doxorubicin), or CDE (cyclophosphamide, doxorubicin, etoposide) for patients with $CD4^+$ counts >100 cells/mm^3 [42].

Pre-HAART Era

Few studies in the pre-HAART era are distinguished among histological variants of ARLs. To further characterize the clinicopathological features of ARLs, a retrospective analysis of pre-HAART data by Hansen et al. described the strong correlation between Epstein–Barr virus (EBV) in the pathogenesis of BL/BLL [43]. An early study including predominantly BL/BLL histology (60%) evaluated low-dose M-BACOD with concurrent antiviral therapy demonstrating both safety and efficacy with this combination [44]. This study also evaluated multiple clinical factors as prognostic indicators; a previous AIDS diagnosis and $CD4^+$ count were significantly associated with survival. These findings are consistent with other prognostic markers for ARLs from the pre-HAART era.

Post-HAART Era

During the post-HAART era, further treatment approaches have been suggested to target specific histological variants of ARL. BL/BLL has a more aggressive clinical history. Interestingly, these lymphomas tend to occur at relatively higher $CD4^+$ counts with a lower incidence at $CD4^+$ count <50 cells/mm^3 and higher at a $CD4^+$ count >250 cells/mm^3 [45]. As HIV infection and $CD4^+$ counts respond to the appropriate antiviral therapy, the incidence of BL has remained constant, while the incidence of other ARL is decreasing [14]. As with DLBCL, in the post-HAART era, histology and tumor-related factors remain of most prognostic significance. Several studies have demonstrated improved long-term survival in BL/BLL patients with shorter more intensive chemotherapy that targets these tumor biology-specific factors. The clinical stage, IPI score, and histology continue to be of most prognostic significance in these ARLs [46, 47].

Primary CNS Lymphoma

PCNSL is a rare lymphoma that affects primarily the CNS without evidence of systemic involvement. Classically, PCNSL has been associated with advanced HIV infection and is commonly seen in individuals with CD4 counts <50 cells/mm^3. In the pre-HAART era, PCNSL accounted for up to 10–20% of all the cases of ARL. With the advent of HAART, the incidence of PCNSL in HIV-infected individuals has decreased [48, 49]; however, the risk of developing PCNSL in HIV-positive individuals remains several thousand-fold higher than the general population. Clinically, patients can present with a wide variety of clinical symptoms such as seizures, headaches, altered mental status, diplopia, dysphagia, and vertigo, among others. The diagnosis is suspected based on clinical symptoms and confirmed by imaging; brain MRI or contrast-enhanced CT shows a ring-enhancing lesion within the white matter. To confirm the diagnosis, a brain biopsy is necessary since other lesions such as cerebral toxoplasmosis can have a similar radiological appearance. Pathologically, most of HIV-associated PCNSL cases show DLBCL morphology [50], although more rare histology subtypes such as T-cell lymphoma or plasmablastic lymphoma have also been described. It is important to note the strong association with EBV infection in patients with HIV-associated PCNSL [51]. The treatment usually requires chemotherapeutic agents with a good CNS distribution, such as methotrexate, which is given intravenously at high doses, in combination with leucovorin. Regimens directed against systemic DLBCL, such as CHOP, will not achieve therapeutic levels within the CNS. Surgery is usually ineffective to completely eradicate the disease. Radiation therapy and steroids can induce short-lived responses with relapses seen up to 90% of the times. Novel approaches combining chemotherapy and radiation therapy are associated with longer survival but can induce dementia or leukoencephalopathy in up to 50% of the patients. The rarity of HIV-associated PCNSL has precluded development of large prospective trials to further characterize treatment of this ARL.

Prognostic Factors in HIV-Associated PCNSL

Given the severe immunosuppression associated with PCNSL, the observed poor overall survival is not surprising. If left untreated, PCNSL is associated with a median survival of 2.5 months. Median survival can improve to 4 months with radiation therapy and up to 12–18 months with chemotherapy. In the pre-HAART era, patients with HIV-associated PCNSL had shorter survival than their immunocompetent counterparts; however, in the post-HAART era, this difference, although smaller, still remains. A large study using SEER data between 1973 and 2004 identified approximately 2,500 PCNSL patients (825 were HIV-positive) [52]. The strongest prognostic factor for survival was HIV-positive status; HIV-positive patients had a median OS of 2 months, compared to 12 months in immunocompetent patients.

Similarly, a recent retrospective study compared the survival of 41 HIV-positive and 45 HIV-negative patients with a pathological or radiological diagnosis of PCNSL [53]. When evaluating patients who received treatment for PCNSL, the median OS of HIV-positive patients was 4 months compared to 15 months in HIV-positive patients ($p=0.03$). In HIV-positive patients treated for PCNSL, the use of HAART and a KPS >70 were associated with a longer survival (7 and 9 months, respectively). At least two separate studies have evaluated the role of immune response to HAART in patients with HIV-associated PCNSL [54, 55]. Both studies found that an immune response to HAART, defined as an increase in the CD4+ counts during therapy for PCNSL, is associated with a markedly improved survival. However, these are small studies of 29 and 25 patients, respectively. Finally, in a retrospective study on 111 patients with PCNSL, HAART and the use of radiation therapy to levels >30 Gy were associated with an improved survival [56].

In conclusion, little is known on prognostic factors for survival in patients with HIV-associated PCNSL. HAART has decreased the incidence of PCNSL and seemed to have mildly improved outcomes; however, the prognosis in HIV-positive patients remains poorer than immunocompetent patients with PCNSL.

Plasmablastic Lymphoma

PBL is a rare lymphoma accounting for 2–3% of all ARLs and, according to the 2008 WHO classification, is one of the ARL more commonly seen in HIV/AIDS patients [57]. To date, there have been no more than 200 cases of HIV-associated PBL reported in the literature. Given its rarity, no prospective trials have been done exclusively in patients with PBL, and most of the data are case reports or case series [58]. The median age at presentation is 38 years with a clear male predominance (7:1) and a median CD4+ count of 178 cells/mm^3. Fifty percent of patients present with advanced clinical stages and 58% with involvement of extra-oral sites. The cell of origin is thought to be a post-germinal-center, terminally differentiated, activated B cells, probably in transition from immunoblast to plasma cell. PBL represents a diagnostic challenge due to the lack of expression of CD45 and CD20 and its plasmablastic morphology; however, immunoglobulin gene rearrangements can be seen in a majority of cases as a reflection of their B-cell lineage. Additionally, there is a universal expression of markers of plasmacytic differentiation, such as CD38, CD138, or MUM-1/IRF-4 [57]. EBV genome demonstrated by expression of EBV-encoded RNA (EBER) can be found in the nucleus of the malignant cells up to 74% of the cases [58]. PBL also represents a therapeutic challenge as it is associated with higher rates of relapse and death associated with disease progression, and a median overall survival of 14–15 months, despite an initial 55% CR rate to chemotherapy [59, 60]. Current guidelines recommend initiation or adjustment of HAART along with the use of intensive regimens more akin to the treatment of BL (i.e., CODOX-M/IVAC, EPOCH, CDE) than DLBCL (CHOP) [42], although a recent review of the literature failed to show a survival benefit from more intensive therapies [59].

Prognostic Factors in HIV-Associated PBL

Prognostic factors in PBL can be subdivided as HIV related and lymphoma related. A recent comparative study evaluating differences between HIV-positive and HIV-negative PBL patients reported that HIV status per se could be of prognostic value; however, this could be a consequence of an immunological response to HAART seen in HIV-positive patients. In HIV-positive patients, the use of HAART has shown to be of prognostic value in patients with HIV-associated PBL in general (i.e., chemotherapy treated or untreated) [60]. HAART, given prior to or after a diagnosis of PBL, remained as a prognostic factor in patients treated with chemotherapy [59], suggesting that the benefits of HAART could be independent of the benefits of chemotherapy. A number of adverse clinical prognostic factors have been identified in patients with PBL. Among them are advanced clinical stage, extra-oral sites of involvement, lack of use of chemotherapy, lack of response to chemotherapy, bone marrow involvement, and presence of B symptoms [60, 61]. In the multivariate analysis, clinical stage and use of chemotherapy were independent factors for PBL patients [60]. In HIV-associated PBL patients who were treated with chemotherapy, clinical stage and response to chemotherapy were independently associated with survival [59]. Pathological factors could also serve as prognostic markers; subset analyses have identified high proliferation rates (Ki-67 >80%) as a marker of worse survival rates in HIV-associated PBL [59], but this would need further validation. More recently, C-MYC gene rearrangements (chromosome 8), similar to the ones found in BL, have been described recurrently in HIV-associated PBL and have been linked to a worse prognosis [62, 63].

In summary, clinical stage, HAART, and chemotherapy seem to have independent prognostic values in patients with HIV-associated PBL. In patients treated with chemotherapy, the clinical stage and obtaining a complete response seem to be the strongest prognostic factors. The emerging data on C-MYC gene rearrangements, although intriguing, needs further studying.

Primary Effusion Lymphoma

PEL is a rare lymphoma, accounting for approximately 2–4% of all ARLs. According to the 2008 WHO classification, PEL is considered one of the ARLs more specifically seen in HIV/AIDS patients. PEL presents more frequently in men than women with median $CD4^+$ counts ranging between 130 and 200 cells/mm^3. PEL commonly presents in serous body cavities such as pleura or peritoneum, resulting in recurrent effusions, although extracavitary presentations have also been described [64]. Due to this unusual extranodal presentation, patients are by definition considered as stage IV disease. The development of PEL is universally associated with the Kaposi sarcoma herpes virus or human herpes virus 8 (HHV-8) and, to a lesser degree, with EBV. Although proven to be a B-cell lymphoma by molecular techniques, PEL seldom expresses leukocyte or B-cell markers and is usually CD45- and CD20-negative. Given the morphological and molecular features of PEL, the cell of origin is thought to be at a B-cell development stage between an immunoblast and a plasma cell. Current guidelines recommend initiation or adjustment of HAART along with combination chemotherapy regimens such CHOP, CDE, dose-adjusted EPOCH, or CDOP. Given the lack of expression of CD20 by PEL, the administration of rituximab is not recommended [42]. A few studies evaluating intracavitary cidofovir in PEL demonstrated anecdotal success [65].

Prognostic Factors in HIV-Associated PEL

The prognosis of HIV-associated PEL remains poor with median OS rates at 2–3 months if left untreated and 6 months with aggressive therapy in recent case series [66, 67]. Due to its rarity and the lack of PEL-specific prospective studies, there is a paucity of data regarding prognostic factors in HIV-associated PEL. The largest published case series reported clinicopathological data on 28 patients with HIV-associated PEL [66]. In the univariate analysis, a series of clinical factors were associated with a worse OS rate, including age <45 years, absence of HAART prior to lymphoma diagnosis, performance status ECOG >2, thrombocytopenia, hypoalbuminemia, and treatment not including methotrexate. However, in the multivariate analysis, only a performance status >2 and absence of HAART prior to PEL diagnosis were adverse independent prognostic factors. It is important to note the retrospective nature of the data collection, the small sample size, and the lack of uniformity in the therapy of HIV-associated PEL patients in this study. A single institution study from Aviano, Italy, reported data from 16 HHV-8-positive lymphomas found among 327 ARLs [68]. In the univariate survival analysis of all ARLs, HHV-8-positive lymphoma, HHV-8 viral load >40,000 copies/mm^3, and performance status >2 were factors associated with a worse outcome. In the multivariate analysis, HHV-8-positive lymphoma was the only independent factor associated with survival.

In summary, HIV-associated PEL seems to have one of the worst prognoses of all ARLs. The use of HAART along with performance status seems to be associated with survival in these patients.

Peripheral T-Cell Lymphoma

Peripheral T-cell lymphomas (PTCLs) are among the ARLs also seen in immunocompetent individuals. Although PTCL occurs rarely in the setting of HIV infection, the risk of developing PTCL has been reported up to 15-fold the risk of the general population [69]. The current WHO classification includes a large variety of PTCLs. For classification purposes, PTCL can be divided as leukemic (i.e., T-cell large granular lymphocytic leukemia, adult T-cell/leukemia/lymphoma), cutaneous (i.e., mycosis fungoides), and systemic (i.e., anaplastic large cell lymphoma [ALCL] or PTCL, not otherwise specified [PTCL-NOS]) [70]. This section will discuss almost exclusively the status of HIV-associated systemic PTCL. Given the rarity of systemic PTCL in HIV-infected individuals, with no more than 150 cases reported in the literature, no prospective studies have been carried to identify its true incidence or prevalence. The available data rely heavily on case reports and case series [71]. The median age at presentation is 38 years with a male predominance (4–5:1). The median $CD4^+$ count is 130 cells/mm^3. The majority of cases (75%) present with advanced clinical stage (i.e., stage III or IV) and 62% with high-risk age-adjusted IPI scores. Interestingly, 70% of cases had at least one extranodal site affected. Pathologically, the most common PTCL subtypes in HIV-infected individuals were PTCL-NOS and ALCL. The CR rate was 43% with a 5-year OS rate of 32%. No specific chemotherapy regimen is considered standard of care in HIV-associated PTCL; however, these patients should be treated with similar therapies as immunocompetent individuals.

Prognostic Factors in HIV-Associated PTCL

The largest literature search in HIV-associated systemic PTCL gathered clinical and pathological data from 85 cases [71]. In this group of heterogeneously treated patients, the use of HAART and EBV positivity within tumor cells was associated with a better OS rate, while an advanced clinical stage was an adverse prognostic factor. A $CD4^+$ count of <50 cells/mm^3 showed a statistical trend toward a poor prognosis. Of note, no multivariate analysis was performed due to missing data. In a recent case series on 51 patients with HIV-associated systemic PTCL [72], $CD4^+$ count <200 cells/mm^3 and a performance status ECOG >1 were associated with worse OS rates, while the use of HAART showed an association with better prognosis. In a multivariate analysis, performance status and use of HAART were independent prognostic factors. Although not included in the multivariate survival analysis, the use of chemotherapy and obtaining a CR were clearly associated with an improved survival in patients diagnosed with these aggressive lymphomas. Scarce data are available on subtypes of HIV-associated PTCL. In a literature review on 37 patients with a diagnosis of HIV-associated ALCL, in which the large majority of patients did not express ALK, early clinical stage was associated with an improved survival, while the use of HAART showed a trend toward significance [73].

Although data are scant, the use of HAART and performance status seemed to be prognostic factors in HIV-associated PTCL. We were unable to find studies evaluating prognostic factors in patients with leukemic and/or primary cutaneous HIV-associated PTCL.

References

1. Raphael M, Said J, Borisch B et al (2008) Lymphomas associated with HIV infection. In: Swerdlow S, Campo E, Harris N et al (eds) WHO classification of tumours of haematopoeitic and lymphoid tissues. IARC, Lyon, pp 340–342
2. Polesel J, Clifford GM, Rickenbach M et al (2008) Non-Hodgkin lymphoma incidence in the Swiss HIV Cohort Study before and after highly active antiretroviral therapy. AIDS 22(2):301–306
3. Long JL, Engels EA, Moore RD et al (2008) Incidence and outcomes of malignancy in the HAART era in an urban cohort of HIV-infected individuals. AIDS 22(4):489–496
4. Kirk O, Pedersen C, Cozzi-Lepri A et al (2001) Non-Hodgkin lymphoma in HIV-infected patients in the era of highly active antiretroviral therapy. Blood 98(12):3406–3412
5. Pfreundschuh M, Trumper L, Osterborg A et al (2006) CHOP-like chemotherapy plus rituximab versus CHOP-like chemotherapy alone in young patients with good-prognosis diffuse large-B-cell lymphoma: a randomised controlled trial by the MabThera International Trial (MInT) Group. Lancet Oncol 7(5):379–391
6. Boue F, Gabarre J, Gisselbrecht C et al (2006) Phase II trial of CHOP plus rituximab in patients with HIV-associated non-Hodgkin's lymphoma. J Clin Oncol 24(25):4123–4128
7. Mead GM, Sydes MR, Walewski J et al (2002) An international evaluation of CODOX-M and CODOX-M alternating with IVAC in adult Burkitt's lymphoma: results of United Kingdom Lymphoma Group LY06 study. Ann Oncol 13(8):1264–1274
8. Wang ES, Straus DJ, Teruya-Feldstein J et al (2003) Intensive chemotherapy with cyclophosphamide, doxorubicin, high-dose methotrexate/ifosfamide, etoposide, and high-dose cytarabine (CODOX-M/IVAC) for human immunodeficiency virus-associated Burkitt lymphoma. Cancer 98(6):1196–1205
9. Montoto S, Wilson J, Shaw K et al (2010) Excellent immunological recovery following CODOX-M/IVAC, an effective intensive chemotherapy for HIV-associated Burkitt's lymphoma. AIDS 24(6):851–856
10. Kaplan LD, Lee JY, Ambinder RF et al (2005) Rituximab does not improve clinical outcome in a randomized phase 3 trial of CHOP with or without rituximab in patients with HIV-associated non-Hodgkin lymphoma: AIDS-Malignancies Consortium Trial 010. Blood 106(5):1538–1543
11. Hoffmann C, Wolf E, Fatkenheuer G et al (2003) Response to highly active antiretroviral therapy strongly predicts outcome in patients with AIDS-related lymphoma. AIDS 17(10):1521–1529
12. Navarro JT, Ribera JM, Oriol A et al (2003) Improved outcome of AIDS-related lymphoma in patients with virologic response to highly active antiretroviral therapy. J Acquir Immune Defic Syndr 32(3):347–348
13. Navarro JT, Ribera JM, Oriol A et al (2001) Influence of highly active anti-retroviral therapy on response to treatment and survival in patients with acquired immunodeficiency syndrome-related non-Hodgkin's lymphoma treated with cyclophosphamide, hydroxydoxorubicin, vincristine and prednisone. Br J Haematol 112(4):909–915
14. Shiels MS, Pfeiffer RM, Hall HI et al (2011) Proportions of Kaposi sarcoma, selected non-Hodgkin lymphomas, and cervical cancer in the United States occurring in persons with AIDS, 1980–2007. JAMA 305(14):1450–1459
15. Ioachim HL, Cooper MC, Hellman GC (1985) Lymphomas in men at high risk for acquired immune deficiency syndrome (AIDS). A study of 21 cases. Cancer 56(12):2831–2842
16. Levine AM (1992) AIDS-associated malignant lymphoma. Med Clin North Am 76(1):253–268
17. Hagemeister FB, Khetan R, Allen P et al (1994) Stage, serum LDH, and performance status predict disease progression and survival in HIV-associated lymphomas. Ann Oncol 5(Suppl 2):41–46
18. Straus DJ, Huang J, Testa MA et al (1998) Prognostic factors in the treatment of human immunodeficiency virus-associated non-Hodgkin's lymphoma: analysis of AIDS Clinical Trials Group protocol 142-low-dose versus standard-dose m-BACOD plus granulocyte-macrophage colony-stimulating factor. National Institute of Allergy and Infectious Diseases. J Clin Oncol 16(11):3601–3606

19. Weiss R, Huhn D, Mitrou P et al (1998) HIV-related non-Hodgkin's lymphoma: CHOP induction therapy and interferon-alpha-2b/zidovudine maintenance therapy. Leuk Lymphoma 29(1–2): 103–118
20. Newell M, Goldstein D, Milliken S et al (1996) Phase I/II trial of filgrastim (r-metHuG-CSF), CEOP chemotherapy and antiretroviral therapy in HIV-related non-Hodgkin's lymphoma. Ann Oncol 7(10):1029–1036
21. Patarca R, Freidlander A, Harrington WJ et al (1996) Peripheral blood T cell subsets as prognostic indicators of chemotherapy outcome in AIDS patients with large cell lymphoma. AIDS Res Hum Retroviruses 12(8):645–649
22. Kaplan LD, Straus DJ, Testa MA et al (1997) Low-dose compared with standard-dose m-BACOD chemotherapy for non-Hodgkin's lymphoma associated with human immunodeficiency virus infection. National Institute of Allergy and Infectious Diseases AIDS Clinical Trials Group. N Engl J Med 336(23):1641–1648
23. Rossi G, Donisi A, Casari S et al (1998) Effects of recombinant granulocyte colony-stimulating factor (G-CSF) in patients treated with ProMACE-CytaBOM for HIV-related non-Hodgkin's lymphoma (NHL). Haematologica 83(4):317–322
24. The International Non-Hodgkin's Lymphoma Prognostic Factors Project (1993) A predictive model for aggressive non-Hodgkin's lymphoma. N Engl J Med 329(14):987–94
25. Navarro JT, Ribera JM, Oriol A et al (1998) International prognostic index is the best prognostic factor for survival in patients with AIDS-related non-Hodgkin's lymphoma treated with CHOP. A multivariate study of 46 patients. Haematologica 83(6):508–513
26. Bower M, Gazzard B, Mandalia S et al (2005) A prognostic index for systemic AIDS-related non-Hodgkin lymphoma treated in the era of highly active antiretroviral therapy. Ann Intern Med 143(4):265–273
27. Lim ST, Karim R, Nathwani BN et al (2005) AIDS-related Burkitt's lymphoma versus diffuse large-cell lymphoma in the pre-highly active antiretroviral therapy (HAART) and HAART eras: significant differences in survival with standard chemotherapy. J Clin Oncol 23(19):4430–4438
28. National Comprehensive Cancer Network [website]. NCCN Guidelines, version 3.2011 (2011) Burkitt lymphoma. Available at http://www.nccn.org/professionals/physician_gls/pdf/nhl.pdf. Accessed 24 May 2011
29. National Comprehensive Cancer Network [website]. NCCN Guidelines, version 3.2011 (2011) Diffuse large B-cell lymphoma. Available at http://www.nccn.org/professionals/physician_gls/pdf/nhl.pdf. Accessed 24 May 2011
30. Lim ST, Karim R, Tulpule A et al (2005) Prognostic factors in HIV-related diffuse large-cell lymphoma: before versus after highly active antiretroviral therapy. J Clin Oncol 23(33):8477–8482
31. Miralles P, Berenguer J, Ribera JM et al (2007) Prognosis of AIDS-related systemic non-Hodgkin lymphoma treated with chemotherapy and highly active antiretroviral therapy depends exclusively on tumor-related factors. J Acquir Immune Defic Syndr 44(2):167–173
32. Mounier N, Spina M, Gabarre J et al (2006) AIDS-related non-Hodgkin lymphoma: final analysis of 485 patients treated with risk-adapted intensive chemotherapy. Blood 107(10):3832–3840
33. Simcock M, Blasko M, Karrer U et al (2007) Treatment and prognosis of AIDS-related lymphoma in the era of highly active antiretroviral therapy: findings from the Swiss HIV Cohort Study. Antivir Ther 12(6):931–939
34. Navarro JT, Ribera JM, Oriol A et al (2007) Advanced stage is the most important prognostic factor for survival in patients with systemic acquired immunodeficiency syndrome-related non-Hodgkin's Lymphoma treated with CHOP and highly active antiretroviral therapy. Int J Hematol 86(4):337–342
35. Ribera JM, Navarro JT, Oriol A et al (2002) Prognostic impact of highly active antiretroviral therapy in HIV-related Hodgkin's disease. AIDS 16(14):1973–1976
36. Bohlius J, Schmidlin K, Costagliola D et al (2009) Prognosis of HIV-associated non-Hodgkin lymphoma in patients starting combination antiretroviral therapy. AIDS 23(15):2029–2037
37. Sparano JA, Lee JY, Kaplan LD et al (2010) Rituximab plus concurrent infusional EPOCH chemotherapy is highly effective in HIV-associated B-cell non-Hodgkin lymphoma. Blood 115(15):3008–3016

38. Xicoy B, Ribera JM, Mate JL et al (2010) Immunohistochemical expression profile and prognosis in patients with diffuse large B-cell lymphoma with or without human immunodeficiency virus infection. Leuk Lymphoma 51(11):2063–2069
39. Spina M, Jaeger U, Sparano JA et al (2005) Rituximab plus infusional cyclophosphamide, doxorubicin, and etoposide in HIV-associated non-Hodgkin lymphoma: pooled results from 3 phase 2 trials. Blood 105(5):1891–1897
40. Tirelli U, Spina M, Jaeger U et al (2002) Infusional CDE with rituximab for the treatment of human immunodeficiency virus-associated non-Hodgkin's lymphoma: preliminary results of a phase I/II study. Recent Results Cancer Res 159:149–153
41. Navarro JT, Lloveras N, Ribera JM et al (2005) The prognosis of HIV-infected patients with diffuse large B-cell lymphoma treated with chemotherapy and highly active antiretroviral therapy is similar to that of HIV-negative patients receiving chemotherapy. Haematologica 90(5):704–706
42. National Comprehensive Cancer Network [website]. NCCN Guidelines, version 3.2011 (2011) AIDS-related B-cell lymphomas. Available at http://www.nccn.org/professionals/physician_gls/pdf/nhl.pdf. Accessed 24 May 2011
43. Hansen PB, Penkowa M, Kirk O et al (2000) Human immunodeficiency virus-associated malignant lymphoma in eastern Denmark diagnosed from 1990–1996: clinical features, histopathology, and association with Epstein-Barr virus and human herpesvirus-8. Eur J Haematol 64(6):368–375
44. Levine AM, Tulpule A, Espina B et al (1996) Low dose methotrexate, bleomycin, doxorubicin, cyclophosphamide, vincristine, and dexamethasone with zalcitabine in patients with acquired immunodeficiency syndrome-related lymphoma. Effect on human immunodeficiency virus and serum interleukin-6 levels over time. Cancer 78(3):517–526
45. Guech-Ongey M, Simard EP, Anderson WF et al (2010) AIDS-related Burkitt lymphoma in the United States: what do age and CD4 lymphocyte patterns tell us about etiology and/or biology? Blood 116(25):5600–5604
46. Astrow AB, Tarabay G, Salerno VE et al (2003) Long-term survival in patients with human immunodeficiency virus-associated small non-cleaved cell lymphoma: the role for short course intensive chemotherapy. Hematol Oncol 21(3):131–140
47. Hoffmann C, Wolf E, Wyen C et al (2006) AIDS-associated Burkitt or Burkitt-like lymphoma: short intensive polychemotherapy is feasible and effective. Leuk Lymphoma 47(9):1872–1880
48. Sparano JA (2001) Clinical aspects and management of AIDS-related lymphoma. Eur J Cancer 37(10):1296–1305
49. Wolf T, Brodt HR, Fichtlscherer S et al (2005) Changing incidence and prognostic factors of survival in AIDS-related non-Hodgkin's lymphoma in the era of highly active antiretroviral therapy (HAART). Leuk Lymphoma 46(2):207–215
50. Kluin PM, Deckert M, Ferry JA (2008) Primary diffuse large B-cell lymphoma of the CNS. In: Swerdlow S, Campo E, Harris N et al (eds) WHO classification of tumours of haematopoeitic and lymphoid tissues. IARC, Lyon, pp 240–241
51. Morgello S (1992) Epstein-Barr and human immunodeficiency viruses in acquired immunodeficiency syndrome-related primary central nervous system lymphoma. Am J Pathol 141(2):441–450
52. Norden AD, Drappatz J, Wen PY et al (2011) Survival among patients with primary central nervous system lymphoma, 1973–2004. J Neurooncol 101(3):487–493
53. Bayraktar S, Bayraktar UD, Ramos JC et al (2011) Primary CNS lymphoma in HIV positive and negative patients: comparison of clinical characteristics, outcome and prognostic factors. J Neurooncol 101(2):257–265
54. Skiest DJ, Crosby C (2003) Survival is prolonged by highly active antiretroviral therapy in AIDS patients with primary central nervous system lymphoma. AIDS 17(12):1787–1793
55. Hoffmann C, Tabrizian S, Wolf E et al (2001) Survival of AIDS patients with primary central nervous system lymphoma is dramatically improved by HAART-induced immune recovery. AIDS 15(16):2119–2127

56. Newell ME, Hoy JF, Cooper SG et al (2004) Human immunodeficiency virus-related primary central nervous system lymphoma: factors influencing survival in 111 patients. Cancer 100(12):2627–2636
57. Stein H, Harris N, Campo E (2008) Plasmablastic lymphoma. In: Swerdlow S, Campo E, Harris N et al (eds) World Health Organization classification of tumours. Tumours of haematopoietic and lymphoid tissues. IARC, Lyon, pp 256–257
58. Castillo J, Pantanowitz L, Dezube BJ (2008) HIV-associated plasmablastic lymphoma: lessons learned from 112 published cases. Am J Hematol 83(10):804–809
59. Castillo JJ, Winer ES, Stachurski D et al (2010) Prognostic factors in chemotherapy-treated patients with HIV-associated Plasmablastic lymphoma. Oncologist 15(3):293–299
60. Castillo JJ, Winer ES, Stachurski D et al (2010) Clinical and pathological differences between human immunodeficiency virus-positive and human immunodeficiency virus-negative patients with plasmablastic lymphoma. Leuk Lymphoma 51(11):2047–2053
61. Hansra D, Montague N, Stefanovic A et al (2010) Oral and extraoral plasmablastic lymphoma: similarities and differences in clinicopathologic characteristics. Am J Clin Pathol 134(5):710–719
62. Bogusz AM, Seegmiller AC, Garcia R et al (2009) Plasmablastic lymphomas with MYC/IgH rearrangement: report of three cases and review of the literature. Am J Clin Pathol 132(4):597–605
63. Valera A, Balague O, Colomo L et al (2010) IG/MYC rearrangements are the main cytogenetic alteration in plasmablastic lymphomas. Am J Surg Pathol 34(11):1686–1694
64. Said J, Cesarman E (2008) Primary effusion lymphoma. In: Swerdlow S, Campo E, Harris N et al (eds) WHO classification of tumours of haematopoeitic and lymphoid tissues. IARC, Lyon, pp 260–261
65. Boulanger E, Agbalika F, Maarek O et al (2001) A clinical, molecular and cytogenetic study of 12 cases of human herpesvirus 8 associated primary effusion lymphoma in HIV-infected patients. Hematol J 2(3):172–179
66. Boulanger E, Gerard L, Gabarre J et al (2005) Prognostic factors and outcome of human herpesvirus 8-associated primary effusion lymphoma in patients with AIDS. J Clin Oncol 23(19):4372–4380
67. Simonelli C, Tedeschi R, Gloghini A et al (2006) Prognostic factors in human herpesvirus 8-related lymphoproliferative disorders associated with HIV infection. J Clin Oncol 24(1):209, author reply 209–10
68. Simonelli C, Tedeschi R, Gloghini A et al (2009) Plasma HHV-8 viral load in HHV-8-related lymphoproliferative disorders associated with HIV infection. J Med Virol 81(5):888–896
69. Biggar RJ, Engels EA, Frisch M et al (2001) Risk of T-cell lymphomas in persons with AIDS. J Acquir Immune Defic Syndr 26(4):371–376
70. Catovsky D, Muller-Hermelink HK, Ralskiaer E (2008) Mature T- and NK-cell neoplasms, Chapter 11. In: Swerdlow S, Campo E, Harris N, et al (eds) WHO classification of tumours of haematopoeitic and lymphoid tissues. IARC, Lyon, pp 269–319
71. Castillo J, Perez K, Milani C et al (2009) Peripheral T-cell lymphomas in HIV-infected individuals: a comprehensive review. J HIV Ther 14(2):34–40
72. Castillo JJ, Beltran BE, Bibas M et al (2011) Prognostic factors in patients with HIV-associated peripheral T-cell lymphoma: a multicenter study. Am J Hematol 86(3):256–261
73. Perez K, Castillo J, Dezube BJ et al (2010) Human Immunodeficiency Virus-associated anaplastic large cell lymphoma. Leuk Lymphoma 51(3):430–438
74. Sawka CA, Shepherd FA, Franssen E et al (2005) A prospective, non-randomised phase 1-2 trial of VACOP-B with filgrastim support for HIV-related non-Hodgkin's lymphoma. Biotechnol Annu Rev 11:381–9
75. Ribera JM, Oriol A, Morgades M et al (2008) Safety and efficacy of cyclophosphamide, adriamycin, vincristine, prednisone and rituximab in patients with human immunodeficiency virus-associated diffuse large B-cell lymphoma: results of a phase II trial. Br J Haematol 140(4):411–9

Part III
Therapy

Future Directions in Aggressive Lymphomas

Guilherme F. Perini and Luis E. Fayad

Abstract New exciting discoveries have emerged in the field of aggressive lymphomas. A better understanding of the biology of lymphomas has been translated into clinical practice, and new drugs are emerging as a hope for better disease control. In this chapter, we review the new therapies for aggressive lymphomas, like proteasome inhibitors, B-cell receptor signaling inhibitors (Syk, Burton's tyrosine kinase and protein kinase C inhibitors) and mammalian targets of rapamycin. Moreover, a concise review of the new monoclonal antibodies (MoAbs) and their new targets is presented. Immunomodulatory drugs like lenalidomide also have shown potential benefit in patients with aggressive lymphomas. Although more studies are necessary, these drugs will probably be incorporated in the management of aggressive lymphomas, with less toxic, targeted therapy.

The hematological malignancies have long been in the forefront of development of cancer therapies. The association of new discoveries in genetics and molecular biology has contributed to a better understanding of cancer and consequent treatment innovations. Chronic myeloid leukemia (CML) remains a paradigm of the foresaid. From the Philadelphia chromosome, the first chromosome-specific abnormality related to cancer [1], to the consequent discovery of the BCR-ABL, a fusion protein with abnormal kinase activity responsible for the proliferation of myeloid cells [2], a new era in cancer biology has emerged. Not long, patients with CML could benefit from these discoveries: imatinib (Gleevec®), a selective inhibitor of tyrosine kinase,

G.F. Perini (✉)
Department of Hematology, Hospital Israelita Albert Einstein,
Avenida Albert Einstein, 627—Morumbi, Sao Paulo 05652-900, Brazil
e-mail: guiperini@einstein.br

L.E. Fayad
Department of Lymphoma/Myeloma, University of Texas M.D Anderson Cancer Center,
Houston, TX, USA

P.J. Quesenberry and J.J. Castillo (eds.), *Non-Hodgkin Lymphoma: Prognostic Factors and Targets*, Cancer Drug Discovery and Development,
DOI 10.1007/978-1-4614-5851-7_10,

has been the first approved molecular targeted therapy in cancer and is now considered standard therapy for patients with CML [3].

New exciting discoveries also emerged in the field of lymphomas. Rituximab (Rituxan®), a chimeric monoclonal antibody targeted at the CD20 epitope present in B cells, has brought to attention the role of immunotherapy in cancer treatment and is now considered essential in the treatment of most B-cell lymphomas [4]. New monoclonal antibodies (MoAb) have been developed for other malignancies, such as acute myeloid leukemia and renal and pulmonary cancer [5, 6]. Conjugation of a radionuclide with MoAbs introduced the conception of radioimmunotherapy, now available for treatment of selected patients with lymphoma [7].

In the past, aggressive lymphomas were considered an obscure disease with a dismal prognosis. Recent discoveries have shed new light, and aggressive lymphomas are now a treatable and curable disease.

New Insights in the Biology of Aggressive Lymphomas

In the past, the diagnosis of lymphoma and cancer in general relied mostly on morphologic features. However, the findings of recurrent cytogenetic abnormalities and consequent molecular alterations, urged the need of more refined diagnosis. Mantle cell lymphoma, for example, is now recognized as a molecular-defined lymphoma, with over expression of cyclin D1, a consequence of the t(11;14) present in malignant cells [8]. In contrast, the diagnosis of diffuse large B-cell lymphoma (DLBCL), the most common subtype of lymphoma, remains confined to morphological and immunohistochemical findings. Consequently, it is reasonable to conclude that different types of DLBCL, with diverse molecular alterations and clinical behavior, are diagnosed and treated the same.

An area of great interest in recent research is the attempt to divide different subtypes of DLBCL [9]. Recently, great interest have been directed to subtypes of aggressive DLBCL-associated MYC rearrangements. Overexpression of *c*-MYC drives cell proliferation and the expression of other genes involved in cell growth, and patients with DLBCL with c-MYC expression usually have high-grade morphologic features that morphologically resemble Burkitt lymphoma (BL) [10]. A subgroup of patients also presents concurrent translocations involving the BCL-2 gene. This subtype of lymphomas, so-called "double hit" DLBCL, usually present with very aggressive disease, with bone marrow involvement, elevated lactate dehydrogenase levels, and multiple extranodal sites [11, 12]. Patients seldom respond to chemotherapy, and those who achieve a response subsequently suffer an early relapse [13]. Studies are being conducted to evaluate the role of intensified chemotherapy in this subset of patients.

Gene profile expression studies have contributed to a better understanding and separation of at least two subtypes of DLBCL: germinal center B-cell (GCB) and activated B-cell (ABC) lymphomas [14]. When the clinical outcome of the cases was examined, cases with the GBC signature had a significantly better prognosis than the cases that expresses the ABC signature [15]. Although the initial studies were conducted in the era pre-rituximab, subsequent studies confirmed the prognostic value of the GCB-cell signature [16]. Subsequent studies have focused on the genes expressed in the GCB or ABC subtypes. High expression of a proliferation signature and low expression of major histocompatibility complex signature are associated with poor survival. Interestingly, studies focusing on the lymph node stromal signature disclosed a potential prognostic value [17]. High expression of stromal signatures associated with extracellular matrix deposition and tissue inflammation (stromal I signature) is associated with better outcome than cases with high expression of signatures associated with angiogenesis (stromal II signature) [18]. Other studies on subsets of DLBCL based on site of presentation also show different patterns of gene expression.

Although these studies have shown the potential of gene expression to define oncogenic pathways, it has yet to be translated in clinical practice. However, new studies have shown that a subset of DLBCL may benefit from a specific therapy. For instance, the Biocoral study, a post hoc study of biological variables of the CORAL study, has shown that patients with relapsed DLBCL with GCB phenotype have better outcomes when treated with R-DHAP instead of R-ICE [19].

Imaging in Aggressive Lymphomas

The traditional approach to treatment monitoring through imaging has relied on anatomical changes assessing tumor size before and after treatment. This approach has proven through time to be rather problematic. The rate of structural regression of tumors after chemotherapy depends on several factors in the host, as well as the amount of fibrosis present in the tumor. Moreover, the response criteria universally adopted are somewhat arbitrary, and a consistent correlation between tumor response and patient survival has not been demonstrated.

Over 50 years ago, Otto Heinrich Warburg discovered that malignant cancers ferment glucose to lactic acid much more rapidly than most normal cells [20]. The latter, known as the "Warburg effect," is the basis for the use of fluorine-18 fluorodeoxyglucose ([^{18}F]FDG) positron emission tomography (PET-CT) for the staging and treatment monitoring of a variety of cancers [21–23]. The first reports of PET-CT for lymphoma imaging were published more than 20 years ago, and during the last decade, PET-CT has been introduced into all of the steps of lymphoma management.

In aggressive lymphomas, PET-CT has proved to be highly sensitive in determining sites of disease [24, 25]. Several studies have demonstrated the superiority of PET-CT for monitoring treatment of aggressive NHL [24–26]. Patients with a negative PET-CT after treatment have better progression-free survival [27]. However, the role of interim PET-CT in DLBCL patients is controversial, with studies showing conflicting results [28, 29]. Outside clinical trials, interim PET-CT is not recommended in patients with DLBCL.

Recent trials are now focusing on PET-CT-tailored strategies. The Groupe d'Etude des Lymphomes de l'Adulte (GELA) is currently conducting a phase III trial of salvage autologous stem cell transplantation (ASCT) if PET results are positive after two cycles of R-CHOP [30]. In the same manner, the British Columbia Cancer Agency is testing four cycles of R-ICE if PET results are positive after four cycles of R-CHOP [31]. The Alberta Cancer Board also conducted a trial of PET-CT-guided treatment and preliminary results suggest that high-dose therapy with R-DICEP and ASCT may improve EFS for poor prognosis DLBCL with interim positive PET-CT [32].

New Treatments in Aggressive Lymphomas

The development of new drugs as well as incorporation of drugs already developed for other malignancies shows promising results in aggressive results.

Proteasome Inhibitors

The proteasome is a multi-subunit protease complex responsible for the elimination of intracellular proteins tagged for degradation [33]. The ubiquitin-proteasome pathway controls protein function through the degradation of polyubiquitinated intracellular proteins, involved in cell cycle regulation, transcription factor activation, and apoptosis [34, 35]. Diverse types of cancer cells undergo apoptosis in response to proteasome inhibition, and many proteins involved in lymphomagenesis are regulated by the proteasome pathway, including cyclins, NF-κB and p53 [36–38].

NF-κB is a family of proteins that control genes implicated in cell activation, proliferation, and apoptosis [39]. Several studies have implicated increased NF-κB activity in different lymphomas, such as MALT lymphomas [40], peripheral T-cell lymphoma [41], and activated B cell-like DLBCL [42]. Bortezomib (Velcade®), a 20S proteasome subunit inhibitor approved for the treatment of relapsed refractory multiple myeloma, has also shown activity in NHL [43]. A phase II trial of 155 pretreated patients with MCL receiving bortezomib (PINNACLE) reported an ORR of 31%, with 14 patients with CR/Cru [44]. Based on this trial, bortezomib is now approved for patients with relapsed/refractory MCL. The role of bortezomib in association with standard chemotherapy for untreated patients with MCL is being evaluated.

Bortezomib has also been studied in patients with DLBCL, with modest activity as a single agent. The association of bortezomib with standard R-CHOP (BR-CHOP) therapy was evaluated in a phase II prospective trial with 76 patients with DLBCL and MCL (40 patients with DLBCL). BR-CHOP resulted in an intent-to-treat response of 88% [45]. The addition of bortezomib in salvage therapy of patients with DLBCL has also been evaluated. Relapsed patients with ABC subtype of DLBCL were treated with bortezomib in combination with dose-adjusted EPOCH chemotherapy. The ORR was 83%, with an OS of 10.8 months [46]. Two prospective trials (LYM2034 and PYRAMID) are assessing the role of bortezomib combined with chemotherapy in upfront therapy of patients with non-GCB DLBCL.

B-Cell Receptor Signaling Inhibitors

B-cell receptor (BCR) plays an important role in normal B-cell development. Progenitor B cells only differentiate into mature B cells if they express a functional BCR, and those B cells that fail to express a BCR undergo apoptosis. Antigen BCR ligation activates a family of tyrosine kinases, named Scr protein kinases. These tyrosine kinases consequently recruit Syk, another tyrosine kinase responsible for activation of several other molecules, including protein kinase C (PKC), phosphatidyl-inositol-3-kinase (PI3K) and AKT (also known as protein kinase B) [47]. In DLBCL, a chronically "tonic signaling" has been observed and gene expression profiling studies have shown that some DLBCL have overexpression of the BCR, indicating a dependence on this signaling pathway [48]. New drugs targeting the BCR signaling pathway are being developed.

Syk Inhibitors

In vitro studies have confirmed the presence of deregulated Syk pathway in DLBCL [49]. Furthermore, in vitro inhibition of Syk induced apoptosis of DLBCL cell lines. Syk inhibitors are now testing the possible therapeutic effect of these drugs.

Fostamatinib disodium (R406), an oral ATP-competitive Syk inhibitor, is the first to be tested in clinical trials. In preclinical studies, R406 inhibited the proliferation and induced apoptosis of DLBCL lines with tonic BCR signaling, especially lines with high expression of cell-surface immunoglobulin [48]. A phase I/II trial including 68 patients with relapsed NHL (23 DLCBL) showed promising results, including a 22% clinical response in DLBCL, with four partial responses and one complete response [50]. Adverse events were mild and included fatigue, gastrointestinal symptoms, and myelosuppression. Further studies both as single agent and in combination with other drugs are being conducted. Moreover, it has been demonstrated that some patients with peripheral T-cell lymphoma also have a deregulated Syk pathway [51], and studies are conducted with fostamatinib in these patients.

Bruton Tyrosine Kinase Inhibitors

Bruton agammaglobulinemia, an X-linked agammaglobulinemia first described in 1952, is caused by mutations in the gene coding for Bruton tyrosine kinase (BTK). Patients with Bruton agammaglobulinemia have profound hypogammaglobulinemia, with fewer than 1% of the normal number of B cells, with an immature phenotype [52].

Another approach to interrupting BCR signaling is with BTK inhibitors. BTK is a component of the BCR signaling pathway and is downstream of Syk. BTK is critical to the maturation of pre-B cells to differentiating mature B cells [52]. Findings suggest that BTK may be an essential transducer of signals that govern immunoglobulin rearrangement events and re-expression of the RAG gene products. BTK signaling may also regulate the survival of immature B cells that have performed a successful Ig light chain rearrangement, as well as governing the entrance of B cells in the follicular center [53].

Targeting BTK is a promising new therapeutic approach in NHL. Ibrutinib (PCI-32765), an oral irreversible BTK inhibitor, has been tested in a phase Ib/II follow-up trial in patients with relapsed or refractory chronic lymphocytic leukemia/small lymphocytic lymphoma and showed an ORR of 70%, in a 10 month follow-up [54]. An interim analysis of a phase II study in 48 patients with relapsed/refractory mantle cell lymphoma showed an overall response rate of 67%. Interestingly, patients exposed to bortezomib had higher rates of response (75% vs. 58%) [55].

Ibrutinib has also been tested in patients with relapsed/refractory ABC DLBCL. In an interim analysis of a phase I/II study, eight patients received ibrutinib in a fixed dose of 560 mg daily for 35 days. Two patients achieved CR, and other three patients achieved stable disease (SD), showing that ibrutinib has clinical activity in aggressive lymphomas [56].

PKC Inhibitors

The PKC family is composed of four main members: conventional PKCs (α, β and γ), novel PKCs, atypical PKCs, and PKC-related kinases. PKC-β protein is a critical component of the BCR signaling pathway and is related to cell survival by activation of the NF-κB complex [57]. PCK-β has also been related in VEGF-mediated angiogenesis [58]. Since both NF-κB and VEGF are implicated with DLBCL, PKC-β is an attractive target for development of new drugs.

Enzastaurin is an oral ATP-competitive selective inhibitor of PKC-β that also targets the PI3K-AKT pathway and has shown proapoptotic, antiproliferative, and antiangiogenic activities in several cancer lines [59]. A phase II trial including 55 patients with relapsed DLBCL disclosed a safe toxicity profile, with rare hematological toxicities. The primary endpoint was freedom from progression after two cycles, and 22% of patients achieved this endpoint, including three patients achieving CR lasting more than 20 months [60]. A phase III trial is testing enzaustarin in combination with R-CHOP for first-line treatment of patients with DLBCL. Enzastaurin maintenance is also being tested in high-risk DLBCL patients achieving a CR after R-CHOP treatment [61].

Bryostatin 1 (B-1) is a modulator of the PKC family and has shown antitumor activity in vitro. An immunomodulatory component is also present, with neutrophil and immune cell activation. Studies in patients with CLL or indolent NHLs are being conducted, exploring the effect of B-1 in combination with other cytotoxic agents [62].

Heat Shock Protein Inhibitors

Heat shock proteins (HSP) are cytosolic molecules responsible for chaperoning multiple proteins necessary for cell signaling, proliferation, and survival [63]. In the presence of cellular stress, an increase in the expression of HSP occurs, and HSP bind to client proteins protecting them from degradation and preserving cells from apoptosis [64].

HSP90, a member of the HSP family, is overexpressed in cancer cells and may be involved in the survival advantage of these cells. Moreover, HSP90 is overexpressed in many NHL subsets, including DLBCL, and is related to histological transformation of indolent lymphomas [65]. Geldanamycin (17-allylamino-17-demethoxygeldanamycin [17-AAG]) is the first HSP90 inhibitor tested in humans. It has shown to induce cell cycle arrest and apoptosis through the downregulation of cyclin-dependent kinase 1 and AKT and the activation of caspase 9 in MCL cell lines [66]. A number of phase I trials with 17-AAG and similars have shown some activity in melanoma [67], myeloma [68], or breast cancer [69]. Phase I studies in patients with relapsed or refractory NHL are ongoing.

Mammalian Target of Rapamycin Inhibitors

Mammalian target of rapamycin (mTOR) is a kinase involved in regulation of proliferation, cell growth, and apoptosis. The activation of the PI3K-AKT-mTOR pathway promotes the translation of proteins that regulate cell cycle, in particular the eukaryotic initiation factor 4E-binding protein 1 and the p70S6 kinase, responsible for the translation of cyclin D1, c-MYC, and Stat3 proteins, all involved in the pathogenesis of NHL [70]. The PI3K pathway is constitutively activated in the majority of B-cell lymphomas, as manifested by phosphorylation of S6K and 4E-BP1 [71]. Moreover, mTOR inhibitors can decrease the expression of cyclin D1 and cyclin/cyclin-dependent kinases, an interesting property for the treatment of MCL [72].

Two rapamycin analogs, temsirolimus and everolimus, have proved to produce growth inhibition in a broad range of tumor models, including lymphoma. Rapamycin and temsirolimus have demonstrated antitumor activity in vitro against a variety of lymphoma cell lines, especially in MCL cells [73]. In a phase II trial with 35 patients with relapsed/refractory MCL, temsirolimus was delivered as a weekly 250 mg intravenous infusion, and showed an ORR of 38%, including 1 CR [74]. The most significant myelosuppression was thrombocytopenia, and the study was repeated with additional patients receiving 25 mg temsirolimus intravenously every week. An ORR of 41% was observed, with lower incidence of thrombocytopenia.

A phase III trial, comparing temsirolimus with investigator's choice of conventional chemotherapy for patients with relapsed/refractory MCL showed better PFS and ORR in patients treated with temsirolimus [75]. In another phase II trial, temsirolimus was combined with rituximab in 71 patients with MCL exposed to rituximab.

The ORR was 48%, with 20% (14 of 71) complete responses, and 28% (20 of 71) partial responses [76]. A phase I trial for new, untreated MCL patients is being conducted, combining rituximab, temsirolimus, and cladribine for patients not transplant eligible.

Everolimus, an oral mTORC1 inhibitor, has also shown antitumor effects. Preclinical studies have shown that everolimus inhibits phosphorylation of mTOR substrates and induces G1 arrest [77]. Moreover, everolimus can sensitize MCL cells to cytotoxic agents, including doxorubicin and bortezomib. Hodgkin lymphoma cells also show activation of the PI3K pathway and are sensitive to everolimus [78]. A phase II trial evaluated everolimus in 37 patients with refractory/relapsed aggressive NHL, including 20 patients with DLBCL and 14 with MCL. The ORR was 32%, with a median duration of response of 3.1 months [79]. Everolimus was well tolerated, despite mild hematological toxicity. Subsequent studies have demonstrated positive results in patients with CLL/SLL [80] and Waldenstrom macroglobulinemia [81]. mTOR inhibitors also have activity in relapsed, aggressive lymphomas. In a phase II study, 47 patients with relapsed DLBCL were treated with single-agent everolimus with an ORR of 30%. Interestingly, an ORR of 63% was observed in relapsed T-cell NHL [82].

In conclusion, the mTOR inhibitors temsirolimus and everolimus have modest single-agent activity in NHL, CLL/SLL, Hodgkin lymphoma, and Waldenstrom macroglobulinemia. These agents are now being tested in larger single-agent studies as consolidation after induction therapy for DLBCL, as treatment for new untreated Waldenstrom macroglobulinemia, relapsed Hodgkin lymphoma, and in combination with chemoimmunotherapy for untreated MCL.

Histone Deacetylase Inhibitors

Histones are small basic proteins that form the nucleosome core by binding to DNA. Histone acetylation is relevant in diverse cellular mechanisms, including chromatin assembly, DNA repair, and gene expression. In a general way, histone acetylation is linked to a relaxed chromatin status, with activation of transcriptional activity. Histone deacetylation, however, causes condensation of the chromatin and repression of transcriptional activity [83]. An imbalance in these mechanisms is involved in the pathogenesis of different tumors. In NHL, the frequent translocation affecting the BCL6 gene activates the HDAC-containing complex and inhibits transcription and differentiation of germinal center B cells [84].

Several histone deacetylase inhibitors (HDAC) are available for treatment of hematological malignancies. Vorinostat (Zolinza®, SAHA) is a HDAC inhibitor approved for the treatment of relapsed cutaneous T-cell lymphomas [85]. A phase II trial of vorinostat in 18 patients with relapsed DLBCL showed modest activity, with only one patient achieving CR [86].

MGCD0103 (mocetinostat) is an oral HDAC inhibitor under study. An interim analysis of a phase II trial in 50 patients with relapsed/refractory DLCBL and FL reported an ORR of 23.5% in DLBCL, with one CR and three PR [87]. Mocetinostat is also being evaluated for patients with HL. Panobinostat, a novel HDAC, inhibits proliferation and induces apoptosis in tumor cell lines. Interestingly, a synergic effect with mTOR inhibitors has been demonstrated [88], and phase I/II trials of panobinostat associated with everolimus are being conducted for patients with relapsed/refractory NHL.

Immunomodulatory Drugs

Immunomodulatory drugs (IMiDs) are a group of compounds structurally and functionally related to thalidomide, an oral sedative with anti-inflammatory properties. Thalidomide interferes with tumor microenvironment and inhibits tumor necrosis factor TNF-α through degradation of its mRNA, as well as IL-6, IL-1, E-selectin, L-selectin, and GM-CSF [89, 90]. Thalidome also stimulates T-cell lymphocytes, inducing proliferation, cytokine production, and cytotoxic activity and upregulates natural killer (NK) cell activity [91]. Furthermore, thalidomide exhibits antiangiogenenic properties, by decreasing expression of vascular endothelial growth factor (VEGF) [92].

Lenalidomide (Revlimid®), a less toxic and more potent IMiD, is extensively used in multiple myeloma [93, 94], and recent clinical studies show promising results in NHL. A phase II trial of single-agent lenalidomide included 49 patients with aggressive NHL, including MCL and DLBCL. The ORR was 35% in all patients and 28% in DLBCL patients [95]. Patients with MCL also showed responses with lenalidomide in combination with rituximab [96]. A phase I/II trial combining lenalidomide with standard R-CHOP (R2-CHOP) in aggressive lymphoma patients has shown a secure toxicity profile, with no major effects or hematological recovery delays. Moreover, for 30 patients evaluable for response, the overall and complete response rate was 100% and 83%, respectively [97]. Lenalidomide may also have distinct activity depending on the GBC/ABC phenotype. In a retrospective study of patients treated with salvage lenalidomide, the overall response rate in patients with non-GCB subtype was superior to the GCB phenotype [98].

Novel Monoclonal Antibodies

Since the introduction of rituximab in the treatment of lymphomas, research has focused on the development of novel monoclonal antibodies. Strategies have been divided in two different groups: improving anti-CD20 activity and development of new targets for immunotherapy.

New Anti-CD20 MoAbs

Ofatumumab (Arzerra®), a fully human IgG anti-CD20 antibody, targets a different epitope within the CD20 molecule, responsible for different therapeutic properties. Compared with rituximab, ofatumumab binds in a region closer to cell membrane, improving binding stability [99]. Moreover, stronger complement-dependent cell lysis (CDC) is observed with ofatumumab, with similar antibody-dependent cellular toxicity (ADCC) [100]. Ofatumumab was tested as monotherapy in patients with FL in a phase I/II trial, with ORR of 13% and an ORR of 22% in patients refractory to rituximab [101]. These encouraging results led to a trial in heavily pretreated patients with relapsed/refractory aggressive B-cell NHL, most of them preexposed to rituximab. Overall response rates reached 11% (three complete responses and six partial responses) [102].

Veltuzumab is also a second-generation of anti-CD20 MoAbs, developed to improve the efficacy of rituximab. Veltuzumab is a humanized antibody with structural differences compared with rituximab and shows similar in vitro CDC and ADCC properties, with a slower dissociation from the CD20 epitope. Moreover, veltuzumab has shown enhanced tumor B-cell depletion compared with rituximab. A recent phase I/II study in patients with relapsed/refractory different subtypes of NHL showed an ORR of 44 and 27% CR [103]. Interestingly, in the DLBCL patients, a PR of 43% was observed, all of them previously treated with R-CHOP.

Obinutuzumab (GA101), a humanized anti-CD20, has specific modifications in the Fc and hinge regions, leading to a high binding affinity to a distinct CD20 epitope and significant increase in FcgRIII receptor binding. These particular alterations result in a superior ADCC and reduced CDC activity. Moreover, obinutuzumab is thought to increase signaling in target cells, activating apoptotic pathways. A superior antitumor activity of GA101 over rituximab has been suggested by studies in animal models of lymphoma [104]. A phase I/II trial of GA101 in relapsed patients with NHL, mostly FL, showed a safe toxicity profile, with ORR of 58% in 12 patients (three CRs and four PRs). In a study with 40 relapsed/refractory aggressive lymphoma patients, an ORR of 30% was observed in DLBCL patients [105].

New Targeted MoAbs

Epratuzumab is a humanized IgG1 anti-CD22 antibody, a protein expressed on the membrane of normal and malignant B cells. CD22 is internalized when it interacts with its natural ligand, and its precise role in B cells is unclear. Epratuzumab shows ADCC and CDC activities, and a phase I/II trial with epratuzumab associated with rituximab showed impressive results in patients with indolent NHL, including CR in patients previously exposed to rituximab. A multicenter phase II trial combining epratuzumab with standard R-CHOP was conducted in patients with DLBCL. Seventy-eight eligible patients were treated with ER-CHOP, with ORR of 95 and 73% CR [106].

Galiximab is a new chimeric IgG MoAb directed against CD80, with synergy effects with rituximab. CD80 is a T-cell co-stimulatory molecule expressed in normal and malignant B cells, and cross-linking of CD80 induces caspase-dependent apoptosis in lymphoma cell lines. Clinical activity of galiximab has been proved mostly in FL, with phase I/II study showing ORR of 64% when associated with rituximab [107].

SGN-40 (dacetuzumab) is also a new and promising MoAb. CD40 is a critical molecule of the TNF family, involved in normal B-cell activation, proliferation, and differentiation. Preclinical studies in human lymphoma cells have shown ADCC activity, as well as cell growth inhibition and apoptosis promotion. After a phase I trial with 35 patients with NHL reporting a safe profile and clinical activity [108], two phase II trials are ongoing with patients with relapsed DLBCL, either as single agent or in combination with chemotherapy. Hence, a phase 1 clinical trial of SGN-40 in combination with rituximab and gemcitabine showed multiple responses in patients with relapsed DLBCL [109].

Blinatumomab is a bi-specific antibody targeting CD19 (B-cell marker) and CD3 (a T-cell engager). Upon binding and engaging both cells, the B cell is stimulated to growth arrest and apoptosis, and T cell is driven to proliferate. In a phase I study with 12 patients with lymphoma, 11 patients had an objective response, and at least half of the responders remained in response at 1 year out of therapy [110].

Inotuzumab ozogamicin is an antibody against CD22 conjugated with calicheamicin, a cytotoxic agent. In a phase I study, responses of 39% were observed in patients with lymphoma, including a 15% response in DLBCL patients. A combination of rituximab with inotuzumab ozogamicin has been tested in patients with recurrent DLBCL, with an ORR of 80%. However, in rituximab-refractory patients, the ORR was much lower (20%) [111].

Conclusion

It has been said that normal lymphocyte differentiation is, in some sense, a disaster waiting to happen [112]. The consequence of this "disaster" is the outbreak of clonal, unorganized, and rapid multiplying malignant B cells. For many years, the use of drugs with cytotoxic effect remained the principle of lymphoma therapy. Outstanding results were achieved with this strategy in some NHL, and a relatively significant proportion of patients could be cured. However, toxicity and late side effects compromised the majority of patients.

Modern oncology is one of the most fascinating areas or research in present years. Knowledge from basic sciences has progressively been translated in clinical outsets. Less toxic, targeted therapy has emerged as a promising approach in lymphoma patients. The understanding of molecular pathways involved in the pathogenesis and clinical behavior of lymphomas has served as foundation for new drug development. Many patients, including the considered nonfit ones, may rely on these new drugs for disease control.

References

1. Nowell PC, Hungerford DA (1960) A minute chromosome in human chronic granulocytic leukemia. Science 132:1497
2. Lugo TG, Pendergast AM, Muller AJ, Witte ON (1990) Tyrosine kinase activity and transformation potency of bcr-abl oncogene products. Science 247:1079–1082
3. Druker BJ, Talpaz M, Resta D et al (2001) Efficacy and safety of a specific inhibitor of the Bcr-Abl tyrosine kinase in chronic myeloid leukemia. N Engl J Med 344:1031–1037
4. Coiffier B, Haioun C, Ketterer N et al (1998) Rituximab (anti-CD20 monoclonal antibody) for the treatment of patients with relapsing or refractory aggressive lymphoma: a multicenter phase II study. Blood 92:1927–1932
5. Sievers EL, Larson RA, Stadtmauer EA, the Mylotarg Study Group et al (2001) Efficacy and safety of gemtuzumab ozogamicin in patients with CD33-positive acute myeloid leukemia in first relapse. J Clin Oncol 19:3244–3254
6. Scott AM, Wolchok JD, Old LJ (2012) Antibody therapy of cancer. Nat Rev Cancer 12(4):278–287
7. Wiseman GA, Gordon LI, Multani PS et al (2002) Ibritumomab tiuxetan radioimmunotherapy for patients with relapsed or refractory non-Hodgkin's lymphoma and mild thrombocytopenia: a phase II multicenter trial. Blood 99:4336–4342
8. Jaffe ES, Harris NL, Stein H, Vardiman JW (eds) (2008) World Health Organization classification of tumors: tumours of the haematopoietic and lymphoid tissues. International Agency for Research on Cancer (IARC) Press, Lyon, France, pp 17–44
9. Au WY, Horsman DE, Gascoyne RD, Viswanatha DS, Klasa RJ, Connors JM (2004) The spectrum of lymphoma with 8q24 aberrations: a clinical, pathological and cytogenetic study of 87 consecutive cases. Leuk Lymphoma 45:519–528
10. Kramer MH, Hermans J, Wijburg E, Philippo K, Geelen E, van Krieken JH et al (1998) Clinical relevance of BCL2, BCL6, and MYC rearrangements in diffuse large B-cell lymphoma. Blood 92:3152–3162
11. Le Gouill S, Talmant P, Touzeau C, Moreau A, Garand R, Juge-Morineau N et al (2007) The clinical presentation and prognosis of diffuse large B-cell lymphoma with t(14;18) and 8q24/c-MYC rearrangement. Haematologica 92:1335–1342
12. Kanungo A, Medeiros LJ, Abruzzo LV, Lin P (2006) Lymphoid neoplasms associated with concurrent t(14;18) and 8q24/c-MYC translocation generally have a poor prognosis. Mod Pathol 19:25–33
13. Niitsu N, Okamoto M, Hirano M (2009) Clinical features and prognosis of de novo diffuse large B-cell lymphoma with t(14;18) and 8q24/c-MYC translocations. Leukemia 23:777–783
14. Alizadeh AA, Eisen MB, Davis RE et al (2000) Distinct types of diffuse large B-cell lymphoma identified by gene expression profiling. Nature 403:503–511
15. Rosenwald A, Wright G, Chan WC et al (2002) The use of molecular profiling to predict survival after chemotherapy for diffuse large-B-cell lymphoma. N Engl J Med 346:1937–1947
16. Friedberg JW (2011) New strategies in diffuse large B-cell lymphoma: translating findings from gene expression analyses into clinical practice. Clin Cancer Res 17(19):6112–6117
17. Orsborne C, Byers R (2011) Impact of gene expression profiling in lymphoma diagnosis and prognosis. Histopathology 58(1):106–127
18. Lenz G, Wright G, Dave SS et al (2008) Lymphoma/leukemia molecular profiling project. Stromal gene signatures in large-B-cell lymphomas. N Engl J Med 359(22):2313–2323
19. Thieblemont C, Briere J, Mounier N et al (2011) The germinal center/activated B-cell subclassification has a prognostic impact for response to salvage therapy in relapsed/refractory diffuse large B-cell lymphoma: a bio-CORAL study. J Clin Oncol 29(31):4079–4087
20. Warburg O, Geissler AW, Lorenz S (1967) [On growth of cancer cells in media in which glucose is replaced by galactose]. Hoppe Seylers Z Physiol Chem 348(12):1686–1687

21. Histed SN, Lindenberg ML, Mena E, Turkbey B, Choyke PL, Kurdziel KA (2012) Review of functional/anatomical imaging in oncology. Nucl Med Commun 33(4):349–361
22. Miller JC, Fischman AJ, Aquino SL, Blake MA, Thrall JH, Lee SI (2007) FDG-PET CT for tumor imaging. J Am Coll Radiol 4(4):256–259
23. Blodgett TM, Meltzer CC, Townsend DW (2007) PET/CT: form and function. Radiology 242(2):360–385
24. Cheson BD (2011) Role of functional imaging in the management of lymphoma. J Clin Oncol 29(14):1844–1854
25. Cheson BD, Pfistner B, Juweid ME et al (2007) Revised response criteria for malignant lymphoma. J Clin Oncol 25(5):579–586
26. Juweid ME, Stroobants S, Hoekstra OS et al (2007) Use of positron emission tomography for response assessment of lymphoma: consensus of the Imaging Subcommittee of International Harmonization Project in Lymphoma. J Clin Oncol 25(5):571–578
27. Spaepen K, Stroobants S, Dupont P et al (2001) Prognostic value of positron emission tomography (PET) with fluorine-18 fluorodeoxyglucose ((18F)FDG) after first line chemotherapy in non-Hodgkin's lymphoma: is (18)FDG-PET a valid alternative to conventional diagnostic method? J Clin Oncol 19(2):4141–4149
28. Spaepen K, Stroobants S, Dupont P et al (2002) Early restaging positron emission tomography with (18)-fluorodeoxyglucose predicts outcome in patients with aggressive non-Hodgkin lymphoma. Ann Oncol 13(9):1356–1363
29. Itti E, Lin C, Dupuis J et al (2009) Prognostic value of interim 18F-FDG PET in patients with diffuse large B-cell lymphoma: SUV-based assessment at 4 cycles of chemotherapy. J Nucl Med 50(4):527–533
30. A study of two associations of rituximab and chemotherapy, with a PET-driven strategy, in lymphoma (LNH2007-3B). ClinicalTrials.gov. http://www.clinicaltrials.gov/ct2/show/NCT00498043. (2007) Last accessed on 07 Jan 2011.
31. Tailoring treatment for B cell non-Hodgkin's lymphoma based on PET scan results mid treatment. ClinicalTrials.gov. http://www.clinicaltrials.gov/ct2/show/NCT00324467. (2006) Last accessed 09 Jan 2010.
32. Stewart DA, Duggan P, Bahlis NJ et al (2009) Interim restaging FDG-PET/CT to guide use of high dose sequential induction therapy with rituximab-dose-intensive cyclophosphamide, etoposide, cisplatin (RDICEP) and rituximab-carmustine, etoposide, cytarabine, melphalan (RBEAM) and autologous stem cell transplantation (ASCT) for poor prognosis diffuse large b-cell lymphoma (DLBCL). ClinicalTrials. Gov Identifier: NCT00530179. Blood 114:3414 (ASH Annual Meeting Abstracts)
33. Bhaumik SR, Malik S (2008) Diverse regulatory mechanisms of eukaryotic transcriptional activation by the proteasome complex. Crit Rev Biochem Mol Biol 43:419–433
34. Frankland-Searby S, Bhaumik SR (2012) The 26S proteasome complex: an attractive target for cancer therapy. Biochim Biophys Acta 1825(1):64–76
35. Sterz J, von Metzler I, Hahne JC et al (2008) The potential of proteasome inhibitors in cancer therapy. Expert Opin Investig Drugs 17(6):879–895
36. Voorhees PM, Dees EC, O'Neil B, Orlowski RZ (2003) The proteasome as a target for cancer therapy. Clin Cancer Res 9:6316–6325
37. Adams J, Palombella VJ, Sausville EA et al (1999) Proteasome inhibitors: a novel class of potent and effective antitumor agents. Cancer Res 59:2615–2622
38. Salvat C, Aquaviva C, Jariel-Encontre I et al (1999) Are there multiple proteolytic pathways contributing to c-Fos, c-Jun and p53 protein degradation in vivo? Mol Biol Rep 26:45–51
39. Karin M, Cao Y, Greten FR, Li ZW (2002) NF-kappaB in cancer: from innocent bystander to major culprit. Nat Rev Cancer 2:301–310
40. Hosokawa Y, Seto M (2004) Nuclear factor kappaB activation and antiapoptosis in mucosa-associated lymphoid tissue lymphoma. Int J Hematol 80(3):215–223
41. Martínez-Delgado B, Cuadros M, Honrado E et al (2005) Differential expression of NF-kappaB pathway genes among peripheral T-cell lymphomas. Leukemia 19(12):2254–2263

42. Calado DP, Zhang B, Srinivasan L et al (2010) Constitutive canonical NF-κB activation cooperates with disruption of BLIMP1 in the pathogenesis of activated B cell-like diffuse large cell lymphoma. Cancer Cell 18(6):580–589
43. Goy A, Younes A, McLaughlin P et al (2005) Phase II study of proteasome inhibitor bortezomib in relapsed or refractory B-cell non-Hodgkin's lymphoma. J Clin Oncol 23:667–675
44. Fisher RI, Bernstein SH, Kahl BS et al (2006) Multicenter phase II study of bortezomib in patients with relapsed or refractory mantle cell lymphoma. J Clin Oncol 24(30):4867–4874
45. Ruan J, Martin P, Furman RR, Lee SM, Cheung K, Vose JM, Lacasce A, Morrison J, Elstrom R, Ely S, Chadburn A, Cesarman E, Coleman M, Leonard JP (2011) Bortezomib plus CHOP-rituximab for previously untreated diffuse large B-cell lymphoma and mantle cell lymphoma. J Clin Oncol 29(6):690–697
46. Dunleavy K, Pittaluga S, Czuczman MS, Dave SS, Wright G, Grant N, Shovlin M, Jaffe ES, Janik JE, Staudt LM, Wilson WH (2009) Differential efficacy of bortezomib plus chemotherapy within molecular subtypes of diffuse large B-cell lymphoma. Blood 113(24): 6069–6076
47. Gururajan M, Jennings CD, Bondada S (2006) Cutting edge: constitutive B cell receptor signaling is critical for basal growth of B lymphoma. J Immunol 176:5715–5719
48. Chen L, Monti S, Juszczynski P et al (2008) SYK-dependent tonic B-cell receptor signaling is a rational treatment target in diffuse large B-cell lymphoma. Blood 111:2230–2237
49. Chen L, Juszczynski P, Takeyama K, Aguiar RC, Shipp MA (2006) Protein tyrosine phosphatase receptor-type O truncated (PTPROt) regulates SYK phosphorylation, proximal B-cell receptor signaling, and cellular proliferation. Blood 108:3428–3433
50. Friedberg JW, Sharman J, Sweetenham J et al (2010) Inhibition of Syk with fostamatinib disodium has significant clinical activity in non-Hodgkin lymphoma and chronic lymphocytic leukemia. Blood 115:2578–2585
51. Feldman AL, Sun DX, Law ME et al (2008) Overexpression of Syk tyrosine kinase in peripheral T-cell lymphomas. Leukemia 22:1139–1143
52. Vihinen M, Mattsson PT, Smith CI (2000) Bruton tyrosine kinase (BTK) in X-linked agammaglobulinemia (XLA). Front Biosci 5:D917–D928
53. Winer ES, Ingham RR, Castillo JJ (2012) PCI-32765: a novel Bruton's tyrosine kinase inhibitor for the treatment of lymphoid malignancies. Expert Opin Investig Drugs 21(3):355–361
54. Byrd JC, Blum KA, Burger JA et al (2011) Activity and tolerability of the Bruton's tyrosine kinase (Btk) inhibitor PCI-32765 in patients with chronic lymphocytic leukemia/small lymphocytic lymphoma (CLL/SLL): interim results of a phase Ib/II study. J Clin Oncol 29(suppl):6508
55. Wang L, Martin P, Blum KA et al (2011) The Bruton's tyrosine kinase inhibitor PCI-32765 is highly active as single-agent therapy in previously-treated mantle cell lymphoma (MCL): preliminary results of a phase II trial. Blood 118:442
56. Staudt LM, Dunleavy K, Buggy JJ et al (2011) The Bruton's tyrosine kinase (Btk) inhibitor PCI-32765 modulates chronic active BCR signaling and induces tumor regression in relapsed/refractory ABC DLBCL. Blood 118:2716
57. Goekjian PG, Jirousek MR (2001) Protein kinase C inhibitors as novel anticancer drugs. Expert Opin Investig Drugs 10:2117–2140
58. McMahon G (2000) VEGF receptor signaling in tumor angiogenesis. Oncologist 5(Suppl 1):3–10
59. Ma S, Rosen ST (2007) Enzastaurin. Curr Opin Oncol 19:590–595
60. Robertson MJ, Kahl BS, Vose JM et al (2007) Phase II study of enzastaurin, a protein kinase C beta inhibitor, in patients with relapsed or refractory diffuse large B-cell lymphoma. J Clin Oncol 25:1741–1746
61. Hagemeister FB (2010) Maintenance and consolidation strategies in non-Hodgkin's lymphoma: a review of the data. Curr Oncol Rep 12(6):395–401

62. Kortmansky J, Schwartz GK (2003) Bryostatin-1: a novel PKC inhibitor in clinical development. Cancer Invest 21(6):924–936
63. Whitesell L, Lindquist SL (2005) HSP90 and the chaperoning of cancer. Nat Rev Cancer 5:761–772
64. Jolly C, Morimoto RI (2000) Role of the heat shock response and molecular chaperones in oncogenesis and cell death. J Natl Cancer Inst 92:1564–1572
65. Valbuena JR, Rassidakis GZ, Lin P et al (2005) Expression of heat-shock protein-90 in non-Hodgkin's lymphomas. Mod Pathol 18:1343–1349
66. Georgakis GV, Li Y, Younes A (2006) The heat shock protein 90 inhibitor 17-AAG induces cell cycle arrest and apoptosis in mantle cell lymphoma cell lines by depleting cyclin D1, Akt, Bid and activating caspase 9. Br J Haematol 135:68–71
67. Solit DB, Chiosis G (2008) Development and application of Hsp90 inhibitors. Drug Discov Today 13:38–43
68. Richardson PG, Chanan-Khan A, Lonial S, Krishman A, Carroll M, Cropp GF, Kersey K, Abitar M, Johnson RG, Hannah AL et al (2007) Tanespimycin (T)+bortezomib (BZ) in multiple myeloma (MM): confirmation of the recommended dose using a novel formulation. Blood 110:1165, ASH Annual Meeting Abstracts
69. Modi S, Stopeck AT, Gordon MS, Mendelson D, Solit DB, Bagatell R, Ma W, Wheler J, Rosen N, Norton L et al (2007) Combination of trastuzumab and tanespimycin (17-AAG, KOS-953) is safe and active in trastuzumab-refractory HER-2 overexpressing breast cancer: a phase I dose-escalation study. J Clin Oncol 25:5410–5417
70. Paez J, Sellers WR (2003) PI3K/PTEN/AKT pathway. A critical mediator of oncogenic signaling. Cancer Treat Res 115:145–167
71. Wlodarski P, Kasprzycka M, Liu X et al (2005) Activation of mammalian target of rapamycin in transformed B lymphocytes is nutrient dependent but independent of Akt, mitogen-activated protein kinase/extracellular signal-regulated kinase, insulin growth factor-I, and serum. Cancer Res 65:7800–7808
72. Bertoni F, Zucca E, Cotter FE (2004) Molecular basis of mantle cell lymphoma. Br J Haematol 124:130–140
73. Bjornsti MA, Houghton PJ (2004) The TOR pathway: a target for cancer therapy. Nat Rev Cancer 4:335–348
74. Witzig TE, Geyer SM, Ghobrial I et al (2005) Phase II trial of single-agent temsirolimus (CCI-779) for relapsed mantle cell lymphoma. J Clin Oncol 23:5347–5356
75. Hess G, Herbrecht R, Romaguera J et al (2009) Phase III study to evaluate temsirolimus compared with investigator's choice therapy for the treatment of relapsed or refractory mantle cell lymphoma. J Clin Oncol 27:3822–3829
76. Ansell SM, Tang H, Kurtin P et al (2009) A phase II study of temsirolimus (CCI-779) in combination with rituximab in patients with relapsed or refractory mantle cell lymphoma [Abstract]. Blood 114:166
77. Haritunians T, Mori A, O'Kelly J, Luong QT, Giles FJ, Koeffler HP (2007) Antiproliferative activity of RAD001 (everolimus) as a single agent and combined with other agents in mantle cell lymphoma. Leukemia 21:333–339
78. Jundt F, Raetzel N, Muller C et al (2005) A rapamycin derivative (everolimus) controls proliferation through down-regulation of truncated CCAAT enhancer binding protein beta and NF- {kappa}B activity in Hodgkin and anaplastic large cell lymphomas. Blood 106: 1801–1807
79. Reeder CB, Gornet MK, Habermann TM et al (2007) A phase II trial of the oral mTOR inhibitor everolimus (RAD001) in relapsed aggressive non-Hodgkin lymphoma (NHL). Blood 110:Abstract 121
80. Zent CS, LaPlant BR, Johnston PB et al (2010) The treatment of recurrent/refractory chronic lymphocytic leukemia/small lymphocytic lymphoma (CLL) with everolimus results in clinical responses and mobilization of CLL cells into the circulation. Cancer 116:2201–2207

81. Ghobrial IM, Gertz M, Laplant B et al (2010) Phase II trial of the oral mammalian target of rapamycin inhibitor everolimus in relapsed or refractory Waldenstrom macroglobulinemia. J Clin Oncol 28:1408–1414
82. Witzig TE, Habermann TM, Reeder C et al (2009) A phase II trial of the oral mtor inhibitor everolimus in relapsed non-Hodgkin's lymphoma and Hodgkin disease [Abstract]. Haematologia 94(Suppl 2):436
83. Menhert JM, Kelly WK (2007) Histone deacetylase inhibitors: biology and mechanism of action. Cancer J 13:23–29
84. Shaffer AL, Yu X, He Y et al (2000) BCL-6 represses genes that function in lymphocyte differentiation, inflammation, and cell cycle control. Immunity 13:199–212
85. Olsen EA, Kim YH, Kuzel TM et al (2007) Phase IIB multicenter trial of Vorinostat in patients with persistent, progressive, or treatment refractory cutaneous T-cell lymphoma. J Clin Oncol 25:3109–3115
86. Crump M, Coiffier B, Jacobsen ED et al (2008) Phase II trial of oral vorinostat (suberoylanilide hydroxamic acid) in relapsed diffuse large-B-cell lymphoma. Ann Oncol 19:964–969
87. Crump M, Andreadis C, Assouline S et al (2008) Treatment of relapsed or refractory non-Hodgkin lymphoma with the oral isotype-selective histone deacetylase inhibitor MGCD0103: interim results from a phase II study. J Clin Oncol 26(15 suppl):Abstract 8528
88. Lemoine M, Derenzini E, Buglio D, Medeiros LJ, Davis RE, Zhang J, Ji Y, Younes A (2012) The pan-deacetylase inhibitor panobinostat induces cell death and synergizes with everolimus in Hodgkin lymphoma cell lines. Blood 26:119(17):4017–4025
89. Corral LG, Muller GW, Moreira AL et al (1996) Selection of novel analogs of thalidomide with enhanced tumor necrosis factor alpha inhibitory activity. Mol Med 2:506–515
90. Corral LG, Haslett PA, Muller GW et al (1999) Differential cytokine modulation and T cell activation by two distinct classes of thalidomide analogues that are potent inhibitors of TNF-alpha. J Immunol 163:380–386
91. Haslett PA, Corral LG, Albert M et al (1998) Thalidomide costimulates primary human T lymphocytes, preferentially inducing proliferation, cytokine production, and cytotoxic responses in the CD8+ subset. J Exp Med 187:1885–1982
92. Gupta D, Treon SP, Shima Y et al (2001) Adherence of multiple myeloma cells to bone marrow stromal cells upregulates vascular endothelial growth factor secretion: therapeutic applications. Leukemia 15:1950–1961
93. Weber D, Chen C, Niesviyky R et al (2006) Lenalidomide plus high-dose dexamethasone versus dexamethasone alone for relapsed or refractory multiple myeloma (MM): results of North American phase III study (MM-009). J Clin Oncol 24:427s
94. Dimopoulos MA, Spenser A, Attal M et al (2005) Study of lenalidomide plus dexamethasone versus dexamethasone alone in relapsed or refractory multiple myeloma (MM): results of phase III study (MM-010). Proc Am Soc Hematol 106:6
95. Witzig TE, Vose JM, Zinzani PL et al (2011) An international phase II trial of single-agent lenalidomide for relapsed or refractory aggressive B-cell non-Hodgkin's lymphoma. Ann Oncol 22(7):1622–1627
96. Wang M, Fayad L, Hagemeister F et al (2007) A phase I/II study of lenalidomide in combination with rituximab in relapsed/refractory mantle cell lymphoma with early evidence of efficacy. J Clin Oncol 25(18 suppl):Abstract 8030
97. Nowakowski GS, Reeder CB, LaPlant B et al (2011) Combination of lenalidomide with R-CHOP (R2CHOP) as an initial therapy in aggressive lymphomas: a phase I/II study. J Clin Oncol 29(suppl):Abstract 8015
98. Hernandez-Ilizaliturri FJ, Deeb G, Zinzani PL et al (2011) Higher response to lenalidomide in elapsed/refractory diffuse large B-cell lymphoma in nongerminal center B-cell-like than in germinal center B-cell-like phenotype. Cancer 117(22):5058–5066
99. Nightingale G (2011) Ofatumumab: a novel anti-CD20 monoclonal antibody for treatment of refractory chronic lymphocytic leukemia. Ann Pharmacother 45(10):1248–1255
100. Sanford M, McCormack PL (2010) Ofatumumab. Drugs 70(8):1013–1019

101. Czuczman MS, Fayad L, Delwail V et al (2012) Ofatumumab monotherapy in rituximab-refractory follicular lymphoma: results from a multicenter study. Blood 119(16):3698–3704
102. Coiffier B, Bosly A, Wu KL et al (2010) Ofatumumab monotherapy for treatment of patients with relapsed/progressive diffuse large B cell lymphoma: results from a multicenter phase II study. Blood 116:Abstract 3955
103. Morschhauser F, Leonard JP, Fayad L et al (2009) Humanized anti-CD20 antibody, veltuzumab, in refractory/recurrent non-Hodgkin's lymphoma: phase I/II results. J Clin Oncol 27(20):3346–3353
104. Mössner E, Brünker P, Moser S et al (2010) Increasing the efficacy of CD20 antibody therapy through the engineering of a new type II anti-CD20 antibody with enhanced direct and immune effector cell-mediated B-cell cytotoxicity. Blood 115(22):4393–4402
105. Cartron G, Thieblemont C, Solal-Celigny P et al (2010) Promising efficacy with the new anti-CD20 antibody GA101 in heavily pre-treated NHL patients—first results from a phase II study in patients with relapsed/refractory DLBCL and MCL. Blood 116(21):2878 (ASH Annual Meeting Abstracts)
106. Micallef IN, Maurer MJ, Wiseman GA et al (2011) Epratuzumab with rituximab, cyclophosphamide, doxorubicin, vincristine, and prednisone chemotherapy in patients with previously untreated diffuse large B-cell lymphoma. Blood 118(15):4053–4061
107. Bhat S, Czuczman MS (2010) Galiximab: a review. Expert Opin Biol Ther 10(3):451–458
108. Advani R, Forero-Torres A, Furman RR et al (2009) Phase I study of the humanized anti-CD40 monoclonal antibody dacetuzumab in refractory or recurrent non-Hodgkin's lymphoma. J Clin Oncol 27(26):4371–4377
109. Forero-Torres A, Bartlett NL, Nasta SD et al (2009) A phase 1b clinical trial of dacetuzumab in combination with rituximab and gemcitabine: multiple responses observed in patients with relapsed diffuse large b-cell lymphoma. Blood 114:586 (ASH Annual Meeting Abstracts)
110. Nagorsen D, Zugmaier G, Viardot A et al (2009) Confirmation of safety, efficacy and response duration in non-Hodgkin lymphoma patients treated with 60 μg/m2/d of BiTE® antibody Blinatumomab. Blood 114:2723 (ASH Annual Meeting Abstracts)
111. Dang NH, Smith MR, Offner F et al (2009) Anti-CD22 Immunoconjugate inotuzumab ozogamicin (CMC-544)+rituximab: clinical activity including survival in patients with recurrent/refractory follicular or 'aggressive' lymphoma. Blood 114:584 (ASH Annual Meeting Abstracts)
112. Shaffer AL, Rosenwald A, Staudt LM (2002) Lymphoid malignancies: the dark side of B-cell differentiation. Nat Rev Immunol 2(12):920–932

New Monoclonal Antibodies for Indolent Non-Hodgkin Lymphoma

Tadeusz Robak

Abstract Over the last few years, several new monoclonal antibodies (mAbs) directed against lymphoid cells have been developed and investigated in indolent non-Hodgkin lymphoma (NHL). New generations of anti-CD20 mAbs were engineered to have augmented antitumor activity by increasing complement-dependent cytotoxicity or antibody-dependent cellular cytotoxicity and increased Fc binding affinity for the low-affinity variants of the FcγRIIIa receptor on immune effector cells. The second-generation mAbs are humanized or fully human to reduce immunogenicity. They include ofatumumab, veltuzumab, and ocrelizumab. The third-generation mAbs, including AME133v, Pro13192, and GA-101, are also humanized, but, in comparison with the second-generation mAbs, they also have an engineered Fc region designed to increase their effector functions. Some other new mAbs are also active in indolent NHL. These treatments include epratuzumab, apolizumab, galiximab, anti-TRAIL receptors mAbs, and anti-CD40 mAbs. Small modular immunopharmaceuticals (SMIP) that retain Fc-mediated effector functions have been also developed and investigated in preclinical studies and clinical trials. The SMIP molecules include TRU-015 (anti-CD20) and TRU-016 (anti-CD37). In addition, zanolimumab is a promising new antibody for the treatment of T CD4+ cell malignancies.

T. Robak (✉)
Department of Hematology, Medical University of Lodz, Copernicus Memorial Hospital, 93-510 Lodz, Ul. Ciolkowskiego 2, Lodz, Poland
e-mail: robaktad@csk.umed.lodz.pl

P.J. Quesenberry and J.J. Castillo (eds.), *Non-Hodgkin Lymphoma: Prognostic Factors and Targets*, Cancer Drug Discovery and Development,
DOI 10.1007/978-1-4614-5851-7_11,

Table 1 Novel anti-CD20 monoclonal antibodies

MoAb	Target	Antibody characteristics
Ocrelizumab	CD20	Type I, 2nd generation, humanized IgG1; binding to different CD20 epitope than rituximab; enhanced ADCC and reduced CDC; enhanced affinity for FcγRIIIa RIIIa
Veltuzumab (IMMU-106, hA20)	CD20	Type I, 2nd generation, humanized IgG1; binding to different CD20 epitope than rituximab; enhanced ADCC and reduced CDC, enhanced affinity for FcγRIIIa RIIIa
Ofatumumab (HuMax-CD20, Arzerra)	CD20	Type I, 2nd generation, human IgG1, binding to different CD20 epitope than rituximab, more effective at CDC and less at ADCC than rituximab
GA-101 (RO5072759)	CD20	Type II, 3rd generation, humanized IgG1, superior ADCC than rituximab and superior direct cell killing
AME-133 (Obinutuzumab, LY2469298)	CD20	Type I, 3rd generation, humanized fusion IgG1; enhanced affinity for FcγRIIIa, superior ADCC
PRO131921	CD20	Type I, 3rd generation, humanized fusion IgG1, improved binding to FcγRIIIa, better ADCC, superior antitumor efficacy
TRU-015	CD20	Antibody-based single-chain polypeptide (SMIP) derived humanized fusion protein; CDC, ADCC and apoptosis induction

Introduction

Rituximab (Rituxan, Mabthera, F. Hoffmann–La Roche), anti-CD20 monoclonal antibody (mAb), was approved by the FDA in 1997 for the treatment of non-Hodgkin lymphoma (NHL). This drug, especially when combined with chemotherapy, has a significant impact in the treatment of B-cell lymphoid malignancies [1]. However, rituximab is only partially effective in NHL, exposing an obvious need to develop new, more specific and active agents. Recently, several new anti-CD20 mAbs have recently been developed (Table 1). In addition, other aAbs targeting B- and T-cell surface molecules are also being evaluated in preclinical and clinical studies (Table 2, Fig. 1). Several of them are under investigation in patients with lymphoid malignancies in phase I/II clinical trials, as single agents or in combination with other drugs (Table 3) [2, 3].

Anti-CD20 Monoclonal Antibodies

New generations of anti-CD20 mAbs have been developed recently (Fig. 1; Table 1) [4, 5]. They were engineered to have augmented antitumor activity by increasing complement-dependent cytotoxicity (CDC) or antibody-dependent cellular cytotoxicity (ADCC) and increased Fc binding affinity for the low-affinity variants of the FcγRIIIa receptor (CD16) on immune effector cells [6].

Table 2 Novel monoclonal antibodies potentially useful for indolent non Hodgkin lymphoma therapy

MoAb	Target	Antibody characteristics
Epratuzumab (hLL2)	CD22	Recombinant, humanized $IgG_{1-\kappa}$; activity mediated through ADCC, reduced CDC
Inotuzumab ozogamicin t(CMC-544)	CD22	Humanized IgG4 covalently linked to calicheamicin, binds to DNA, causes DNA-strand breaks and apoptosis
BL-22 (RFB4 (dsFv)-PE38)	CD22	Recombinant immunotoxin consisting of the Fv portion of the anti-CD22 antibody RFB4 fused to a fragment of *Pseudomonas* exotoxin-A
Moxetumomab pasudotox (CAT-8015, HA22)	CD22	Anti-CD22 antibody fused to the modified form of *Pseudomonas* exotoxin-A (PE38); greater affinity for CD22 than BL-22
Apolizumab (HU1D10, Remitogen)	HLA-DRβ	Humanized IgG1 inducing ADCC, CDC, and apoptosis
Milatuzumab (IMMU-115)	CD74	Humanized IgG1 inducing ADCC, CDC, and apoptosis
Lucatumumab (HCD122, CHIR-0.12.12)	CD40	Human IgG1, blocking interaction of CD40 and its ligand on malignant cells, ADCC induction
Dacetuzumab (SGN-40)	CD40	Humanized IgG1, apoptosis, and ADCC induction
Galiximab (B 7.1; IDEC-114)	CD80	Chimeric IgG1 antibody with human constant regions and primate (cynomologous macaque) variable regions; ADCC induction
TRU-016	CD37	Antibody-based single-chain polypeptide (SMIP derived humanized fusion protein); induction of apoptosis directly via binding to the CD37 receptor, CDC and ADCC induction
Blinatumomab (MT-103)	CD19/CD3	Bispecific, T cell engaging antibody, effectively redirected T cells for selective lysis of CD19+ B cells
XmAb5574	CD19	Humanized antibody with a modified Fc domain
Mapatumumab (HGS-ETR1)	TRAIL-R1	Fully human IgG1 inducing apoptosis
Lexatumumab	TRAIL-R2	Fully human IgG1 inducing apoptosis
Conatumumab(AMG 655)	TRAIL-R2	Fully human IgG1 inducing apoptosis
Spilizumab (MEDI-507)	CD2	Humanized anti-CD2 IgG1κ, ADCC induction
Zanolimumab(HuMax-CD4)	CD4	Human IgG1κ, exerts its action through inhibition of CD4+ T-cell signaling and decreasing T-cell activation

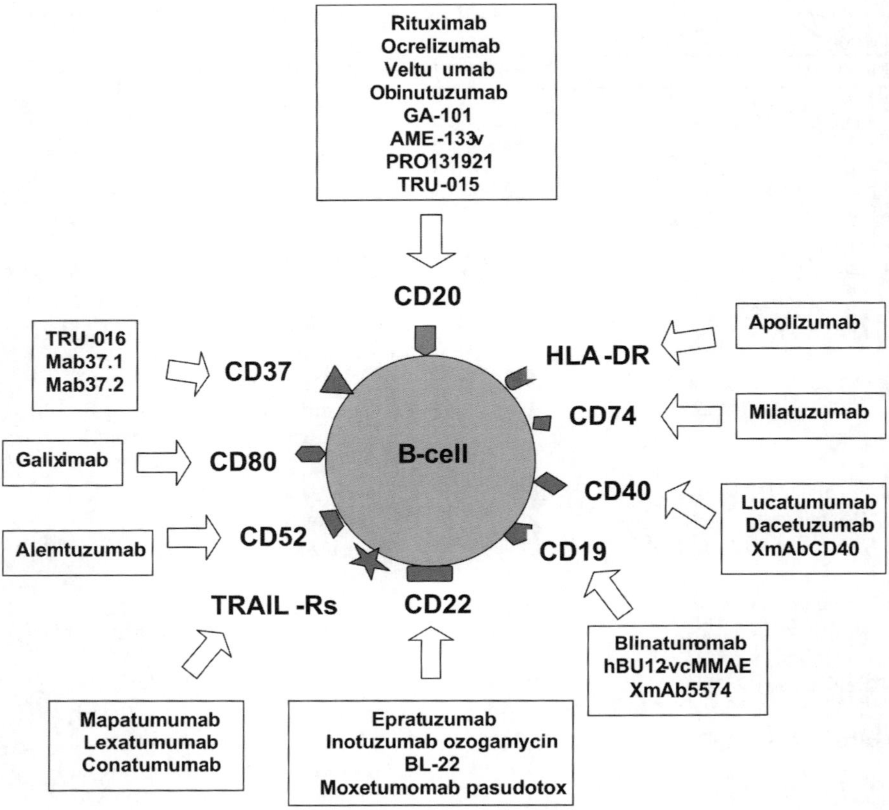

Fig. 1 B-cell surface antigen targets for therapeutic monoclonal antibodies

Second-Generation Anti-CD20 Monoclonal Antibodies

The second-generation mAbs are humanized or fully human to reduce immunogenicity but with an unmodified Fc region. They include ocrelizumab, veltuzumab, and ofatumumab.

Ocrelizumab

Ocrelizumab (Genentech Inc./Biogen Idec Inc./Chugai Pharmaceutical Co. Ltd/ Roche Holding Ag) is a type 1, humanized, anti-CD20, IgG1 mAb that leads to enhanced ADCC and reduced CDC activities compared with rituximab [7]. This agent has the potential for enhanced efficacy in NHL compared with rituximab due to increased binding affinity for the low-affinity variants of the FcγRIIIa receptor on

Table 3 Clinical trials of novel monoclonal antibodies (mAbs) in indolent non-Hodgkin lymphoma

Study	Monoclonal antibody	Diagnosis	Study phase	Number of pts	Response
Morschhauser et al. [9]	Ocrelizumab	Relapsed/refractory FL	I/II	47	OR: 36% CR/CRu: 13%
Morschhauser et al. [14]	Veltuzumab	Relapsed/refractory NHL	I/II	82 (55 FL)	OR in FL: 44% CR in FL: 27%
Negrea et al. [13]	Veltuzumab	Untreated or relapsed NHL or CLL	I/II	26	NHL: CR + Cru + PR: 53% (8/15) CLL-OR: 0
Hagenbeek et al. [15]	Ofatumumab	Relapsed/refractory FL	I/II	40	OR: 20–63%
Hagenbeek et al. [18]	Ofatumumab	Refractory to rituximab FL	III	116	OR: 11%
Salles et al. [21]	GA-101	Relapsed/refractory NHL	I/IIa	24[a]	CR: 19% PR: 25%
Salles et al. [22]	GA-101	Relapsed/refractory NHL	I	21	OR: 43% 5 CR/CRu, 4 PR
Friedberg et al. [34]	PRO131921	Relapsed/refractory indolent NHL	I	24 (22 FL)	PR: 6 pts
Leonard et al. [30]	Epratuzumab	Recurrent indolent NHL	I/II	55	OR: 18% CR: 3 pts
Advani et al. [35]	Inotuzumab ozogamicin	Relapsed/refractory NHL	I	79 (35FL)	OR: 39% (68% for FL treated with MTD)
Czuczman et al. [53]	Galiximab	Relapsed/refractory FL	I/II	35	OR: 11% (2CR, 2PR)
Younes et al. [68]	Mapatumumab	Relapsed/refractory NHL	Ib/II	40 (17FL)	OR: 3 pts CR: 2 pts
Viardot et al. [61]	Blinatumomab	Relapsed NHL	I	22 (12FL)	OR: 82% CR + Cru: 45%
Kim et al. [77]	Zanolimumab	Refraktory CTCL	II	46	OR: 15 pts

[a]Complete data available on the first 12 patients

CR complete response, *CRu* CR unconfirmed, *CTCL* cutaneous T-cell lymphoma, *FL* follicular lymphoma, *NHL* non-Hodgkin lymphoma, *OR* overall response, *pt* patient, *PR* partial response immune effector cells [8]. Ocrelizumab binds to a different, but overlapping, epitope of the extracellular domain of CD20 as compared with rituximab. In a dose-escalation study, a total of 47 patients with relapsed/refractory follicular lymphoma (FL) following prior rituximab-containing therapy received infusions of ocrelizumab every 3 weeks at 200, 375, and 750 mg/m^2 for up to eight doses [9]. The overall response (OR) rate was 38%, including 13% complete response (CR) or CR unconfirmed (CRu). The median progression-free survival (PFS) was 11.4 months. The most common adverse events (AEs) were infusion-related reactions observed in 74% of the patients.

Veltuzumab

Veltuzumab (IMMU-106, hA20; Immunomedics Inc., Morris Plains, NJ) is a type 1, humanized, anti-CD20, IgG1 mAb with complementarity-determining regions (CDRs) similar to rituximab [10]. This mAb is generated using the same human immunoglobulin as the anti-CD22 mAb epratuzumab and has a >90% humanized framework. It is also very similar to rituximab in terms of antigen binding, specificity binding, and dissociation constant [11]. Veltuzumab differs from rituximab by one amino acid (Asp101 instead of Asn101) in the CDR3 region of the variable heavy chain. This antibody has enhanced binding avidities and a stronger effect on CDC compared with rituximab in selected cell lines [12]. When compared with rituximab, veltuzumab had significantly reduced off-rates in three human lymphoma cell lines tested, as well as increased CDC in one of three cell lines, but no other in vitro differences [10].

Initial clinical studies have shown good safety and efficacy results in NHL patients and have confirmed its effectiveness [9, 13, 14]. Veltuzumab can be given in a shorter infusion time than approved doses of rituximab and can be administered subcutaneously. A phase I/II dose-escalation study was performed in 82 patients with relapsed/refractory NHL including 55 FL and 27 other B-cell lymphomas [14]. Veltuzumab was administered once weekly for 4 weeks at doses ranging from 80 to 750 mg/m^2. In the FL group, 24 (44%) patients had objective response, with 15 (27%) CR or CRu. Median duration of CR was 19.7 months. The drug was generally well tolerated with no grade 3–4 drug-related AEs.

Subcutaneous administration of veltuzumab was also investigated in a multicenter, phase I/II study in previously untreated or relapsed CD20+ indolent NHL or chronic lymphocytic leukemia (CLL) [13]. Twenty-six patients, including 15 NHL and 11 CLL, received subcutaneous veltuzumab 2 weeks apart at dose levels of 80, 160, or 320 mg. In the NHL patients, the objective response rate was 53% (8/15), with a CR rate of 20% (3/15). In NHL, these low subcutaneous doses achieved sustained serum levels with OR rates and durable CR comparable to those seen even with higher intravenous doses. Treatment was well tolerated, with only mild, transient injection-site reactions and tenderness. Further clinical studies of veltuzumab given in intravenous or subcutaneous injection are ongoing, either as a single agent or in combination regimens (ClinicalTrials.gov identifier: NCT00112970; NCT00989586; NCT01147393; NCT00546793).

Ofatumumab

Ofatumumab (HuMax-CD20; Arzerra™, GlaxoSmithKline plc/Genmab A/S) is a fully human, IgG1 mAb recognizing a different CD20 epitope to rituximab and demonstrating a higher cytotoxic potential than rituximab [15, 16]. Ofatumumab is more effective than rituximab at CDC induction and killing target cells [16, 17]. The close binding proximity of ofatumumab to the cell membrane likely results in highly efficient complement deposition on B-cell membranes, without high levels of systemic release of activated complement components.

The results of the first phase I/II clinical trial with ofatumumab in CD20-positive, relapsed, or refractory FL patients have been reported recently [15]. Patients received eight once-weekly infusions of ofatumumab (dose 1, 300 mg; doses 2–8, 500 or 1,000 mg). The OR rate in the 1,000 mg group was 10%, including one CR, and the median PFS was 6.0 months. The OR rate in the total population was 11%, and stable disease was observed in 50% of the patients. Among 27 patients who were refractory to prior rituximab monotherapy, the OR rate was 22%, indicating activity despite refractoriness to rituximab. In another study, patients with rituximab-refractory FL received eight once-weekly infusions of ofatumumab (dose 1, 300 mg; doses 2–8, 500 or 1,000 mg). The OR rate in the 1,000 mg group was 10%, including one CR [18]. Ofatumumab was well tolerated, and no unexpected toxicities were observed.

Third-Generation Anti-CD20 Monoclonal Antibodies

The third-generation mAbs are also humanized, but in comparison with the second-generation mAbs, they also have an engineered Fc region designed to increase their effector functions by increasing binding affinity for the FcγRIIIa receptor [4]. Both polymorphisms in FcγRIIIa and the structure of mAb Fc can impact on the affinity between FcγRIIIa and mAb. The third-generation mAbs include GA-101, AME133v, and Pro131921.

GA-101

GA-101 (RO5072759 Obinutuzumab, Hoffman La Roche and Genentech) is a fully humanized, type II, anti-CD20, IgG1 mAb that differs significantly from other anti-CD20 mAbs [19, 20]. It has been derived from humanization of the parental B-Ly1 mouse antibody and subsequent glycoengineering using GlycoMab® technology. GA-101 was engineered for enhanced ADCC, superior direct cell-killing properties and low CDC activity, in comparison with currently available type I antibodies. GA-101 binds with high affinity to the CD20 epitope, and, as a result, induction of ADCC is 5–100 times greater than rituximab. It also exhibits greater caspase-independent apoptosis induction than rituximab. However, its CDC activity is low.

In a phase I/IIa study, GA-101 was evaluated as a single agent at doses from 50 to 2,000 mg in 24 patients with aggressive and indolent NHL or CLL. The patients had previously received a median of four prior regimens with 95% of them exposed to prior rituximab [21]. GA-101 was administered intravenously as a single agent on days 1, 8, and 22 and subsequently every 3 weeks for a total of nine infusions. The antibody demonstrated a similar safety profile to rituximab. Circulating B-cell depletion occurred rapidly and was sustained in all patients. Overall response was observed in nine (43%) patients, including five CR/CRu and four partial responses (PR). Six patients had an ongoing response ranging from 7.5+ to 17+ months. The pharmacokinetic data collected for GA-101 was reported to be similar to that of rituximab [22]. The most common AEs were grade 1 or 2 infusion-related reactions essentially limited to the first infusion. It is currently being explored as a single agent and in combination with chemotherapy in phase II and III studies in indolent/aggressive NHL and CLL (ClinicalTrials.gov Identifier: NCT00576758; NCT00825149; NCT01010061).

AME133v

AME-133v (LY2469298; Eli Lilly & Company) is a type I, humanized IgG1 mAb with enhanced affinity for CD20 and FcγRIIIa and an enhanced ADCC activity compared with rituximab [4]. In vitro experiments showed that tumor cells coated with this mAb are more effective at activating NK cells at both low and saturating mAb concentrations irrespective of FcγRIIIa polymorphism [23]. When compared with rituximab, AME-133v has a tenfold improved killing of human B cells, suggesting that AME-133v would exhibit greater potency and efficacy than rituximab in the treatment of CD20-positive lymphoid malignancies. This mAb may be particularly useful in patients carrying low-affinity FcγRIIIa genotypes (e.g., *FCGR3A* 158Phe/Phe), who do not respond well to rituximab.

PRO131921

PRO131921 (Genentech, Inc.) is a type 1, humanized 2H7 mAb engineered to have improved binding to FcγRIIIa and better ADCC compared with rituximab [6]. In preclinical in vivo lymphoma models, PRO131921 has superior antitumor efficacy compared with rituximab. In a phase I study, PRO131921 was evaluated in 24 patients with CD20+, relapsed or refractory NHL, including 20 patients with FL [24]. They were treated with PRO131921 at doses of 25–800 mg/m^2 by intravenous infusions once weekly for 4 weeks on days 1, 8, 15, and 22. There were six cases of PR, 13 of stable disease, and three of progressive disease. The most common AEs were grade 1 or 2 chills, fatigue, fever, nausea, dizziness, diarrhea, and hypotension. Pharmacokinetic data for PRO131921 were similar to rituximab. A correlation between higher normalized drug exposure (normalized AUC) and both tumor shrinkage and clinical response was observed.

Small Modular Immunopharmaceuticals

Small modular immunopharmaceutical (SMIP™) molecules are single-chain polypeptides consisting of one binding domain, one hinge domain, and one effector domain [25]. SMIP biopharmaceuticals belong to a novel proprietary biologic compound class that retain Fc-mediated effector functions and are smaller than mAbs.

TRU-015

The TRU-015 SMIP molecule (CytoxB20G, Trubion Pharmaceuticals Inc. and Pfizer Inc.) is derived from key domains of an anti-CD20 antibody, for the potential intravenous infusion treatment of autoimmune diseases and B-cell lymphoid malignancies. TRU-015 consists of a single-chain Fv specific for CD20 linked to the human IgG1 hinge domain and the heavy-chain constant region domains CH2 and CH3 [26]. It is effective in mediating target cell killing in the mechanism of ADCC but has reduced CDC activity compared with rituximab. TRU-015 also showed direct, pro-apoptotic activity against B-lymphoma cells. At equivalent dose levels, TRU-015 was more effective than rituximab in vivo against large volume Ramos and moderate volume Daudi lymphoma xenograft models and was comparable to rituximab in B-cell depletion in nonhuman primates following single-dose administration [27, 28]. Clinical development efforts for the treatment of lymphoma are ongoing (ClinicalTrials.gov Identifier: NCT00521638).

Anti-CD22 Monoclonal Antibodies

CD22 is a membrane glycophosphoprotein found on nearly all healthy B-lymphocytes and most B-cell lymphomas. Anti-CD22 mAbs induce signal transduction processes and apoptosis in targeted cells.

Epratuzumab

Epratuzumab (Immunomedix, Inc., Moris Plains, NJ, USA) is a humanized anti-CD22 mAb currently in clinical trials for treatment of non-Hodgkin lymphoma and autoimmune disorders [29]. It was derived from the murine IgG2a MoA (LL2) generated against Raji Burkitt lymphoma cells, which acts as an immunomodulatory agent. Epratuzumab induced internalization and signaling of CD22 when tested in vitro on Burkitt B-cell lines and fresh CLL cells and is selectively active against normal and neoplastic B cells [29]. The combination of epratuzumab and rituximab is more effective than rituximab alone in inhibiting proliferation of Daudi Burkitt lymphoma.

In phase I/II trials, patients with NHL were treated with intravenous epratuzumab weekly for 4 weeks at doses of either 120, 240, 360, 480, 600, or 1,000 mg/m^2 [30]. Overall, 24% of FL patients showed an objective response. However, there was no objective response among the group of 12 patients with small lymphocytic lymphoma (SLL). Other studies demonstrated higher efficacy of epratuzumab in combination with rituximab [31, 32].

Inotuzumab Ozogamicin

Inotuzumab ozogamicin (CMC-544, Wyet) is a CD22-targeted cytotoxic agent composed of a humanized IgG4 anti-CD22 antibody covalently linked to calicheamicin, a potent cytotoxic antitumor antibiotic [33]. In various animal models of human B-cell lymphomas (BCL), inotuzumab ozogamicin induced dose-dependent regression of the tumors [34]. In a disseminated BCL model, 60% of inotuzumab ozogamicin-treated mice and 20% of rituximab-treated mice survived for 125 days. In a phase I study, CMC-544 showed significant clinical activity in patients with relapsed/refractory FL and diffused large B-cell lymphoma (DLBCL) with clinically manageable thrombocytopenia as the main toxicity [35]. The OR rate was 39% for the 79 enrolled patients including 68% for patients with FL treated at the maximum tolerated dose (MTD). Median PFS for FL patients was 10 months.

Anti-CD22 Immunotoxins

Two immunotoxins, BL-22 and moxetumomab pasudotox, targeting CD22 have been investigated in indolent lymphoid malignancies.

BL-22

BL-22 (RFB4 (dsFv)-PE38, CAT-3888, GCR-3888; Genencor) is a 63-kDa recombinant immunotoxin containing truncated *Pseudomonas* exotoxin and variable domains from anti-CD22. Sixteen hairy cell leukemia (HCL) patients who were resistant to 2-CdA were included into the study. BL22 at doses between 0.2 and 4.0 mg was administered as a 30 min intravenous infusion every other day to a total of three doses. Of 16 patients treated with this antibody, 11 (69%) had a CR and 2 had a PR. During a median follow-up of 16 months, 3 of the 11 patients who had a CR were retreated with BL22 because of relapse, and all of them had a second CR [36].

Moxetumomab Pasudotox

Moxetumomab pasudotox (CAT-8015, HA22; Medimmune, Inc.) is a new generation of CD22-specific targeted immunotoxin composed of anti-CD22 antibody fused to the modified form of *Pseudomonas* exotoxin [37]. This agent has a novel mechanism of action as compared to other anti-CD22 monoclonal antibodies. Moxetumomab pasudotox is internalized upon binding to CD22, inhibiting protein translation and promoting apoptosis. Preliminary results of moxetumomab pasudotox in patients with refractory/relapsed hairy cell leukemia have been recently reported. A total of 26 patients have received moxetumomab pasudotox to date including 14 treated previously with rituximab. No dose limited toxicity (DLT) has been established so far, and MTD has not been reached. Nineteen patients (73.1%) responded with a CR rate of 34.6% and a PR rate of 38.5%. This data indicates that moxetumomab pasudotox is a promising new agent for patients with HCL and supports further investigation in patients with this disease and other CD22-positive indolent lymphoid malignancies.

Anti-HLA-DR

The human leukocyte antigen-DR (HLA-DR) is one of three polymorphic isotypes of the class II major histocompatibility complex (MHC) antigen. HLA-DR is expressed on most malignant and normal B cells.

Apolizumab

Apolizumab (HU1D10, Remitogen [Protein Design Labs, Fermont, CA], anti-MHC-II) is a humanized IgG1 antibody specific for a polymorphic determinant found on the HLA-DRβ chain. Apolizumab can induce apoptosis in CLL cells and other NHL cells [38]. In addition, this mAb induces ADCC and CDC based on expression of target antigen and alters the cell membrane polarization and permeability [39]. Rech et al. reported the results of a pilot study evaluating the effectiveness and toxicity of apolizumab with granulocyte colony-stimulating factor (G-CSF) in the treatment of refractory or relapsed NHL patients [40]. The doses of apolizumab ranged from 0.15 to 1.5 mg/m^2. The combination was clinically well tolerated with only two patients experiencing grade 3/4 hematological toxicity. Two patients with FL obtained prolonged stabilization lasting 12 and 36 months. However, given the toxicity and low efficacy in NHL, further development of apolizumab was discontinued.

Anti-CD74 Monoclonal Antibodies

CD74 is a type II trans membrane glycoprotein that functions as a MHC class II molecule [41]. The selective expression of this molecule on NHL cells and fast internalization provides an attractive target for antibody-based therapy.

Milatuzumab

Milatuzumab (hLL1, IMMU-115, Immunomedics, Inc.) is a humanized LL1 mAb (IgG1κ) investigated as a novel therapeutic approach for the therapy of CD74-expressing malignancies, such as NHL and multiple myeloma (MM) [42]. Preclinical studies of milatuzumab have shown its therapeutic activity in B-cell malignancies. A high therapeutic index was achieved in preclinical models of NHL with a recombinant fusion protein of humanized anti-CD74 and the toxin Ranpirnase and an immunoconjugate composed of doxorubicin and hLL1 (hLL1-dox, IMMU-110) [43, 44]. Phase I/II trials of milatuzumab in patients with lymphoma are now under way (ClinicalTrials.gov Identifier: NCT00989586, NCT00868478).

Anti-CD40 Monoclonal Antibodies

CD40 is a type-1 transmembrane protein of the tumor necrosis factor receptor superfamily, overexpressed by the malignant B cells [2]. Preclinical and early clinical data with CD40 antibodies have validated CD40 as a target for B-lineage malignancies. Two mAbs directed against CD40 have been developed and investigated in preclinical studies and clinical trials: lucatumumab (HCD122) and dacetuzumab (SGN-40).

Lucatumumab

Lucatumumab (HCD122, CHIR-0.12.12; Novartis Pharmaceuticals) is a fully human anti-CD40 mAb that blocks CD40/CD40L interactions in vitro and inhibits CD40L-induced proliferation of human peripheral blood lymphocytes without disturbing baseline lymphocyte proliferation. Lucatumumab triggers cell lysis via ADCC in cells overexpressing CD40 [45, 46]. A Phase I/II study in adults with NHL who have progressed after at least two prior therapies is currently ongoing (ClinicalTrials.gov Identifier: NCT00670592).

Dacetuzumab (SGN-40)

Dacetuzumab (Seattle Genetics, Inc) is another humanized anti-CD40 IgG1 mAb, which induces ADCC and apoptosis of NHL cells contributing to in vivo antitumor activity observed in human lymphoma xenograft models [47]. Dacetuzumab is able to initiate multiple signaling cascades upon ligation of CD40 on NHL cell lines. Dacetuzumab-mediated cytotoxicity is associated with upregulation of cytotoxic ligands of the tumor necrosis factor (TNF) family including Fas/FasL, TNF-related apoptosis-inducing ligand, and TNFalpha. The toxicity profile and preliminary antitumor activity of dacetuzumab were investigated in phase I study in patients with refractory or recurrent B-cell NHL. Six objective responses were reported including one CR and five PR [48]. No dose dependence of AEs was observed.

XmAbCD40

XmAbCD40 is a humanized anti-CD40 antibody with Fc engineered for increased FcγR binding [45]. XmAbCD40 has significantly enhanced ADCC relative to anti-CD40 IgG1 against B-cell NHL, leukemia, and MM cell lines and against primary tumors. In addition, it significantly inhibited lymphoma growth in disseminated and established mouse xenografts and was more effective than rituximab.

Anti-CD80 Monoclonal Antibodies

CD80 is a member of the B7 family of costimulatory molecules expressed in antigen-presenting cells, normal B cells, and various subtypes of B-cell lymphomas. It is known for its role in regulating T-cell activity and in regulation of normal and malignant B cells [49]. In vitro binding of CD80 by specific monoclonal antibodies results in growth inhibition and apoptosis of normal and malignant B cells [50]. CD80 is an attractive target for mAbs potentially useful in the treatment of lymphoid malignancies.

Galiximab

Galiximab (B 7.1; Biogen Idec Inc., San Diego, CA) is a macaque–human chimeric anti-CD80 monoclonal antibody with human IgG1 constant region and macaque variable region. Preclinical studies on various B-cell lymphoma cell lines indicate that galiximab induces cell lysis in the mechanism of ADCC [51]. Galiximab in combination with rituximab increased ADCC and increased survival over that observed with either drug alone [52]. Early clinical trials seem to confirm high activity and acceptable toxicity of galiximab in lymphoid malignancies in humans [53, 54]. Czuczman et al. [53], in multicenter, dose-escalation phase I/II study, evaluated the safety, pharmacokinetics, and efficacy of galiximab in patients with relapsed or refractory FL. Four patients (11%) responded, including two CR and two PR, and 12 patients (34%) demonstrated a stable condition. The time to best response was delayed in comparison with other mAbs, suggesting an alternative mechanism of action. A total of 22 (60%) of 37 patients experienced adverse events related to galiximab. More recently, Leonard et al. [54] conducted a phase II study to evaluate galiximab in combination with standard doses of rituximab in patients with relapsed FL. Seventy-three patients received rituximab at 375 mg/m^2 and galiximab at doses 125, 250, 375, or 500 mg/m^2. The OR rate at recommended phase II dose of galiximab 500 mg/m^2 was 60%, including 19% CR, 14% unconfirmed CR, and 33% PR. The median progression-free survival was 12.1 months. The most common study-related adverse events were lymphopenia, neutropenia, fatigue, and chills.

Anti-CD37 Monoclonal Antibodies

CD37 is a heavily glycosylated 40–52 kDa tetraspanin transmembrane family protein selectively expressed on normal mature B cells and by most B-cell malignancies [25]. CD37 is upregulated in CLL cells compared with healthy peripheral blood leukocytes, and significant expression has also been detected on neoplastic cells of patients with NHL. Reduced levels have been detected on plasma cells, and non-detectable levels found on CD10+ precursor B cells in the bone marrow. However, it is expressed at a very low density on monocytes, macrophages, neutrophils, T cells, plasma cells, and dendritic cells and is not expressed on erythrocytes, platelets, or NK cells.

TRU-016

TRU-016 (Trubion Pharmaceuticals Inc.) is a new humanized anti-CD37 SMIP protein directed against CD37 [25]. TRU-016 induces apoptosis directly via binding to the CD37 receptor, which results in upregulation of a pro-apoptotic protein, BIM. The drug has a favorable safety profile and significant activity in indolent lymphoid malignancies. In phase I study, TRU-016 encouraged reduction in tumor lymphocyte blood counts, lymph node/spleen size, and improvement in normal hematopoietic function in patients with high-risk CLL [55]. For CLL patients with one or two prior therapies, the OR rate was 44% (7/16). Phase 1/1b study of TRU-016 in patients with previously treated CLL or selected subtypes of NHL is ongoing (ClinicalTrials.gov Identifier: NCT00614042).

MAb 37.1 and MAb 37.2

MAb 37.1 is a chimeric IgG1-type of anti-CD37 molecule which has been Fc engineered to improve ADCC activity. MAb 37.2 is a humanized version of mAb 37.1 [56]. Both antibodies deplete CLL cells in vitro more effectively than rituximab and alemtuzumab. These antibodies should be further investigated in CLL and NHL in clinical trials

Anti-CD19 Monoclonal Antibodies

CD19 is a 95-kDa glycoprotein member of the immunoglobulin (Ig) superfamily expressed from the earliest stages of pre-B-cell development until terminal B-cell differentiation into plasma cells [57]. CD19 represents an attractive immunotherapy target for cancers of lymphoid origin due to its high expression levels on the vast majority of NHL and acute lymphoblastic leukemia cells. This molecule acts as a co-receptor, enhancing signaling and antigen processing by the B-cell receptor complex in response to antigen stimulation.

hBU12-vcMMAE

hBU12-vcMMAE is a novel, humanized anti-CD19 antibody drug conjugate consisting of the tubulin-destabilizing auristatin derivative MMAE and a novel, humanized anti-CD19 antibody [58]. In vitro, hBU12-vcMMAE induced killing of rituximab-sensitive and rituximab-resistant NHL cell lines. However, the activity of hBU12-vcMMAE in NHL patients remains to be determined in clinical trials.

Blinatumomab

Blinatumomab (MT103) is a single-chain bispecific monoclonal antibody constructed with specificity for CD19 and CD3 that can effectively redirect T cells for highly selective lysis of CD19+ target cells. It belongs to the class of bispecific T cell engagers (BiTE®). Blinatumomab is a first antibody, which can potentially engage all cytotoxic T cells within a patient for tumor cell lysis [59]. In an in vitro study, blinatumomab induced a higher degree of lysis of human lymphoma lines than rituximab and was active at a much lower concentration. In addition, the combination of rituximab with blinatumomab enhanced the activity of rituximab, in particular at low effector-to-target cell ratios and at low antibody concentrations [60].

The high single-agent activity of blinatumomab in indolent NHL has been confirmed by a number of studies. In a phase I study, 52 patients (21 with FL, 21 with MCL, and 10 with other subtypes of lymphoma) were treated with blinatumomab at a dose range of 0.5–90 $\mu g/m^2/day$ [61]. Ninety percent of the patients had prior exposure to rituximab and 45% to fludarabine. The medically most important AEs that resulted in permanent discontinuation were CNS events. Eight out of the nine patients with constant dosing showed an objective response. Median duration of response was 26 months.

XmAb5574

XmAb5574 is a humanized anti-CD19 antibody with a modified constant fragment (Fc) domain designed to enhance binding of FcgammaRIIIa [62]. In vitro, the enhanced antibody-dependent cell-mediated ADCC of XmAb5574 is 100–1,000 times greater than that of anti-CD19 IgG1 analogue against a broad range of B-lymphoma cell lines, acute lymphoblastic leukemia, and mantle cell lymphoma cells. The XmAb5574-dependent ADCC is mediated by natural killer (NK) cells through a granzyme B-dependent mechanism. In experiments with CLL cells, NK cell-mediated ADCC with XmAb5574 was enhanced further by lenalidomide [63]. In vivo, XmAb5574 significantly inhibited lymphoma growth in mouse xenograft models and showed more potent antitumor activity than its IgG1 analogue. In nonhuman primates, XmAb5574 infusion caused an immediate and dose-related B-cell depletion in the blood [64]. This antibody warrants further clinical evaluation in CD19-positive lymphoid malignancies.

Monoclonal Antibodies to the TRAIL Receptors

Tumor necrosis factor-related apoptosis-inducing ligand (TRAIL) selectively induces apoptosis in cancer cells by binding to two membrane-bound death receptors, TRAIL-R1 (death receptor 4, DR4) and TRAIL-R2 (death receptor 5, DR5). The TRAIL-R1 is expressed more frequently on the surface of tumor cells than on the surface of normal cells [65]. TRAIL-R1- and TRAIL-R2-induced apoptosis is mediated through activation of both extrinsic and intrinsic intracellular death signaling pathways. Mapatumumab and lexatumumab are fully human agonistic monoclonal antibodies that bind with high affinity to the TRAIL-R1/DR4 and TRAIL-R2/DR5, respectively.

Mapatumumab

Mapatumumab [(HGS-ETR1, TRM-1, Cambridge Antibody Technology (CAT) and Human Genome Sciences, Inc. (HGS)] is a fully human IgG1 monoclonal antibody specific and agonistic to TRAIL-R1/DR4. This antibody induces apoptosis in various tumor cell types, in vitro and in vivo, by binding to TRAIL-R1, leading to activation of the caspase cascade, cleavage of key intracellular signaling components and DNA, and subsequent cell death [66]. Mapatumumab may also activate Fc-mediated antibody effector functions, such as ADCC and CDC [67].

The safety and efficacy of mapatumumab was evaluated in patients with relapsed or refractory NHL [68]. Among 40 patients, six patients experienced tumor shrinkage following mapatumumab therapy and three patients with FL experienced a CR or PR. The median PFS for 17 FL patients was 6 months. Two patients with FL demonstrated durable stable disease after six cycles with a PFS of 24 and 21 months, respectively. The most common AEs possibly related to mapatumumab included nausea, fatigue, diarrhea, anorexia, and pyrexia.

Lexatumumab

Lexatumumab (HGS-ETR2) is also a fully human agonistic mAb to the TRAIL-R2 that activates the extrinsic apoptosis pathway and has potent preclinical antitumor activity. In a phase 1, dose-escalation study, the safety, tolerability, pharmacokinetics, and immunogenicity of lexatumumab were evaluated in patients with advanced solid tumors. This trial has shown that lexatumumab can be safely administered every 14 days at 10 mg/kg. Nine of 31 patients achieved a stable condition [69]. The phase I trial studying the side effects and best dose of lexatumumab, both alone and together with recombinant interferon gamma, in patients with lymphoma who have relapsed or not responded to previous treatment is ongoing (ClinicalTrials.gov Identifier: NCT00428272).

Conatumumab

Conatumumab (AMG 655; Amgen Inc. and Takeda Bio Development Center Ltd) is an investigational, fully human IgG1 monoclonal agonist antibody directed against the extracellular domain of TRAIL-R2 (death receptor 5). Conatumumab mimics the activity of native TRAIL and induces tumor cell apoptosis via caspase activation [70]. Preclinical studies indicate that conatumumab inhibits experimental solid tumor growth in xenograft models and conatumumab enhances the antitumor activity of agents, such as irinotecan and gemcitabine in vivo. Safety and tolerability of this agent was evaluated in patients with advanced solid tumors [71]. Conatumumab was well tolerated and there were no dose-limiting toxicities. An MTD was not reached. The combination of conatumumab with either bortezomib or vorinostat showed antitumor activity in patients with relapsed or refractory lymphoma [72].

Anti-T Cell Monoclonal Antibodies

CD2, CD4, and CD52 are expressed on normal and malignant T cells and are good targets for monoclonal antibodies useful for the treatment of T-cell lymphomas.

Siplizumab

CD2 is a T-cell marker expressed on all mature T cells and most natural killer (NK) cells, although it is highly expressed on activated T cells and less intensively expressed on resting T cells. Siplizumab (MEDI-507, MedImmune, Inc.) is a humanized mAb directed against CD2 that was genetically engineered from the rat version of the mAb (BTI-322) by BioTransplant (Charlestown, MA) for use in the prevention of allograft rejection [73]. The drug was effective in an animal model of adult T-cell leukemia/

lymphoma (ATLL). Survival of the ATL-bearing mice treated with siplizumab was significantly longer as compared with controls ($P<0.0001$) [74]. Preliminary clinical trial results showed similar antineoplastic activity in 29 patients with T-cell malignancies, including 15 patients with ATLL and 7 patients with large granular lymphocyte leukemia [75]. Although initial responses were encouraging, four (13.7%) patients developed EBV-related lymphoproliferative disease (EBV-LPD), and the trial was stopped. However, clinical trial on siplizumab in combination with chemotherapy and rituximab in patients with T-cell or natural killer-cell NHL is ongoing (ClinicalTrials.gov Identifier: NCT00832936).

Zanolimumab

The CD4 molecule is a single-chain transmembrane glycoprotein of 55 kDa that consists of four extracellular Ig-like domains and a short cytoplasmic tail. Zanolimumab (HuMax-CD4; TenX Biopharma, Inc.) is a high affinity fully human monoclonal IgG1κ antibody, targeting the CD4-molecule. Zanolimumab exerts its action through inhibition of CD4+ T cell signaling, induction of Fc-dependent ADCC, and CD4 down-modulation [76]. Phase II studies in early and late stage cutaneous T-cell lymphoma (CTCL) showed that zanolimumab induced a marked clinical effect with early, high, and durable responses [77, 78]. In these trials, 46 patients with treatment refractory CD4(+) mycosis fungoides (MF) or Sézary syndrome (SS) were treated with 17 weekly infusions of zanolimumab at doses of 280, 560, or 980 mg. OR was noted in 13 patients with MF and 2 patients with SS. In the 560 and 980 mg dose groups, a response rate of 56% was obtained with a median response of 81 weeks. At high dose levels, median response duration lasted 20 months (range 8–91 weeks), with low-grade infections and eczematous dermatitis being frequently observed adverse events. The treatment was well tolerated with no dose-related toxicity other than the targeted depletion of peripheral T cells. The efficacy and safety of zanolimumab was also evaluated in 21 patients with relapsed or refractory CD4(+) peripheral T-cell lymphoma (PTCL) of non-cutaneous type [79]. The patients were treated with weekly intravenous infusions of zanolimumab 980 mg for 12 weeks. Objective tumor responses were observed in five (24%) of the patients with two CRu (CR unconfirmed) and three PR. The most frequently reported AEs were rash, pyrexia, and infections.

Conclusions

Monoclonal antibody therapy is one of the most significant advances in the treatment of NHL in the last two decades. Novel monoclonal antibodies alone and in combination with chemotherapy form the basis for innovative therapeutic strategies evaluated in well designed clinical trials.

Acknowledgement This work was supported in part by grants from the Medical University of Lodz (No 503/1-093-01/503-1).

References

1. Keating GM (2010) Rituximab: a review of its use in chronic lymphocytic leukaemia, low-grade or follicular lymphoma and diffuse large B-cell lymphoma. Drugs 70:1445–1476
2. Bhat SA, Czuczman MS (2009) Novel antibodies in the treatment of non-Hodgkin's lymphoma. Neth J Med 67:311–321
3. Robak T (2008) Novel monoclonal antibodies for the treatment of chronic lymphocytic leukemia. Curr Cancer Drug Targets 8:156–171
4. Robak T, Robak E (2011) New anti-CD20 monoclonal antibodies for the treatment of B-cell lymphoid malignancies. BioDrugs 25:13–25
5. Lim SH, Beers SA, French RR et al (2010) Anti-CD20 monoclonal antibodies: historical and future perspectives. Haematologica 95:135–143
6. van Meerten T, Hagenbeek A (2010) CD20-targeted therapy: the next generation of antibodies. Semin Hematol 47:199–210
7. Hutas G (2008) Ocrelizumab, a humanized monoclonal antibody against CD20 for inflammatory disorders and B-cell malignancies. Curr Opin Investig Drugs 9:1206–1215
8. Kausar F, Mustafa K, Sweis G et al (2009) Ocrelizumab: a step forward in the evolution of B-cell therapy. Expert Opin Biol Ther 9:889–895
9. Morschhauser F, Marlton P, Vitolo U et al (2010) Results of a phase I/II study of ocrelizumab, a fully humanized anti-CD20 mAb, in patients with relapsed/refractory follicular lymphoma. Ann Oncol 21:1870–1876
10. Goldenberg DM, Rossi EA, Stein R et al (2009) Properties and structure-function relationships of veltuzumab (hA20), a humanized anti-CD20 monoclonal antibody. Blood 113:1062–1070
11. Stein R, Qu Z, Chen S et al (2004) Characterization of a new humanized anti-CD20 monoclonal antibody, IMMU-106, and its use in combination with the humanized anti-CD22 antibody, epratuzumab, for the therapy of non-Hodgkin's lymphoma. Clin Cancer Res 10:2868–2878
12. Goldenberg DM, Morschhauser F, Wegener WA (2010) Veltuzumab (humanized anti-CD20 monoclonal antibody): characterization, current clinical results, and future prospects. Leuk Lymphoma 51:747–755
13. Negrea OG, Allen SL, Rai KR et al (2009) Subcutaneous injections of low doses of humanized anti-CD20 veltuzumab for treatment of indolent B-cell malignancies [abstract]. Blood 114:3757
14. Morschhauser F, Leonard JP, Fayad L et al (2009) Humanized anti-CD20 antibody, veltuzumab, in refractory/recurrent non-Hodgkin's lymphoma: phase I/II results. J Clin Oncol 27:3346–3353
15. Hagenbeek A, Gadeberg O, Johnson P et al (2008) First clinical use of ofatumumab, a novel fully human anti-CD20 monoclonal antibody in relapsed or refractory follicular lymphoma: results of a phase I/II trial. Blood 111:5486–5495
16. Robak T (2008) Ofatumumab, a human monoclonal antibody for lymphoid malignancies and autoimmune disorders. Curr Opin Mol Ther 10:294–309
17. Teeling JL, Mackus WJ, Wiegman LJ et al (2006) The biological activity of human CD20 monoclonal antibodies is linked to unique epitopes on CD20. J Immunol 177:362–371
18. Hagenbeek A, Fayad L, Delwail V et al (2009) Evaluation of ofatumumab, a novel human CD20 monoclonal antibody, as single agent therapy in rituximab-refractory follicular lymphoma [abstract]. Blood 114:935
19. Robak T (2009) GA-101, a third-generation, humanized and glyco-engineered anti-CD20 mAb for the treatment of B-cell lymphoid malignancies. Curr Opin Investig Drugs 10:588–596
20. Mössner E, Brünker P, Moser S et al (2010) Increasing the efficacy of CD20 antibody therapy through the engineering of a new type II anti-CD20 antibody with enhanced direct and immune effector cell-mediated B-cell cytotoxicity. Blood 115:4393–4402
21. Salles GA, Morschhauser F, Cartron G et al (2008) A phase I/II study of RO5072759 (GA101) in patients with relapsed/refractory CD20+ malignant disease [abstract]. Blood 93:234
22. Salles G, Morschhauser F, Lamy T et al (2009) Phase I study of RO5072759 (GA101) in patients with relapsed/refractory CD20+ non-Hodgkin lymphoma (NHL) [abstract]. Blood 114:1704

23. Bowles JA, Wang SY, Link BK et al (2006) CD20 monoclonal antibody with enhanced affinity for CD16 activates NK cells at lower concentrations and more effectively than rituximab. Blood 108:2648–2654
24. Friedberg JW, Vose JM, Kahl BS et al (2009) A phase I study of PRO131921, a novel anti-CD20 monoclonal antibody in patients with relapsed/refractory CD20+ indolent NHL: correlation between clinical responses and AUC pharmacokinetics [abstract]. Blood 114:3742, ASH Annual Meeting Abstracts
25. Robak T, Robak P, Smolewski P (2009) TRU-016, a humanized anti-CD37 IgG fusion protein for the potential treatment of B-cell malignancies. Curr Opin Investig Drugs 10:1383–1390
26. Hayden-Ledbetter MS, Cerveny CG, Espling E et al (2009) CD20-directed small modular immunopharmaceutical, TRU-015, depletes normal and malignant B cells. Clin Cancer Res 15:2739–2746
27. Barone D, Burge DJ, Baum P et al (2005) Prolonged depletion of circulating B cells in cynomolgus monkeys after a single dose of TRU-015, a novel CD20 directed therapeutic. Ann Rheum Dis 64(suppl 3):159–160
28. Barone D (2005) TRU-015, a novel CD20-directed biologic therapy, demonstrates significant anti-tumor activity in human tumor xenograft models [abstract]. Proc Am Soc Clin Oncol 24:2549
29. Carnahan J, Stein R, Qu Z et al (2007) Epratunuzumab, a CD22-targeting recombinant humanized antibody with a different mode of action from rituximab. Mol Immunol 44:1331–1341
30. Leonard JP, Coleman M, Ketas JC et al (2003) Phase I/II trial of epratuzumab humanized anti-CD22 antibody in indolent non-Hodgkin's lymphoma. J Clin Oncol 21:3051–3059
31. Leonard JP, Coleman M, Ketas JC et al (2005) Combination antibody therapy with epratuzumab and rituximab in relapse or refractory non-Hodgkin's lymphoma. J Clin Oncol 23:5044–5051
32. Strauss SJ, Morschhauser F, Rech J et al (2006) Multicenter phase II trial of immunotherapy with the humanized anti CD-22 antibody epratuzumab in combination with rituximab in refractory or recurrent non-Hodgkin's lymphoma. J Clin Oncol 24:3880–3886
33. Wong BY, Dang NH (2010) Inotuzumab ozogamicin as novel therapy in lymphomas. Expert Opin Biol Ther 10:1251–1258
34. DiJoseph JF, Dougher MM, Kalyandrug LB et al (2006) Antitumor efficacy of a combination of CMC-544 (inotuzumab ozogamicin), a CD22-targeted cytotoxic immunoconjugate of calicheamicin, and rituximab against non-Hodgkin's B-cell lymphoma. Clin Cancer Res 12:242–249
35. Advani A, Coiffier B, Czuczman MS et al (2010) Safety, pharmacokinetics, and preliminary clinical activity of inotuzumab ozogamicin, a novel immunoconjugate for the treatment of B-cell non-Hodgkin's lymphoma: results of a phase I study. J Clin Oncol 28:2085–2093
36. Kreitman RJ, Wilson WH, Bergeron K et al (2001) Efficacy of the anti-CD22 recombinant immunotoxin BL22 in chemotherapy-resistant hairy-cell leukemia. N Engl J Med 345:241–247
37. Kreitman RJ, Tallman MS, Coutre S et al (2009) Phase I dose-escalation study of CAT-8015 (HA22), a CD22-specific targeted immunotoxin, in relapsed or refractory hairy cell leukemia. Blood 114:888, ASH Annual Meeting Abstracts
38. Mone AP, Huang P, Pelicano H et al (2004) HU1D10 induces apoptosis concurrent with activation of the AKT survival pathway in human chronic lymphocytic leukemia cells. Blood 103:1846–1854
39. Hill ML, Weiner GJ, Link BK (2005) *In vitro* activity of the humanized anti-HLA-DR antibodies KRN848 and apolizumab in non-Hodgkin's lymphoma cell lines. Blood 106(Suppl 1): Abstract 4826
40. Rech J, Repp R, Rech D et al (2006) A humanized HLA-DR antibody (Hu1D10, apolizumab) in combination with granulocyte colony-stimulating factor (filgrastim) for the treatment of non-Hodgkin's lymphoma: a pilot study. Leuk Lymphoma 47:2147–2154
41. Stein R, Mattes MJ, Cardillo TM et al (2007) CD74: a new candidate target for the immunotherapy of B-cell neoplasms. Clin Cancer Res 13(18 Pt 2):5556s–5563s
42. Mark T, Martin P, Leonard JP, Niesvizky R et al (2009) Milatuzumab: a promising new agent for the treatment of lymphoid malignancies. Expert Opin Investig Drugs 18:99–104

43. Sapra P, Stein R, Pickett J et al (2005) Anti-CD74 antibody-doxorubicin conjugate, IMMU-110, in a human multiple myeloma xenograft and in monkeys. Clin Cancer Res 11:5257–5264
44. Chang CH, Sapra P et al (2005) Effective therapy of human lymphoma xenografts with a novel recombinant ribonuclease/anti-CD74 humanized IgG4 antibody immunotoxin. Blood 106:4308–4314
45. Horton HM, Bernett MJ, Peipp M et al (2010) Fc-engineered anti-CD40 antibody enhances multiple effector functions and exhibits potent in vitro and in vivo antitumor activity against hematologic malignancies. Blood 116:3004–3012
46. Luqman M, Klabunde S, Lin K et al (2008) The antileukemia activity of a human anti-CD40 antagonist antibody, HCD122, on human chronic lymphocytic leukemia cells. Blood 112:711–720
47. Law CL, Gordon KA, Collier J et al (2005) Preclinical antilymphoma activity of a humanized anti-CD40 monoclonal antibody, SGN-40. Cancer Res 65:8331–8339
48. Advani R, Forero-Torres A, Furman RR et al (2009) Phase I study of the humanized anti-CD40 monoclonal antibody dacetuzumab in refractory or recurrent non-Hodgkin's lymphoma. J Clin Oncol 27:4371–4377
49. Suvas S, Singh V, Sahdev S et al (2002) Distinct role of CD80 and CD86 in the regulation of the activation of B-cell and B-cell lymphoma. J Biol Chem 277:7766–7775
50. Bhat S, Czuczman MS (2010) Galiximab: a review. Expert Opin Biol Ther 10:451–458
51. Vinjamaram S, Czuczman MS, Hernandez-Ilizaliturri FJ (2008) The use of galiximab in non-Hodgkin lymphoma. Clin Lymphoma Myeloma 8:277–282
52. Hariharan K, Anderson D, Leigh B et al (2001) Therapeutic activity of IDEC-114 (anti-CD80) and rituximab (Rituxan) in B cell lymphoma. Blood 98(Suppl 1):Abstract 2549
53. Czuczman MS, Thall A, Witzig TE et al (2005) Phase I/II study of galiximab, an anti-CD80 antibody, for relapsed or refractory follicular lymphoma. J Clin Oncol 23:4390–4398
54. Leonard J, Friedberg J, Younes A et al (2007) A phase I/II study of galiximab (an anti-CD80 monoclonal antibody) in combination with rituximab for relapsed or refractory follicular lymphoma. Ann Oncol 18:1216–1223
55. Furman RR, Andritos L, Flinn IW et al (2010) Phase 1 dose escalation study of TRU-016, an anti-CD37 SMIPTM protein in relapsed and refractory CLL [Abstract 56]. Blood 116(Suppl):31
56. Zenz T, Volden M, Mast T et al (2010) Exceptional in vitro activity of CD37 antibodies in CLL [Abstract 2460]. Blood 116:1021
57. Fearon DT, Carroll MC (2000) Regulation of B lymphocyte responses to foreign and self-antigens by the CD19/CD21 complex. Annu Rev Immunol 18:393–422
58. Gerber HP, Kung-Sutherland M, Stone I et al (2009) Potent antitumor activity of the anti-CD19 auristatin antibody drug conjugate hBU12-vcMMAE against rituximab-sensitive and -resistant lymphomas. Blood 113:4352–4361
59. Bargou R, Leo E, Zugmaier G et al (2008) Tumor regression in cancer patients by very low doses of T cell engaging antibody. Science 321:974–977
60. Nagorsen D, Bargou R, Ruttinger D et al (2009) Immunotherapy of lymphoma and leukemia with T-cell engaging BiTE antibody blinatumomab. Leuk Lymphoma 50:886–891
61. Viardot A, Goebeer M, Sheele JS et al (2010) Treatment of patients with non-Hodgkin lymphoma (NHL) with CD19/CD3 bispecific antibody blinatumomab (MT103): double-step dose increase to continuous infusion of 60 μg/m^2/d is tolerable and highly effective [Abstract 2880]. Blood 116:1186
62. Horton HM, Bernett MJ, Pong E et al (2008) Potent in vitro and in vivo activity of an Fc-engineered anti-CD19 monoclonal antibody against lymphoma and leukemia. Cancer Res 68:8049–8057
63. Awan FT, Lapalombella R, Trotta R et al (2010) CD19 targeting of chronic lymphocytic leukemia with a novel Fc-domain-engineered monoclonal antibody. Blood 115:1204–1213
64. Zalevsky J, Leung IW, Karki S et al (2009) The impact of Fc engineering on an anti-CD19 antibody: increased Fcgamma receptor affinity enhances B-cell clearing in nonhuman primates. Blood 113:3735–3743
65. Humphreys RC, Halpern W (2008) TRAIL receptors: targets for cancer therapy. Adv Exp Med Biol 615:127–158

66. Pukac L, Kanakaraj P, Humphreys R et al (2005) HGS-ETR1, a fully human TRAIL-receptor 1 monoclonal antibody, induces cell death in multiple tumour types in vitro and in vivo. Br J Cancer 92:1430–1441
67. Maddipatla S, Hernandez-Ilizaliturri FJ, Knight J, Czuczman MS (2007) Augmented antitumor activity against B-cell lymphoma by a combination of monoclonal antibodies targeting TRAIL-R1 and CD20. Clin Cancer Res 13:4556–4564
68. Younes A, Vose JM, Zelenetz AD et al (2010) A Phase 1b/2 trial of mapatumumab in patients with relapsed/refractory non-Hodgkin's lymphoma. Br J Cancer 103:1783–1787
69. Wakelee HA, Patnaik A, Sikic BI et al (2010) Phase I and pharmacokinetic study of lexatumumab (HGS-ETR2) given every 2 weeks in patients with advanced solid tumors. Ann Oncol 21(2):376–381
70. Kaplan-Lefko PJ, Graves JD, Zoog SJ et al (2010) Conatumumab, a fully human agonist antibody to death receptor 5, induces apoptosis via caspase activation in multiple tumor types. Cancer Biol Ther 9:618–631
71. Herbst RS, Kurzrock R, Hong DS et al (2010) A first-in-human study of conatumumab in adult patients with advanced solid tumors. Clin Cancer Res 16:5883–5891
72. Younes A, Kirschbaum M, Sokol L et al (2009) Safety and tolerability of conatumumab in combination with bortezomib or vorinostat in patients with relapsed or refractory lymphoma. Blood 114:1708
73. Branco L, Barren P, Mao SY et al (1999) Selective deletion of antigen-specific, activated T cells by a humanized MAB to CD2 (MEDI-507) is mediated by NK cells. Transplantation 68:1588–1596
74. Zhang Z, Zhang M, Ravetch JV et al (2003) Effective therapy for a murine model of adult T-cell leukemia with the humanized anti-CD2 monoclonal antibody, MEDI-507. Blood 102:284–288
75. O'Mahony D, Morris JC, Stetler-Stevenson M et al (2009) EBV-related lymphoproliferative disease complicating therapy with the anti-CD2 monoclonal antibody, siplizumab, in patients with T-cell malignancies. Clin Cancer Res 15:2514–2522
76. Ruuls SR, Lammerts van Bueren JJ, van de Winkel JG et al (2008) Novel human antibody therapeutics: the age of the Umabs. Biotechnol J 3:1157–1171
77. Kim YH, Duvic M, Obitz E, Gniadecki R et al (2007) Clinical efficacy of zanolimumab (HuMax-CD4): two phase 2 studies in refractory cutaneous T-cell lymphoma. Blood 109:4655–4662
78. Mestel DS, Beyer M, Möbs M et al (2008) Zanolimumab, a human monoclonal antibody targeting CD4 in the treatment of mycosis fungoides and Sézary syndrome. Expert Opin Biol Ther 8:1929–1939
79. d'Amore F, Radford J, Relander T et al (2010) Phase II trial of zanolimumab (HuMax-CD4) in relapsed or refractory non-cutaneous peripheral T cell lymphoma. Br J Haematol 150:565–573

Current Therapies for T-cell Lymphomas

Francine M. Foss

Abstract Peripheral T-cell lymphomas (PTCL) are a heterogeneous group of clinically aggressive diseases associated with poor outcome. One of the difficulties in classifying and studying treatment options in clinical trials is the rarity of these subtypes. The International T-cell Lymphoma Project has identified that the outcomes for the majority of the different subtypes of PTCL are poor using conventional lymphoma therapies. Recently, aggressive first-line strategies including consolidation with stem cell transplantation have led to improved survival in selected patients, but the majority of patients either fail to respond to therapy or are not candidates for stem cell transplantation. Novel approaches have included new classes of drug and biological agents, including antifolates, immunoconjugates, histone deacetylase (HDAC) inhibitors, monoclonal antibodies, nucleoside analogs, proteasome inhibitors, and signal transduction inhibitors. Molecular profiling has led to identification of relevant pathways for future novel approaches.

Introduction

The aggressive T-cell lymphomas are a diverse group of disorders that are associated with a poor prognosis (Fig. 1). Classification of PTCL is complex and has been further hampered by a paucity of molecular markers. The World Health Organization classification of non-Hodgkin's lymphomas includes many a number of subtypes of aggressive T-cell lymphomas (Table 1) characterized based primarily on their clinical and histopathologic features and subgroups them into the cutaneous, nodal, extranodal, and leukemic groups [1].

F.M. Foss, M.D. (✉)
Clinical Investigations, Hematologic Malignancies, Yale Cancer Center,
Yale University School of Medicine, 333 Cedar Street, FMP 112,
PO Box 208032, New Haven, CT 06520-8032, USA
e-mail: francine.foss@yale.edu

P.J. Quesenberry and J.J. Castillo (eds.), *Non-Hodgkin Lymphoma: Prognostic Factors and Targets*, Cancer Drug Discovery and Development,
DOI 10.1007/978-1-4614-5851-7_12, © Springer Science+Business Media New York 2013

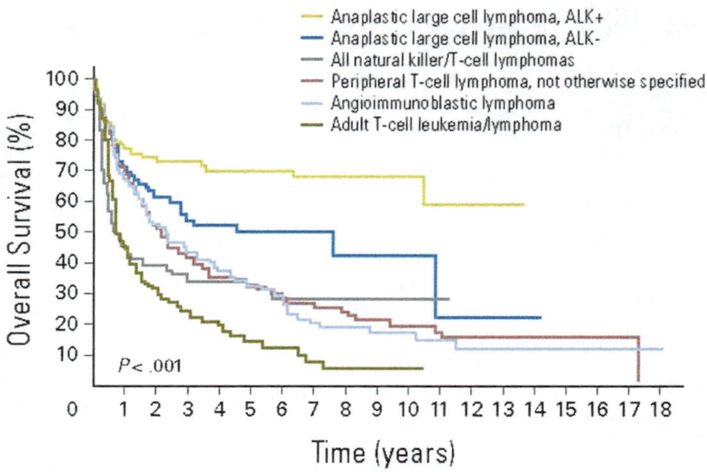

Fig. 1 Overall survival of patients with the common subtypes of PTCL. Vose et al. (International T-cell Lymphoma Project), J Clin Oncol 2008; 26:4124–4130. Figure 2A p 4127

The nodal lymphoma group includes PTCL, not otherwise specified (PTCL-NOS), anaplastic large cell lymphoma (ALCL), and angioimmunoblastic T-cell lymphoma (AITL). ALCL is further separated into the ALK^+ and ALK^- entities. According to the International PTCL study, PTCL-NOS accounts for 26% of cases, AITL accounts for 18.5%, anaplastic lymphoma kinase (ALK)-positive ALCL accounts for 6.6% and ALK-negative ALCL for 5.5% of cases [2].

The extranodal T-cell lymphomas comprise a group of less well understood diseases identified based on their tissue trophism. Hepatosplenic gamma-delta T-cell comprises 1.4% of cases and is characterized by gamma-delta T-cell infiltration of the liver, spleen, and bone marrow sinusoids. Outcomes are poor with a median survival of less than 2 years. Enteropathy-associated T-cell lymphoma (EATL) accounts for 4.7% of cases and is comprised of two morphologic variants, the pleomorphic type, associated with celiac disease and usually $CD3^+$, $CD7^+$, and $CD56^-$, and the monomorphic type, which is $CD56^+$ and often not associated with celiac disease [3]. Subcutaneous panniculitis-like T-cell lymphomas (SPTCL) constitute only 0.9% of PTCL and presents with subcutaneous nodules that are typically $CD3^+$, $CD4^-$, and $CD8^+$, with TCR-[alpha]/[beta]$^+$ expression. The cutaneous panniculitis-like T-cell lymphomas with TCR-[gamma]/[delta]$^+$ expression have now been reclassified as cutaneous gamma/delta T-cell lymphoma [21]. NK-cell lymphomas include extranodal NK/T-cell lymphoma, nasal type, blastic NK-cell lymphoma, and aggressive NK-cell leukemia account for 10.4% of PTCL cases. EBV has been implicated and found in the tumor cells of nasal/NK-cell lymphomas and aggressive NK-cell leukemia [4].

The leukemic group of T-cell lymphomas consists of adult T-cell lymphoma (ATLL) associated with human T-lymphotropic virus type I (HTLV-1), T-cell chronic large granular lymphocytic (LGL) leukemia, aggressive NK-cell leukemia, and T-cell prolymphocytic leukemia. LGL leukemia often has an indolent clinical course and is associated with neutropenia, while aggressive NK cell leukemia and

Table 1 The WHO classification for PTCLs was updated in 2008

Old WHO classification [7]	New WHO classification [9]
Precursor T-cell lymphoma	
• T-lymphoblastic lymphoma/leukemia	
Mature T-cell lymphomas	
• T-cell prolymphocytic leukemia	T-cell prolymphocytic leukemia
• T-cell granular lymphocytic leukemia	T-cell large granular lymphocytic leukemia
• Aggressive NK-cell leukemia	Aggressive NK-cell leukemia
	Indolent large granular NK-cell lymphoproliferative disorder (provisional)
• Adult T-cell lymphoma/leukemia (HTLV1+)	Adult T-cell leukemia/lymphoma
• Extranodal NK/T-cell lymphoma, nasal type	Extranodal NK/T-cell lymphoma, nasal type
• Enteropathy-type T-cell lymphoma	Enteropathy-associated T-cell lymphoma
• Hepatosplenanic T-cell lymphoma	Hepatosplenic T-cell lymphoma
• Subcutaneous panniculitis-like T-cell lymphoma	Subcutaneous panniculitis-like T-cell l ymphoma (αβ only)
	Primary cutaneous γδ T-cell lymphoma
• Mycosis fungoides/Sézary syndrome	Mycosis fungoides & Sézary syndrome
• Anaplastic large-cell lymphoma, systemic or cutaneous	Anaplastic large cell lymphoma—ALK$^+$
	Anaplastic large cell lymphoma—ALK$^-$ (provisional)
• Peripheral T-cell lymphoma, unspecified	Peripheral T-cell lymphoma, not otherwise specified
• Angioimmunoblastic T-cell lymphoma	Angioimmunoblastic T-cell lymphoma
	Primary cutaneous CD30$^+$ T-cell LPD
	• LYP and primary cutaneous ALC
	Primary cutaneous CD4$^+$ small/medium T-cell lymphoma (provisional)
	Primary cutaneous CD8$^+$ aggressive epidermotropic cytotoxic T-cell lymphoma (provisional)
	Systemic EBV + T-cell LPD of childhood
	Hydroa vacciniforme-like lymphoma

The new classification expanded some existing disease types and added several new provisional diseases

ATLL often have a poor outcome even with systemic therapy. HTLV-1-associated lymphomas include acute ATLL, which presents predominantly with a leukemic component, smoldering ATLL, which is characterized by small numbers of circulating leukemia cells without nodal involvement, lymphomatous ATLL, which presents with lymphadenopathy without leukemic involvement, and chronic ATLL, which is characterized by skin lesions, leukemic, nodal, and visceral disease without hypercalcemia, gastrointestinal involvement, bone, or central nervous system (CNS) disease. HTLV-1 infection is prevalent in Japan and the Caribbean basin, but only a small proportion of patients carrying the virus develop a malignancy.

The cutaneous group of T-cell lymphomas includes mycosis fungoides (MF) and the Sezary syndrome (SS) and variants of MF, which often have an indolent clinical course. Large cell transformation may occur in patients with MF or SS and this is often associated with a poor outcome. The primary CD30$^+$ cutaneous disorders include cutaneous anaplastic large cell lymphoma, which is characteristically ALK-negative is often localized to the skin and is treated locally. The pleomorphic CD4$^+$ T-cell lymphomas are a group of disorders resembling PTCL-NOS but occurring only in the skin with no systemic manifestations and are often treated with local irradiation with no systemic recurrence in the majority of cases.

Therapeutic Approaches for Aggressive T-Cell Lymphomas

Standard First-Line Therapy

T-cell lymphomas have traditionally been treated much like the B-cell lymphomas with CHOP based regimens. Outcomes using this approach have been reviewed in a retrospective meta-analysis of 2,912 patients treated with cyclophosphamide, doxorubicin, vincristine, and prednisone (CHOP) or CHOP-like regimens which reported a 5-year overall survival (OS) of 37% [5]. Results using other more aggressive regimens have been reported in a retrospective study from MD Anderson Cancer Center including hyperfractionated cyclophosphamide, vincristine, doxorubicin and dexamethasone (HyperCVAD) and etoposide, cisplatin, cytarabine, and prednisone (ESHAP) in 135 patients with PTCL. Among those patients with non-ALCL disease, there was no significant difference in outcome between those treated with CHOP vs. the more aggressive regimens (3-year OS: 43% vs. 49%) [6].

In a prospective study by Mercadal et al., a Mega-CHOP/ESHAP regimen (cyclophosphamide 2,000 mg/m(2)/day, adriamycin 90 mg/m(2)/day, vincristine and prednisone alternating with three courses of ESHAP) was used followed by autologous stem cell transplant for patients achieving remission [7]. Of 41 patients enrolled, only 68% completed the planned treatment with 20 complete responses (CR) and four partial responses. The outcome of the 16 patients who showed primary refractoriness to Mega-CHOP/ESHAP was extremely poor, with a median OS of 8 months. Overall, the CR rate in this study (50%) was not better than with CHOP alone, suggesting no advantage to this more aggressive approach.

Recently the German High Grade Non-Hodgkin's Lymphoma Study group explored the use of dose intensive CHOP or the addition of etoposide to CHOP for aggressive lymphomas. They reported results for patients with aggressive T-cell lymphomas treated on seven trials with six to eight courses of CHOP or CHOEP (CHOP plus etoposide) [8]. Of 343 T-cell patients enrolled in these studies, 70 had PTCL-NOS, 28 had AITL, 78 had ALK-positive ALCL, and 113 had ALK-negative ALCL. As an aggregate, the younger patients demonstrated an improvement in even-free survival (EFS) for both etoposide-containing regimens (75% vs. 51%) compared to the non-etoposide regimens, but there was no OS difference. The positive effect of etoposide on EFS was seen only in the most favorable ALK-positive patients and not in patients with PTCL-NOS or AITL, in whom there was no statistically significant difference between the etoposide and non-etoposide regimens. For the elderly patients, neither shortening of the time interval between cycles from 3 to 2 weeks (CHOP-21 vs. CHOP-14), administration of eight instead of six courses of CHOP-14, nor the addition of etoposide (CHOEP) significantly improved EFS or OS, but toxicity was increased. Patients with a favorable International Prognostic Index (IPI) score of 0–1 had a 3-year EFS above 50%, compared to 34% for those with IPI of two or greater. The conclusions from this study, which is one of the largest randomized studies of first-line regimens for aggressive lymphomas, is that younger patients may benefit from the addition of etoposide in terms of response rate and EFS, which would therefore potentially allow more patients to undergo a consolidation autologous stem cell transplant in first remission. The standard for elderly patients remains six cycles of CHOP. Finally, the excellent outcomes in patients with low IPI suggest that this group may do well and should be distinguished from the intermediate and high IPI patients.

When the German study group explored the results of a more dose intense regimen, Mega-CHOEP, results were inferior to those of standard dose CHOP or CHOEP. Of 33 patients treated, the 3-year event-free survival was only 26%, and the regimen was associated with more toxicity.

Another more intensive regimen, ACVBP (doxorubicin 75 mg/m^2 D1, cyclophosphamide 1,200 mg/m^2 D1, vindesine 2 mg/m^2 D1 and D5, bleomycin 10 mg D1 and D5 and prednisone D1 to D5), followed by a sequential consolidation consisting of methotrexate (two courses), etoposide + ifosfamide (four courses) and cytarabine (two courses) at 2 weeks intervals, was evaluated in aggressive T-cell lymphoma by the GELA. In a randomized study reported by Tilly et al., there was a benefit to the more aggressive regimen compared to CHOP [9]. Subsequently, the addition of bortezomib on days 1 and 5 of each ACVBP cycle and then days 1, 8, and 15 every 4 weeks as a consolidation showed no further benefit [10]. Of 57 patients enrolled, 46 patients responded, 28 patients completed the consolidation phase of the study, and 39% of patients died from lymphoma.

Another alternative first-line regimen, etoposide, ifosfamide, cisplatin alternating with doxorubicin, bleomycin, vinblastine, dacarbazine (VIP-reinforced-ABVD; VIP-rABVD) was compared to CHOP-21 in 88 patients with PTCL [11]. The Groupe Ouest Est d'Etude des Leucemies et Autres Maladies du Sang (GOELAMS) treated 88 patients with this regimen and reported a 2-year EFS of 41% vs. 45% for the more aggressive regimen compared to CHOP-21 with a similar median OS of 42 months for each of the arms.

New Combination Therapies for PTCL

CHOP-Based Regimens

Based on the demonstration that 40% of PTCL cases have been shown to express CD52 by immunohistochemistry, alemtuzumab has been used as a single agent in relapsed PTCL and in combination with chemotherapy in the front line [12].

One phase II study by Kim et al. enrolled 20 patients treated with CHOP combined with intravenous alemtuzumab in 3-week cycles (cycle 1: 10 mg on day 1, 20 mg on day 2; subsequent cycles: 30 mg on day 1) as frontline therapy [13]. All patients received trimethoprim/sulfamethoxazole and acyclovir prophylaxis during the study and up to a minimum of 2 months following discontinuation of the alemtuzumab. Responses were seen in all ten patients with PTCL-NOS, 1 of 3 with extranodal NK/T cell lymphoma, 2 of 3 with AITL, and 1 of 2 with ALK-negative ALCL and SPTCL, respectively. Toxicity was high, with 90% of patients experiencing grade 4 neutropenia and 5 of 20 with cytomegalovirus (CMV) reactivation. Additionally, there were two treatment-related deaths. In another study by Gallamini et al., alemtuzumab was given subcutaneously at a dose of 30 mg on day 1 in cycles 1–4 of CHOP in the first cohort of patients and then for all eight courses in the second cohort [14]. Of 24 evaluable patients, 71% had CR, including all six with AITL, all three with ALK-negative ALCL, 7 of 14 with PTCL-NOS, and one with EATL. The incidence of neutropenia remained high at 34% of the treatment cycles, but CMV reactivation was lower at 9%. Serious infections included one patient with Jacob-Creutzfeldt virus and two with aspergillosis. The overall median duration of response was 11 months.

Another phase I study evaluated alemtuzumab combined with dose-adjusted EPOCH (infusional etoposide, prednisone, vincristine, cyclophosphamide, doxorubicin) in patients with aggressive T-cell lymphomas [15]. In this study, alemtuzumab was administered at doses of 30, 60, or 90 mg prior to each EPOCH cycle. Significant bone marrow aplasia occurred in two of three patients at both the 60 and 90 mg dose groups; therefore, phase II study accrual is continuing at the 30 mg dose of alemtuzumab. Infections were reported in 11 of 14 patients from bacterial, fungal, and viral pathogens.

Based on these results, the alemtuzumab-CHOP combination is being compared to CHOP-21 in by the Nordic Lymphoma Group and the German High Grade Lymphoma Groups (the ACT Trial). Patients over age 60 are randomized and followed until progression. Patients under age 60 are randomized to either six cycles of CHOP-14 or four cycles of alemtuzumab-CHOP-14 and two cycles of CHOP-14 without alemtuzumab vs. six cycles of CHOP-14. Patients in remission will then undergo an autologous stem cell transplant.

Another targeted agent that has been combined with CHOP in first-line therapy for PTCL is denileukin diftitox, a fusion protein which combines the interleukin-2 gene with diphtheria toxin, thereby delivering the active toxin moiety to lymphoma cells expressing the interleukin-2 receptor. Denileukin diftitox has shown activity in relapsed aggressive T-cell lymphomas, with a response rate of 48% in 27 heavily pretreated patients [16]. A multicenter prospective phase II trial was conducted to combine denileukin diftitox with CHOP in 49 untreated patients with aggressive PTCL subtypes [17]. In this study, denileukin diftitox was administered at a dose of 18 μg/kg/day on days 1 and 2 and CHOP was given on day 3; this was followed by growth factor support on day 4 every 21 days. Histologic subtypes included: ALCL 8, AILT 10, PTCL-NOS 19, EATL 3, SPTCL 5, NK/T 1, hepatosplenic TCL 1. The median cycles was six with seven patients completing only one cycle of therapy; three patients died with progressive disease (PD) after cycle 1, and four patients were taken off study for toxicity. The overall response rate (ORR) in 47 patients was 68% with 57% CR. In the efficacy-evaluable patients (≥2 cycles completed) the ORR was 86% (CR 75%). The median progression-free survival (PFS) was 12 months and 2-year estimated OS was 60%. The median response duration for the 33 responders was 29 months. The most frequent grade 3 or 4 adverse events were bone marrow suppression and febrile neutropenia. There was no prolonged immunosuppression, and no opportunistic infections were observed.

The combination of CHOP with rituximab was explored by the GELA group in elderly patients (age 59–79) with AITL in an attempt to target non-neoplastic B-lymphocytes which may provide paracrine growth factors to the malignant T-cells. Twenty-five patients aged 59–79 years with newly diagnosed AITL received eight cycles of rituximab (375 mg/m^2 at day 1 of each cycle) and CHOP (R-CHOP21). Most of the patients had advanced disease (stage IV: 92% and B symptoms: 68%). Twenty-one patients completed all eight cycles. The overall response rate was 80%, with 44% achieving a complete response. With a median follow up of 24 months, the progression free survival was 42% and the 2-year-OS was 62%, which was no different than with CHOP alone in this population.

The anti-VEGF receptor monoclonal antibody, bevacizumab has also been combined with CHOP as first-line therapy for PTCL. Several PTCL subytpes, especially AITL and PTCL-NOS demonstrate overexpression of angiogenic factors, such as vascular endothelial growth factor (VEGF). At least one relapsed AITL patient has achieved a CR following treatment with bevacizumab [18]. A combination of CHOP and bevacizumab has been studied in patients with PTCL or NK-cell neoplasms by the Eastern Cooperative Oncology Group. Patients received bevacizumab at a dose of 15 mg/kg on day 1 followed by maintenance bevacizumab. However, this trial has been suspended when a preliminary analysis reported a high incidence of cardiac events related to the therapy, including four cases of congestive heart failure [19].

Gemcitabine-Based Regimens

Because results with CHOP and traditional anthracycline regimens have overall been inferior, other non-anthracycline regimens have been used in first-line therapy. Gemcitabine is an agent which is not metabolized by the multidrug resistance p-glycoprotein pathway and which has demonstrated efficacy in T-cell lymphomas as a single agent [20]. Zinzani reported results from 19 patients with cutaneous T-cell lymphoma (CTCL) and 20 patients with PTCL who received gemcitabine at a dose of 1,200 mg/m^2 on days 1, 8, and 15 every 28 days. The overall response rate was 51%; MF patients had a CR rate of 16% and a PR rate of 32%, while PTCL patients had a CR rate of 30% and a PR rate of 25%. Gemcitabine combined with cisplatin (GEM-P, gemcitabine 1,000 mg/m^2 days 1, 8, and 15, cisplatin 100 mg/m^2 on day 8) was reported to demonstrate a response rate of 73% and grade 3 or 4 neutropenia in 41% of patients [21]. The combination of vinorelbine 25 mg/m^2 and gemcitabine 1,000 mg/m^2 on days 1 and 8 of each 21-day cycle was also found to be active, with a 70% response rate in a pilot study [22]. The incorporation of gemcitabine into a CHOP-based regimen (CHOP-EG, CHOP plus etoposide and gemcitabine) was also explored [23]. The regimen consisted of CHOP plus etoposide 100 mg/m^2 day 1 and gemcitabine 600 mg/m^2 every 21 days. Of 26 enrolled patients, the overall response rate was 76.9% and median event free survival was 7 months. The most severe adverse event was grade 4 neutropenia in 14 patients (53.8%) and febrile neutropenia in four patients (15.4%). While active, this regimen did not appear to be superior to studies with CHOEP and incidence of myelosuppression was higher.

The Southwest Oncology Group has recently completed a study of gemcitabine, cisplatin, etoposide, and methylprednisolone (PEGS) for patients with untreated or relapsed PTCL. The majority of the patients (79%) were untreated at the time of study entry. The 1 year event-free survival was reported to be 38%. Another regimen incorporating gemcitabine was the GIVOX regimen (gemcitabine, ifosfamide, and oxaliplatin). In a group of high risk PTCL patients, the response rate was 86% with 67% CR and the 5-year EFS was 49%. Toxicities were primarily hematologic, with grade 4 thrombocytopenia and anemia occurring in 38% and 24% of patients respectively. Overall, gemcitabine based regimens have not been shown to have superior outcomes when compared to CHOP-based therapies but there are no randomized trials comparing these two approaches.

Transplantation as a Consolidation Therapy

Because of the historically poor outcomes and high relapse rates after first-line chemotherapy in aggressive T-cell lymphomas, the role of autologous or allogeneic stem cell transplantation in first remission has been explored in a number of small series and more recently in prospective nonrandomized trials. The largest studies from the Nordic and German study groups report overall EFS ranging from 30 to 50% and transplant rates of 40–70% based on intent to treat analysis. The Nordic group reported results from 160 patients treated with an etoposide-based regimen (CHOEP-14) followed by carmustine, etoposide, cytarabine, and melphalan (BEAM) conditioning [24]. At a median follow up of 4 years, the OS was 50% and the PFS was 48%. Outcome results were similar for each of the nodal subtypes of PTCL. In the German study reported by Reimer et al., 83 patients were treated with CHOP×4, followed by Dexa-BEAM or ESHAP [25]. The conditioning regimen for the transplant included total body irradiation along with cyclophosphamide. In this study, the CR rate to CHOP was 39%, and only 66% of patients were able to be transplanted. At a mean follow up of 33 months, the OS was 48%, and the EFS was 53%. Comparison of these two different approaches suggests that there may be no benefit for total body irradiation in this setting, and BEAM or chemotherapy based conditioning regimens remain the standard.

Novel Therapies for T-Cell Lymphomas

A number of novel agents have been used in T-cell lymphomas and have shown efficacy (Table 2). Monoclonal antibodies and fusion toxins targeting surface epitopes have been the most successful, including alemtuzumab and denileukin difititox. Other novel classes of drugs, including the HDAC inhibitors and pralatrexate have recently been FDA-approved for patients with relapsed and refractory disease. Response rates have been similar for many of the novel agents when used in the relapsed and refractory setting (Table 3). Pathway targeted agents have recently been explored in T-cell lymphomas and studies are underway to determine their efficacy as single agents and in combination with cytotoxic therapy.

Monoclonal Antibodies and Immunoconjugates

Siplizumab, an antibody targeting CD2, has shown activity in early studies in patients with aggressive T-cell malignancies. In a phase I trial in patients with CD2-expressing hematologic malignancies, there were two CR in patients with LGL, three partial responses (PRs) in patients with ATLL, and one PR in a patient with CTCL [26, 27]. A subsequent dose escalation study produced a PR in a patient with NK-cell LGL and a CR in a PTCL patient. Several cases of EBV-associated lymphoproliferative disease occurred, so subsequent trials with siplizumab have combined the antibody with rituximab to prevent EBV emergence [27].

Another humanized antibody, zanolimumab, an anti-CD4 antibody, has been shown to be active in both cutaneous and systemic aggressive T-cell lymphomas [28]. In a study of 21 PTCL patients, there were clinical responses in 24% [29].

LMB-2 is another agent targeting the CD25 component of the interleukin-2 receptor. LMB-2 consists of a single chain antibody (anti-CD25) conjugated to *Pseudomonas* toxin. LMB-2 has shown clinical activity in phase II trials in B-cell chronic lymphocytic leukemia, CTCL, and hairy cell leukemia. ATLL is the PTCL subtype that is most sensitive to LMB-2, but clinical responses have been limited to a rapid disease progression after >95% tumor reduction and immunogenic reactions [30]. A phase II clinical trial combines LMB-2 with fludarabine and cyclophosphamide.

The CD30 receptor, which is expressed on the anaplastic large cell lymphomas as well as a subset of other aggressive T-cell lymphomas, has been targeted with both monoclonal antibodies and, more recently, with an immunoconjugate, SGN35. Two anti-CD30 MAbs, iratumumab and SGN-30, have shown efficacy as single agents in patients with relapsed and refractory $CD30^+$ ALCL [31, 32]. In vitro studies further demonstrated additive or synergistic effects when the antibodies were combined with conventional chemotherapy [33].

SGN-35 is an immunoconjugate consisting of the SGN-30 antibody and monomethyl auristatin, a microtubule inhibitor [34, 35]. In vitro studies demonstrated the efficacy of this agent in CD30 expressing anaplastic large cell lymphoma cell lines and in malignant leukemia cells from patients with HTLV-1-associated

Table 2 Novel agents in use or trials in PTCL[a]

Type of agent	Name	Description	Disease(s)
Antifolates	Pralatrexate	10-deazaminopoterin	PTCL, CTCL
Conjugates	LMB-2	Anti-Tac (anti-CD25) fused to *Pseudomonas* toxin	CTCL, PTCL (esp ATL)
	Denileukin diftitox	IL-2 targeting domain fused with diphtheria toxin	CTCL, PTCL
	Brentuximab vedotin	CD30 antibody conjugated to monomethylauristan-E	$CD30^+$ T-cell lymphoma
HDAC inhibitors	Belinostat	PXD101	CTCL, PTCL
	Panobinostat	LBH589	CTCL, ATL
	Romidepsin	Depsipeptide	CTCL, PTCL
	Vorinostat	Suberoylanilide hydroxamic acid (SAHA)	CTCL
Immunomodulatory agents	Lenalidomide	Derivative of thalidomide	PTCL, CTCL
Immunosuppressive agents	Cyclosporine	Inhibitor of the NF-AT transcription complex	AITL
Monoclonal antibodies	Alemtuzumab	Anti-CD52	PTCL
	Bevacizumab	Anti-VEGF	PTCL (esp AITL), NK-cell
	Iratumumab	Anti-CD30	$CD30^+$ ALCL
	KW-0761	Anti-CCR4	ATL, PTCL
	SGN-30	Anti-CD30	$CD30^+$ ALCL
	Siplizumab	Anti-CD2	PTCL, NK-cell, ATL
	Zanolimumab	Anti-CD4	CTCL, PTCL
Nucleoside analogs	Cladribine	Purine nucleoside analog	PTCL
	Clofarabine	Purine nucleoside analog	PTCL, NK-cell
	Fludarabine	Purine nucleoside analog	PTCL, CTCL
	Forodesine	Metabolic enzyme inhibitor	PTCL, CTCL
	Gemcitabine	Pyrimidine nucleoside analog	PTCL
	Nelarabine	Purine nucleoside analog	T-ALL, T-NHL
	Pentostatin	Metabolic enzyme inhibitor	PTCL
Proteasome inhibitors	Bortezomib	Proteasome inhibitor	CTCL
Signaling inhibitors	Enzastaurin	Selective inhibitor of protein kinase C	PTCL, CTCL
	R788	Syk inhibitor	PTCL

AITL angioimmunoblostic T-cell lymphoma, *ALL* acute lymphoblastic leukemia, *ATL* adult T-cell leukemia-lymphoma, *CTCL* cutaneous T-cell lymphoma, *esp* especially, *IL-2* interleukin-2, *MAb* monoclonal antibody, *NHL* non-Hodgkin's lymphoma, *Ph* phase, *PTCL* peripheral T-cell lymphoma
[a]There are several other experimental agents in various stages of clinical trials for T-cell lymphoma

ATLL [36, 37]. In phase I studies, SGN-35 demonstrated significant clinical activity in relapsed/refractory systemic ALCL [38, 39]. In these trials, 86% of patients (6/7) had documented CR. Subsequently, a phase II multicenter registration trial of brentuximab vedotin was conducted in patients with relapsed or refractory ALCL. The overall response rate was 86% (50 of 58 patients), with CR in 53%. Pts received

Table 3 Response rates for new therapies in T-cell lymphoma

Drug	Author, year	No of PTCL pts	Response duration	ORR
Alemtuzumab	Enblad *Blood 2004*	14	2, 6, 12 months	5/14
	Zinzani *2005*	10	7 months	6/10
Gemcitabine	Zinzani *Ann Oncol 2010*	20	15–60 months (only CCRs)	55%
Zanolimumab	D'amore *BJH 2010*	21		27%
Lenalidomide	Dueck *Cancer* 2010	23	OS: 241 days	7/23
Denileukin	Dang *Br J Haematol 2004*	27	PFS: 6 months	13/27
Pentostatin	Tsimberidiou *Cancer 2004*	42	4.5 months	55%
Brentuximab vedotin	Shustov *ASH 2010*	58 (ALCL)	EFS: 1.2 months	1/8
Pralatrexate	O'Connor *JCO 2011*	115 (109)	DOR: 10.1 months PFS: 3.5 months	32/109
Romidepsin	Piekarz *Blood 2011*	45	DOR 8.9 months (CR:29.7 months)	17/45
	Coiffier et al., *ICML 2011*	130	DOR: 17 months	34/130

brentuximab vedotin 1.8 mg/kg q3 weeks for up to 16 cycles. Pts had received a median of two (range 1–6) prior systemic therapies, 62% of pts had primary refractory disease, 50% were refractory to their most recent prior therapy, and 22% had never responded to any prior therapy. Peripheral sensory neuropathy was the most frequent side effect and occurred in 36% of patients. Baed on these findings, brentixumab vedotin has been recently approved in patients with relapsed $CD30^+$ systemic ALCL. The use of brentuximab vedotin along with chemotherapy as first-line treatment for systemic ALCL is under investigation.

Histone Deacetylase Inhibitors

HDAC inhibitors are potent inducers of protein and histone acetylation and modulate expression of a number of cellular genes and pathways. HDAC and histone acetyltransferases regulate chromatin structure and function by removal and addition, respectively, of the acetyl group from the lysine residues of core nucleosomal histones, thus regulating gene expression [40]. HDAC inhibitors increase the acetylation of histones, as well as other nuclear factors. A number of clinical pathways have been shown to be modulated by HDAC agents, including apoptosis and cell survival pathways, angiogenesis pathways, and cell cycle genes. HDAC inhibitors have demonstrated significant clinical activity in T cell lymphomas and two of these agents, vorinostat and romidepsin, are FDA approved. The first agent in clinical trials was vorinostat (SAHA). Early studies with vorinostat demonstrated activity in patients with CTCL. A Phase II study in relapsed and refractory CTCL patients showed that a dose of 400 mg daily was well tolerated [41]. A subsequent study of oral vorinostat capsules at a dose of 400 mg daily demonstrated an ORR of 30% with one CR in a patient with advanced tumor stage CTCL [42].

Romidepsin is an intravenous HDAC inhibitor which is administered at a dose of 14 mg/m^2 weekly for 3 weeks on a 4 week cycle. In a Phase II study of relapsed and refractory CTCL patients, an overall response rate of 34% was reported [43]. The median response duration was 15 months (range 1–20+) and median time to progression was 8.3 months in early and 6.4 months in more advanced disease.

Romidepsin was subsequently explored in patients with relapsed and refractory PTCL. A multicenter phase II study was initiated by the group at the NCI, which enrolled 43 heavily pretreated patients (mean of 3.9 prior therapies). The ORR was 39% [44]. The median response duration was 8.3 months (range 1.6 months to 4.8+ years). A multicenter, multinational phase IIB registration study of romidepsin at the same dose and schedule in relapsed and refractory PTCL enrolled 130 patients with a median of two prior therapies. The ORR in this trial was 26% with 15% CR by radiographic documentation. Twenty-one patients (16%) had received a prior transplant and 49 patients (38%) were refractory to their most recent therapy. ORR and median DOR were similar across subtypes. The median duration of response for all responders was 28 months. Disease control rate including stable disease was 46%. Toxicities included gastrointestinal and constitutional events and thrombocytopenia.

Belinostat, a hydroxamic acid-derived HDACi, has been studied in both intravenous and oral formulations. Belinostat was administered intravenously at 1,000 mg/m^2/ daily for 5 days every 3 weeks in 53 patients including 19 with refractory PTCL and 29 with refractory CTCL [45]. The ORR in PTCL was 32% with two CR and a median response duration of 8.9+ months, and 14% in CTCL, with a response duration of 9.1 months. A multicenter phase II registration trial of belinostat in relapsed PTCL patients has been completed.

Additive and synergistic activity has been demonstrated in vitro for combinations of HDAC inhibitors with a number of agents, including topoisomerase inhibitors, bortezomib, and cytotoxic chemotherapy drugs and clinical trials are underway to explore the activity of these combinations in T-cell lymphomas. In one study, the combination of HDAC inhibitors and hypomethylating agents has been shown to be synergistic in vitro [46].

Pralatrexate

Pralatrexate is a novel folate antagonist whose activity is associated with binding to the reduced folate carrier. In a phase I/II dose escalation trial of pralatrexate in refractory lymphoma patients, the response rate was 54% for patients with T-cell lymphomas [47, 48]. These encouraging results led to the PROPEL trial, a multicenter phase II trial of pralatrexate in relapsed and refractory PTCL. The trial enrolled 111 patients who were treated with pralatrexate weekly for 6 weeks on a 7-week cycle. The median prior to therapies was three, and 63% of patients had no response to their last line of therapy. The ORR was 29% and the median response duration was 10.1 months [49]. Five patients with relapsed/refractory PTCL who responded to single-agent pralatrexate were able to undergo a curative stem cell transplant. Drug-related adverse events included mucositis in 70% of patients and thrombocytopenia in 40%. The incidence of mucositis with pralatrexate is ameliorated to some degree by the administration of cobalamin and folic acid during the course of therapy [50]. A number of recent studies have explored the potential synergy between pralatrexate and other active agents in T-cell lymphoma.

Immunomodulators and Immunosuppressants

Cyclosporine is an immunosuppressive agent that inhibits the NF-AT transcription complex, which activates the genes encoding cytokines and cell surface molecules involved in cell-to-cell communication and death. An early study exploring the activity of cyclosporine in CTCL and aggressive T-cell lymphomas demonstrated only modest activity [51]. A more recent study of cyclosporine was conducted in patients with AITL because this subtype of T-cell lymphoma is characterized by immune dysregulation, Cyclosporine was administered to 12 patients [52]. Two-thirds (thee CRs, five PRs) of the patients responded, but there were four deaths. A phase II trial of cyclosporine in AITL was conducted by the Eastern Cooperative Oncology Group but closed early due to slow accrual.

Other immune modulating and antiangiogenic agents, including bevacizumab, rituximab, lenalidomide, and thalidomide, are also being explored as single agents and in combination with chemotherapy. A phase II study of lenalidomide at a dose of 25 mg/m^2 daily for 21 days of a 28 day cycle was conducted in 24 relapsed PTCL patients [53]. The ORR was 30% with a PFS of 95 days. Toxicities included neutropenia and thrombocytopenia in 20% and 33% of patients, respectively. Combinations with lenalidomide are currently being planned.

Nucleoside Analogs

Deoxycoformycin (pentostatin) and forodesine are nucleoside analogs which have shown activity in both cutaneous and aggressive T-cell malignancies. Deoxycoformycin is an inhibitor of adenosine deaminase and as such it does not incorporate into DNA, unlike the other nucleoside analogs. Pentostatin increases the deoxyadenosine triphosphate pool, which leads to apoptosis in T-cells. A study conducted at MD Anderson Cancer Center reported an ORR of 71% in 24 patients with cutaneous T-cell lymphoma [54]. In the largest reported experience with pentostatin reported from the Royal Marsden, 145 patients with postthymic T-cell malignancies were given pentostatin intravenously at 4 mg/m^2/week for the first

4 weeks and then every 2 weeks until maximal response. The ORR was 32%, with marked variation according to diagnosis. The best responses occurred in patients with SS (62%) and T-PLL (45%), with CRs in three of 16 patients with SS and five of 55 patients with T-PLL. In contrast, no responses were documented in 13 patients with other types of cutaneous T-cell lymphoma, including five MF. Two of five patients with LGL had a CR and two of four with SS had a PR. A low response rate was observed in 27 patients with PTCL (19%) and in 25 with ATLL (12%) [55, 56].

Forodesine (BCX-1777, Immucillin H, 1-(9-deazahypoxanthin)-1,4-dideoxy-1,4-imino-D-ribitol) is another novel nucleoside [57]. Forodesine blocks purine nucleoside phosphorylase (PNP), preventing plasma dGuo from being cleaved to Gu, leading to accumulation of dGTP, which leads to inhibition of ribonucleotide reductase and apoptosis. A phase I/II study of oral forodesine in relapsed and refractory CTCL patients reported a 53% overall response rate, and a phase II trial has been completed [58].

Proteasome Inhibitors

Bortezomib, a proteasome inhibitor, has been well tolerated and active as a single agent in relapsed or refractory CTCL patients [59]. In a phase II study of bortezomib in relapsed CTCL or PTCL patients, the ORR was 67% with two CR and no grade 4 toxicity [59]. Bortezomib was also shown to potentially synergize with pralatrexate in an in-vitro system [60].

Signaling Inhibitors

Enzastaurin is a selective inhibitor of protein kinase C (PKC), which acts in part through the AKT pathway. By targeting the PI3K/AKT pathways, enzastaurin inhibits cell proliferation, induces tumor cell apoptosis, and suppresses tumor-induced angiogenesis in CTCL cell lines [61]. Enzastaurin is currently being explored in two phase II trials: one for patients with several types of lymphoma, including PTCL and CTCL, and another for relapsed CTCL patients.

The PI3 kinase inhibitors are another class of agents which may have therapeutic efficacy in T-celll malignancies. PI3K-δ has demonstrated a role in receptor and cytokine signaling and is important for T-cell function including proliferation, activation, and differentiation [62]. The PI3K-δisoform-specific inhibitor CAL-101 (GS-1101) has demonstrated clinical activity in patients with hematologic malignancies. In heavily pre-treated patients with refractory CLL and bulky lymphadenopathy, single agent CAL-101 was highly active and clinically efficacious, providing a durable clinical benefit [63]. Studies to explore the role of PI3 kinase inhibitors in T-cell lymphomas are underway.

Treatment Approaches for Individual Subtypes

NK/T Cell Lymphomas

One of the most difficult subtypes of PTCL to treat is NK/T-cell lymphoma. Patients with this subtype have responded poorly to anthracycline containing regimens. Patients with localized disease (Stage I, II) tend to do very well with a combination of chemotherapy and involved field radiation. The radiotherapy is an important component of management of localized NK/T cell lymphomas and has been administered both before and after cytotoxic chemotherapy. However, once the disease becomes more advanced, outcomes are relatively poor, with 2-year OS rates of 0% for those with disseminated disease [64]. Further, the CR rate for patients with advanced-stage NK/T-cell lymphoma treated with CHOP-like regimens is relatively low, with a 5-year OS rate of <10% [5]. A regimen of ifosfamide, methotrexate, etoposide, and prednisolone proved to be more effective with a 79% CR rate in early stage patients, but the CR rate was only 13% in advanced stage patients [65]. Furthermore, the relapse rate was high in both groups. The combination of CHOP and etoposide demonstrated a CR rate of 45% with a 3-year OS rate of 59% for nasal-type NK-cell lymphoma [66].

Recently, two groups have explored the activity of asparaginase-containing regimens. The combination of L-asparaginase with dexamethasone and methotrexate induced an overall response rate of 67% and a CR rate of 50% in a study of relapsed or refractory patients [67]. In another study, with an asparaginase, methotrexate, and dexamethasone regimen, response were seen in 14 of 18 evaluable patients after three cycles with 61% CR [68]. Based on these encouraging results, an asparaginase-containing regimen, SMILE, was studied as first-line therapy in patients with advanced NK/T-cell lymphomas by the NK Study Group. The SMILE regimen consists of methotrexate, etoposide, ifosfamide, dexamethasone, and L-asparaginase. Of 39 patients enrolled, 21 were newly diagnosed, 13 relapsed, and 5 had primary refractory disease [69]. Of 29 patients who completed the therapy, the overall response rate was 74%, with 38% CR. The incidence of myelosuppression was high, with Grade 3 or 4 infections in 41% of patients. Nevertheless, this regimen has been adopted by many centers for this group of difficult patients.

HTLV-1-Associated T-Cell Leukemia/Lymphoma

For patients with ATLL, results with conventional chemotherapy regimens have been uniformly poor. A phase III Japanese study evaluated a combination regimen of VCAP (vincristine, cyclophosphamide, doxorubicin, and prednisone), AMP (doxorubicin, ranimustine, and prednisone), and VECP (vindesine, etoposide, carboplatin, and prednisone) against CHOP-14 in ATLL [70]. The study demonstrated superiority for VCAP-AMP-VECP for newly diagnosed aggressive ATLL patients.

A phase II study is in preparation to investigate the ability of allogeneic stem cell transplant after induction with the VCAP-AMP-VECP regimen to prolong the median survival time, which is currently 13 months with the VCAP-AMP-VECP regimen.

The use of interferon and zidovudine has been shown to induce responses in up to 50% of patients with acute or lymphomatous ATLL [71] In a recent meta-analysis, 116 patients with acute ATLL, 18 patients with chronic ATLL, 11 patients with smoldering ATLL, and 100 patients with lymphomatous ATLL were evaluated [72]. Five-year OS rates were 46% for 75 patients who received first-line antiviral therapy ($P=0.004$), 20% for 77 patients who received first-line chemotherapy, and 12% for 55 patients who received first-line chemotherapy followed by antiviral therapy. Patients with acute, chronic, and smoldering ATLL significantly benefited from first-line antiviral therapy, whereas patients with lymphomatous ATLL experienced a better outcome with chemotherapy. In acute ATLL, 82% of patients were alive at 5 years with antiviral therapy, and 100% of patients with chronic and smoldering ATL were alive at 5 years. Multivariate analysis showed that first-line antiviral therapy significantly improved OS (hazard ratio, 0.47; 95% CI, 0.27–0.83; $P=0.021$). Prospective studies are underway to explore the use of zidovudine and interferon in smoldering ATLL.

Finally, a humanized anti-CCR4 antibody, KW-0761, has shown promise as a single agent in Japan for the treatment of ATLL. KW-0761 was used for relapsed patients with CCR4-positive ATL and PTCL in a phase I study [73]. The ORR was 31% (5/16; 95% CI, 11–59). There were no dose-limiting toxicities, and no anti-KW-0761 antibodies were detected. A phase II trial for relapsed ATLL patients was recently completed [74]. Of 27 enrolled patients (14 acute, 6 lymphomatous, 7 chronic ATLL), the ORR was 54% with seven CR. Toxicities included cytopenias (lymphopenia 96%, neutropenia 33%), skin rash (52%), and mild transaminitis. KW-0761 is now being combined with CHOP chemotherapy for first-line treatment of patients with ATLL.

Enteropathy-Associated T-Cell Lymphoma

EATL is a rare primary extranodal T-cell lymphoma in characterized by infiltration of malignant T-cell within the gastrointestinal epithelium. EATL represents 4.7% of cases of PTCL around the world and consists of two distinct histopathologic subtypes, EATL type 1, which is associated with a history of celiac sprue, and EATL type 2.

EATL type 1 is more frequent (80–90% of cases) and is a pleomorphic infiltate of anaplastic T-lymphocytes with a phenotype that is $CD3^+$, $CD7^+$, $CD5^-$, $CD8^-$, $CD4^-$, $CD103^+$. The tumor cells may express cytotoxic markers such as TIA-1, and a subset may express CD30. EATL Type 2 occurs sporadically and is composed of monomorphic populations of T-cells, which are characteristically $CD3^+$, $CD8^+$, and $CD56^+$. Chromosomal abnormalities found in EATL include gains at chromosome

9q33-q34 in up to 70% of cases. In the International T-cell Lymphoma Project, 69% of EATL patients had Stage III/IV disease at presentation. Bone marrow involvement was rare and occurred in only 3% of cases, and only 25% of patients had a low IPI (0–1) [75].

Most patients with EATL present with abdominal pain or perforation and are diagnosed at the time of laparotomy. With conventional CHOP chemotherapy, the 5 year OS and PFS were 20% and 4% respectively. Even for the low IPI group, 5-year survival was only 29%. Recent strategies to improve outcomes have included more aggressive treatment regimens and introduction of non-anthracycline-based regimens in the first line. The Nordic group reported results from 21 patients treated with CHOEP-14 followed by stem cell transplant. On that study, 33% of patients never made it to transplant due to progressive disease, and at 45 month follow up, 10 (45%) of patients were still alive [76]. Lennerd et al. have reported the use of CHOP×1 cycle followed by three cycles of non-cross resistant chemotherapy consisting of ifosfamide, etoposide, and epirubicin with intermediate dose methotrexate and then autologous stem cell transplantation. With this regimen, they have reported a response rate of 69% with a 5-year survival of 60%. Thus far there has been no data comparing outcomes with autologous vs. allogeneic stem cell transplantation in EATL, but patients with high IPI should be considered for clinical trials testing this approach. There is little data on efficacy of salvage therapy in EATL, so the treatment focus should be on effective first-line therapy followed by a consolidation with stem cell transplantation.

Subcutaneous Panniculitis-Like T-Cell Lymphoma

SPTCL is characterized by infiltration of malignant T-lymphocytes in subcutaneous tissue, often rimming the fat lobules. Although SPTCL has been recognized as a distinctive entity in the category of peripheral T-cell lymphoma in the WHO classification, its diagnostic criteria has been redefined by the recent WHO-European Organization for Research and Treatment of Cancer (EORTC) classification for primary cutaneous lymphomas. The term SPTCL is now restricted to primary tumors expressing the alpha/beta T-cell receptor phenotype. These lymphomas are usually CD3(+), CD4(−), CD8(+), and CD56(−), and usually have an indolent clinical course. The tumors expressing the gamma/delta phenotype have been reclassified as primary cutaneous gamma/delta T-cell lymphoma (PCGD-TCL).

SPTCL usually presents with one or multiple subcutaneous nodules involving one or multiple areas of the body and may be associated with fevers, weight loss, and pancytopenia. The pancytopenia is often cytokine mediated, as bone marrow involvement is rare [77, 78]. The hemophagocytic syndrome may occur in up to one third of patients and in some cases may be fulminant. The clinical course for patients with SPTCL has been highly variable, due in part to the small number of cases reported and to the fact that until recently the distinction between the alpha/beta and gamma/delta subtypes had not been uniformly made at diagnosis. Kong et al. have reviewed 22 cases of SPTCL in Asia and have identified angioinvasion as a poor prognostic marker [79].

PCGD-TCL accounts for less than 1% of all cutaneous TCL and presents as diffuse skin involvement with disseminated lesions that mainly affect the extremities and frequently are associated with ulceration and necrosis. The phenotype of PCGD patients is $CD3^+$, $CD8^-$ with expression of cytotoxic markers in most cases (TIA-1, granzyme B, perforin). Unlike alpha/beta SPTCL, dissemination to other extranodal sites is frequently, and the majority of patients present with B-symptoms.

A retrospective review by Willemze and colleagues and the EORTC Cutaneous Lymphoma Group describes clinical features and outcomes of 63 patients with SPTCL and 20 with PCGD-TCL based on careful pathological review of the cases [80]. The median age was younger (39 years vs. 59 years) for the SPTCL patients, and there was no difference in the frequency of B-symptoms or bone marrow involvement between the groups. There was a higher frequency of hemophagocytic syndrome in the PCGD-CTL group compared to the SPTCL group (45% vs. 17%). When treatment and outcomes were reviewed, it was noted that 50–70% of patients received CHOP like regimens, 10–38% had immunosuppressive therapies, and a small number were treated with radiation or local excision of the nodules. With initial therapy, 80% of patients in the SPTCL group had a response, compared to 65% in the PCGD group. The 5-year OS for the SPTCL patients was 82% vs. 11% for the PCGD patients.

Treatment approaches for SPTCL and PCGD-TCL have not been clearly established. In the retrospective EORTC review, half of the patients were treated with aggressive chemotherapy and several had autologous stem cell transplantation as a consolidation. One third of the patients were treated with single agent therapies such as methotrexate, prednisone, cyclosporine, chlorambucil, or cyclophosphamide. Sixteen of 24 had a complete response, but nine of these relapsed and five subsequently had a durable response on reinstitution of the same therapy. Eight of the patients received CHOP in relapse and three had a CR. Of five patients presenting with a solitary skin relapse, all were treated with local therapy (radiotherapy or surgery) and are in remission. In the PCGD group, 14 of 20 patients received multiagent chemotherapy and only three had a CR; one patient went on to allogeneic transplant and had a CR after transplant. Seven patients developed visceral disease and at 12 months, 15 of 20 had died of hemophagocytic syndrome or progressive disease.

Other case reports and small series have described responses in SPTCL and PCGD-TCL patients. In one single institution review of ten consecutive patients, three (two SPTCL and one PCGD-TCL) were treated initially with denileukin diftitox; one each with SPTCL and PCGD- TCL disease had PR on therapy and have been maintained without PD [81]. Seven patients were treated with cytotoxic chemotherapy regimens. Four of seven achieved a remission after EPOCH (2), denileukin diftitox-CHOP (1) or pentostatin/cyclophosphamide followed by alemtuzumab (1). Four patients (one with refractory SPTCL, two with refractory PCGD- TCL and one with PCGD- TCL in first CR after denileukin diftitox-CHOP) underwent allogeneic hematopoietic stem cell transplantation (HSCT) from matched-related donors. Two patients are alive six and 13 months after HSCT with no evidence of disease; one patient died in CR from infectious complications of

HSCT, and one relapsed 6 months after HSCT and died from PD. At a median follow up of 3 years from diagnosis, eight patients (80%) are alive, including the two patients with SPTCL and six of eight patents with PCGD- TCL. In patients who were refractory to CHOP in one series, response to cyclosporine was reported in four [82]. Another report has demonstrated the efficacy of a fludarabine-based regimen in one patient with aggressive disease [83].

On the basis of these findings, the treatment approach to PCGD-TCL should be similar to that of other aggressive poor prognosis T-cell lymphomas and should include multiagent chemotherapy followed by stem cell transplantation from an allogeneic donor if one is available. Patients with SPTCL with a benign clinical behavior may be managed with single agent therapies. For those with progressive or disseminated disease or with the hemophagocytic syndrome, multiagents chemotherapy followed by autologous stem cell transplantation should be considered.

The Role of Transplantation in Aggressive T-Cell Lymphomas

Several retrospective studies suggest that there are populations of patients with PTCL that will benefit from transplantation. The National Cancer Consortium Network (NCCN) guideline includes transplant as an option for consolidation after first remission in patients with histologies other than ALK-positive ALCL with advanced stage disease. The role of autologous transplantation in relapsed or primary refractory disease is less well defined. Disease status at transplant is a major predictor of success, with inferior results reported for patients who are not chemosensitive. In several reports, only 25–30% of refractory patients benefit from this approach. In the studies where 5-year outcomes are reported, OS average 34%. The single center experience at Stanford reported only a modest benefit after autologous transplant (5-year OS of 36%) for patients with relapsed disease and a 5-year OS of 76% in patients transplanted in first remission.

A prospective study from Germany using chemotherapy and up-front autologous transplantation for PTCL has demonstrated that a significant number of patients were never able to be transplanted due to progression of disease on first-line therapy. The treatment regimen consisted of 4–6 cycles of CHOP, followed by either dexaBEAM or ESHAP. Patients in complete or partial remission then underwent myeloablative chemoradiotherapy and autologous stem cell transplant. Two thirds (66%) of the patients were chemosensitive and went on to autologous stem cell transplant. At a median follow-up time of 33 months, the estimated 3-year OS and PFS for patients in complete response were 48% and 36%, respectively. Patients who did not experience a response to chemotherapy and therefore did not undergo autologous stem cell transplant had a very poor outcome, with a median survival of less than 2 years.

There are currently no randomized studies comparing outcomes between autologous and allogeneic transplant approaches. The Nordic and German lymphoma groups are launching a large, prospective randomized trial to compare the different strategies as consolidation after first-line therapy. In a retrospective single-institution study that compared autologous and allogeneic transplant, outcomes for autologous transplant were best when conducted in first remission, and allogeneic transplant was better for patients with resistant or relapsed disease. Further prospective studies are needed to define which subsets of PTCL patients will optimally benefit from allogeneic or autologous stem cell transplant [84–88].

Evidence-Based Treatment Approaches for PTCL

Because of the inferior outcomes with CHOP-based regimens, novel strategies are needed for patients with aggressive T-cell lymphomas. The NCCN has established evidence-based treatment approaches for T-cell lymphoma and stratifies patients based on stage. For early stage patients with localized disease, chemotherapy should be followed by involved field radiotherapy. It is recommended that all patients except for those with low IPI be consolidated with autologous stem cell transplant. ALK-positive ALCL is identified as the one subtype, which has an excellent outcome and should not be transplanted in first remission. Recent data suggest that ALK-positive patients with high IPI could be an exception to this rule. In prospective trials where up to 40% of patients do not undergo a complete remission and therefore cannot be consolidated with transplant, new approaches are necessary.

Selection of first-line therapy based on histopathologic features has not yet been widely employed but should be considered. For nodal T-cell lymphomas (PTCL-NOS, AITL, ALCL) the standard regimen used is a CHOP-based therapy. For extra-nodal subtypes, regimens may be individualized. For SPTCL, distinction should be made between the alpha-beta type and the gamma-delta type, which is now included in the category of cutaneous gamma-delta T-cell lymphoma. The alpha-beta patients may be treated with single-agent therapies or combination chemotherapy and generally have an excellent outcome. The cutaneous gamma-delta T-cell lymphomas overall do poorly and should be treated with aggressive chemotherapy followed by transplantation. Likewise, hepatosplenic and intestinal T-cell lymphomas have a poor outcome. In one study, 26 enteropathy-associated T-cell lymphoma patients were treated with CHOP then methotrexate alternating with ifosfamide, etoposide, and epirubicin.[128] Patients who achieved CR went on to transplant ($n=33$). For the transplanted EATL, the PFS and OS were 52% and 60%, respectively. NK/T-cell lymphoma patients have also had inferior outcomes with CHOP-based regimens, and consideration of alternative regimens such as SMILE and asparaginase combinations should be strongly considered for these patients.

The role of autologous vs. allogeneic stem cell transplantation in patients with poor prognosis subtypes such as NK/T cell and gamma-delta T-cell lymphomas has not been ascertained. In retrospective series, results with these subtypes are inferior to those of the more common PTCL-NOS and AITL subtypes after autologous transplantation. Therefore, consolidation with allogeneic stem cell transplantation should be considered in patients who have appropriate donors.

References

1. (1997) The Non-Hodgkin's Lymphoma Classification Project. A clinical evaluation of the International Lymphoma Study Group classification of non-Hodgkin's lymphoma. Blood 89:3909–3918
2. Vose J, Armitage J, Weisenburger D et al (2008) The International T-Cell Lymphoma Project. International peripheral T-cell and natural killer/T-cell lymphoma study: pathology findings and clinical outcomes. J Clin Oncol 26:4124–4130
3. Zettl A, deLeeuw R, Haralambieva E, Mueller-Hermelink HK (2007) Enteropathy-type T-cell lymphoma. Am J Clin Pathol 127:701–706
4. Jung CK, Lee KY, Kim Y et al (2001) Epstein-Barr virus infection, drug resistance and prognosis in Korean T- and NK-cell lymphomas. Pathol Int 51:355–363
5. Abouyabis AN, Shenoy PJ, Lechowicz MJ, Flowers CR (2008) Incidence and outcomes of the peripheral T-cell lymphoma subtypes in the United States. Leuk Lymphoma 49:2099–2107
6. Escalon MP, Liu NS, Yang Y et al (2005) Prognostic factors and treatment of patients with T-cell non-Hodgkin lymphoma: the M.D. Anderson Cancer Center experience. Cancer 103:2091–2098
7. Mercadal S, Briones J, Xicoy B et al (2008) Intensive chemotherapy (high-dose CHOP/ ESHAP regimen) followed by autologous stem-cell transplantation in previously untreated patients with peripheral T-cell lymphoma. Ann Oncol 19:958–963
8. Schmitz N, Trumper L, Ziepert M et al (2010) Treatment and prognosis of mature T-cell and NK-cell lymphoma: an analysis of patients with T-cell lymphoma treated in studies of the German High-Grade Non-Hodgkin Lymphoma Study Group. Blood 116:3418–3425
9. Tilly H, Lepage E, Coiffier B et al (2003) Intensive conventional chemotherapy (ACVBP regimen) compared with standard CHOP for poor-prognosis aggressive non-Hodgkin lymphoma. Blood 102:4284–4289
10. Delmer A, Fitoussi O, Gaulard P et al (2009) A phase II study of bortezomib in combination with intensified CHOP-like regimen (ACVBP) in patients with previously untreated T-cell lymphoma: Results of the GELA LNH05-1 T trial. ASCO Meeting Abstracts 27:8554
11. Simon A, Peoch M, Casassus P et al (2010) Upfront VIP-reinforced-ABVD (VIP-rABVD) is not superior to CHOP/21 in newly diagnosed peripheral T cell lymphoma. Results of the randomized phase III trial GOELAMS-LTP95. Br J Haematol 151:159–166
12. Piccaluga PP, Agostinelli C, Righi S, Zinzani PL, Pileri SA (2007) Expression of CD52 in peripheral T-cell lymphoma. Haematologica 92:566–567
13. Kim JG, Sohn SK, Chae YS et al (2007) Alemtuzumab plus CHOP as front-line chemotherapy for patients with peripheral T-cell lymphomas: a phase II study. Cancer Chemother Pharmacol 60:129–134
14. Gallamini A, Zaja F, Patti C et al (2007) Alemtuzumab (Campath-1 H) and CHOP chemotherapy as first-line treatment of peripheral T-cell lymphoma: results of a GITIL (Gruppo Italiano Terapie Innovative nei Linfomi) prospective multicenter trial. Blood 110:2316–2323
15. Janik JEPS et al (2005) A pilot study of campath-1 with dose-adjusted EPOCH in CD52 expressing aggressive T-cell malignancies. Blood 106:33348
16. Dang NH, Pro B, Hagemeister FB et al (2007) Phase II trial of denileukin diftitox for relapsed/ refractory T-cell non-Hodgkin lymphoma. Br J Haematol 136:439–447
17. Foss FM, Sjak-Shie NN, Goy A, Advani R, Jacobsen ED (2010) Phase II study of denileukin diftitox with CHOP chemotherapy in newly-diagnosed PTCL: CONCEPT trial. ASCO Meeting Abstracts 28:8045
18. Bruns I, Fox F, Reinecke P et al (2005) Complete remission in a patient with relapsed angioimmunoblastic T-cell lymphoma following treatment with bevacizumab. Leukemia 19:1993–1995
19. Advani RH, Hong F, Ganjoo KN et al (2009) Cardiac toxicity associated with the anti-VEGF monoclonal antibody bevacizumab (avastin) in combination with CHOP (A-CHOP) chemotherapy

for peripheral T cell lymphoma (PTCL): the ECOG 2404 trial. Blood 114:1671 (ASH Annual Meeting Abstracts)
20. Zinzani PL, Venturini F, Stefoni V et al (2010) Gemcitabine as single agent in pretreated T-cell lymphoma patients: evaluation of the long-term outcome. Ann Oncol 21:860–863
21. Arkenau HT, Chong G, Cunningham D et al (2007) Gemcitabine, cisplatin and methylprednisolone for the treatment of patients with peripheral T-cell lymphoma: the Royal Marsden Hospital experience. Haematologica 92:271–272
22. Spencer A, Reed K, Arthur C (2007) Pilot study of an outpatient-based approach for advanced lymphoma using vinorelbine, gemcitabine and filgrastim. Intern Med J 37:760–766
23. Kim JG, Sohn SK, Chae YS et al (2006) CHOP plus etoposide and gemcitabine (CHOP-EG) as front-line chemotherapy for patients with peripheral T cell lymphomas. Cancer Chemother Pharmacol 58:35–39
24. d'Amore F, Jantunen E, Relander T (2009) Hemopoietic stem cell transplantation in T-cell malignancies: who, when, and how? Curr Hematol Malig Rep 4:236–244
25. Reimer P, Rudiger T, Geissinger E et al (2009) Autologous stem-cell transplantation as first-line therapy in peripheral T-cell lymphomas: results of a prospective multicenter study. J Clin Oncol 27:106–113
26. O'Mahony D, Morris J, Moses L et al (2005) Phase I trial of siplizumab in CD2-positive lymphoproliferative disease. Blood 106:937a
27. O'Mahony D, Morris J, Stetler-Stevenson M et al (2007) EBV-related lymphoproliferative disease complicating therapy with siplizumab, a novel anti-CD2 mediated T- and NK-cell depleting agent, in patients with T-cell malignancies. Blood 110:1043a
28. Casale D, Bartlett N, Hurd D et al (2006) A phase I open label dose escalation study to evaluate MEDI-507 in patients with CD2-positive T-cell lymphoma/leukemia. Blood 108:771a
29. d'Amore F, Radford J, Jerkeman M et al (2007) Zanolimumab (HuMax-CD4™), a fully human monoclonal antibody: efficacy and safety in patients with relapsed or treatment-refractory non-cutaneous CD4+ T-cell lymphoma. Blood 110:999z
30. Kreitman RJ, Wilson WH, White JD et al (2000) Phase I trial of recombinant immunotoxin anti-Tac(Fv)-PE38 (LMB-2) in patients with hematologic malignancies. J Clin Oncol 18(8):1622–1636
31. Forero-Torres A, Leonard JP, Younes A et al (2009) A phase II study of SGN-30 (anti-CD30 mAb) in Hodgkin lymphoma or systemic anaplastic large cell lymphoma. Br J Haematol 146:171–179
32. Ansell SM, Horwitz SM, Engert A et al (2007) Phase I/II study of an anti-CD30 monoclonal antibody (MDX-060) in Hodgkin's lymphoma and anaplastic large-cell lymphoma. J Clin Oncol 25:2764–2769
33. Borchmann P, Treml JF, Hansen H et al (2003) The human anti-CD30 antibody 5 F11 shows in vitro and in vivo activity against malignant lymphoma. Blood 102:3737–3742
34. Francisco JA, Cerveny CG, Meyer DL et al (2003) cAC10-vcMMAE, an anti-CD30-monomethyl auristatin E conjugate with potent and selective antitumor activity. Blood 102:1458–1465
35. Wahl AF, Klussman K, Thompson JD et al (2002) The anti-CD30 monoclonal antibody SGN-30 promotes growth arrest and DNA fragmentation in vitro and affects antitumor activity in models of Hodgkin's disease. Cancer Res 62:3736–3742
36. Maeda N, Muta H, Oflazoglu E, Yoshikai Y (2010) Susceptibility of human T-cell leukemia virus type I-infected cells to humanized anti-CD30 monoclonal antibodies in vitro and in vivo. Cancer Sci 101:224–230
37. Fromm JR, McEarchern JA, Kennedy D, Anju T, Shustov AR, Gopal AK (2010) Preclinical and clinical binding properties, internalization kinetics, and clinicopathological activity of brentuximab vedotin (SGN-35): a novel antibody drug conjugate for anaplastic large cell lymphoma and classical Hodgkin Lymphoma. Blood 116:1789 (ASH Annual Meeting Abstracts)

38. Bartlett NL, Younes A, Carabasi MH et al (2008) A phase 1 multidose study of SGN-30 immunotherapy in patients with refractory or recurrent CD30+ hematologic malignancies. Blood 111:1848–1854
39. Younes A, Bartlett NL, Leonard JP et al (2010) Brentuximab vedotin (SGN-35) for relapsed CD30-positive lymphomas. N Engl J Med 363:1812–1821
40. Martinez-Iglesias O, Ruiz-Llorente L, Sanchez-Martinez R, Garcia L, Zambrano A, Aranda A (2008) Histone deacetylase inhibitors: mechanism of action and therapeutic use in cancer. Clin Transl Oncol 10:395–398
41. Duvic M, Talpur R, Ni X et al (2007) Phase 2 trial of oral vorinostat (suberoylanilide hydroxamic acid, SAHA) for refractory cutaneous T-cell lymphoma (CTCL). Blood 109:31–39
42. Olsen EA, Kim YH, Kuzel TM et al (2007) Phase IIb multicenter trial of vorinostat in patients with persistent, progressive, or treatment refractory cutaneous T-cell lymphoma. J Clin Oncol 25:3109–3115
43. Whittaker SJ, Demierre MF, Kim EJ et al (2010) Final results from a multicenter, international, pivotal study of romidepsin in refractory cutaneous T-cell lymphoma. J Clin Oncol 28:4485–4491
44. Piekarz R, Wright J, Frye R et al (2009) Final results of a phase 2 NCI multicenter study of romidepsin in patients with relapsed peripheral T-cell lymphoma (PTCL). Blood 114:1657 (ASH Annual Meeting Abstracts)
45. Pohlman B, Advani R, Duvic M et al (2009) Final results of a phase II trial of belinostat (PXD101) in patients with recurrent or refractory peripheral or cutaneous T-cell lymphoma. Blood 114:920 (ASH Annual Meeting Abstracts)
46. Marchi E, Bongero DC, Kalac M, Scotto L, O'Connor OA (2010) The combination of histone deacetylase inhibitors and hypomethylating agents exhibits marked synergy in preclinical models of T-cell lymphoma. Blood 116:3937 (ASH Annual Meeting Abstracts)
47. O'Connor OA, Hamlin PA, Portlock C et al (2007) Pralatrexate, a novel class of antifol with high affinity for the reduced folate carrier-type 1, produces marked complete and durable remissions in a diversity of chemotherapy refractory cases of T-cell lymphoma. Br J Haematol 139:425–428
48. O'Connor OA, Horwitz S, Hamlin P et al (2009) Phase II-I-II study of two different doses and schedules of pralatrexate, a high-affinity substrate for the reduced folate carrier, in patients with relapsed or refractory lymphoma reveals marked activity in T-cell malignancies. J Clin Oncol 27:4357–4364
49. O'Connor OA, Pro B, Pinter-Brown L et al (2011) Pralatrexate in patients with relapsed or refractory peripheral T-cell lymphoma: results from the pivotal PROPEL study. J Clin Oncol 29:1182–1189
50. Pro B, Coiffier B, Horwitz SM et al (2009) Correlation between baseline methylmalonic acid status and mucositis severity in the PROPEL study: implications for vitamin prophylaxis. Blood 114:1681 (ASH Annual Meeting Abstracts)
51. Cooper DL, Braverman IM, Sarris AH et al (1993) Cyclosporine treatment of refractory T-cell lymphomas. Cancer 71:2335–2341
52. Advani R, Horwitz S, Zelenetz A, Horning SJ (2007) Angioimmunoblastic T cell lymphoma: treatment experience with cyclosporine. Leuk Lymphoma 48:521–525
53. Dueck GS, Chua N, Prasad A et al (2009) Activity of lenalidomide in a phase II trial for T-cell lymphoma: report on the first 24 cases. ASCO Meeting Abstracts 27:8524
54. Kurzrock R, Pilat S, Duvic M (1999) Pentostatin therapy of T-cell lymphomas with cutaneous manifestations. J Clin Oncol 17:3117–3121
55. Catovsky D (1996) Clinical experience with 2′-deoxycoformycin. Hematol Cell Ther 38(Suppl 2):S103–S107
56. Dearden CE (2006) Role of single-agent purine analogues in therapy of peripheral T-cell lymphomas. Semin Hematol 43:S22–S26

57. Korycka A, Blonski JZ, Robak T (2007) Forodesine (BCX-1777, Immucillin H)–a new purine nucleoside analogue: mechanism of action and potential clinical application. Mini Rev Med Chem 7:976–983
58. Duvic M, Forero-Torres A, Foss F et al (2006) Oral forodesine is clinically active in refractory cutaneous T-cell lymphoma. Results of a phase I/II study. Blood 108:698a
59. Zinzani PL, Musuraca G, Tani M et al (2007) Phase II trial of proteasome inhibitor bortezomib in patients with relapsed or refractory cutaneous T-cell lymphoma. J Clin Oncol 25:4293–4297
60. Marchi E, Paoluzzi L, Venkatraman SE, O'Connor OA (2008) Pralatrexate (PDX) compliments the activity of the proteasome inhibitor bortezomib (B) in in vitro models of lymphoid T-cell malignancies. Blood 112:3619
61. Querfeld C, Rizvi MA, Kuzel TM et al (2006) The selective protein kinase C beta inhibitor enzastaurin induces apoptosis in cutaneous T-cell lymphoma cell lines through the AKT pathway. J Invest Dermatol 126:1641–1647
62. Fung Leung W (2011) Phosphoinositide 3-kinase delta (PI3Kdelta) in leukocyte signaling and function. Cell Signal 23(4):603–608
63. Coutre SE, Byrd JC, Furman RR, Brown JR, Benson DM, Wagner-Johnston ND et al (2011) Phase 1 study of CAL-101, an isoform-selective inhibitor of phosphatidylinositol 3 kinase P110δ, in patients with previously treated chronic lymphocytic leukemia. J Clin Oncol 29:6631
64. Yamaguchi M, Tobinai K, Oguchi M et al (2009) Phase I/II study of concurrent chemoradiotherapy for localized nasal natural killer/T-cell lymphoma: Japan Clinical Oncology Group Study JCOG0211. J Clin Oncol 27:5594–5600
65. Lee KW, Yun T, Kim DW et al (2006) First-line ifosfamide, methotrexate, etoposide and prednisolone chemotherapy +/– radiotherapy is active in stage I/II extranodal NK/T-cell lymphoma. Leuk Lymphoma 47:1274–1282
66. Yong W, Zheng W, Zhu J et al (2006) Midline NK/T-cell lymphoma nasal-type: treatment outcome, the effect of L-asparaginase based regimen, and prognostic factors. Hematol Oncol 24:28–32
67. Yamaguchi M, Suzuki R, Kwong YL et al (2008) Phase I study of dexamethasone, methotrexate, ifosfamide, L-asparaginase, and etoposide (SMILE) chemotherapy for advanced-stage, relapsed or refractory extranodal natural killer (NK)/T-cell lymphoma and leukemia. Cancer Sci 99:1016–1020
68. Jaccard A, Gachard N, Marin B et al (2011) Efficacy of L-asparaginase with methotrexate and dexamethasone (AspaMetDex regimen) in patients with refractory or relapsing extranodal NK/T-cell lymphoma, a phase II study. Blood 117:1834–1839
69. Yamaguchi M, Kwong Y, Maeda Y et al (2010) Phase II study of SMILE chemotherapy for newly-diagnosed stage IV, relapsed or refractory extranodal NK/T-cell lymphoma, nasal type: NKTSG study. ASCO Meeting Abstracts 28:8044
70. Tsukasaki KUA, Fukuda H et al (2007) VCAP-AMP-VECP compared with biweekly CHOP for adult T-cell leukemia-lymphoma: Japan Clinical Oncology Group Study JCOG9801. J Clin Oncol 25:5458–5464
71. Gill PS, Harrington W Jr, Kaplan MH et al (1995) Treatment of adult T-cell leukemia-lymphoma with a combination of interferon alfa and zidovudine. N Eng J Med 332:1744–1748
72. Bazarbachi A, Plumelle Y, Carlos Ramos J et al (2010) Meta-analysis on the use of zidovudine and interferon-alfa in adult T-cell leukemia/lymphoma showing improved survival in the leukemic subtypes. J Clin Oncol 28:4177–4183
73. Yamamoto KUA, Tobinai K et al (2010) Phase I study of KW-0761, a defucosylated humanized anti-CCR4 antibody, in relapsed patients with adult T-cell leukemia-lymphoma and peripheral T-cell lymphoma. J Clin Oncol 28:1591–1598
74. Ishida T, Joh T, Uike N et al (2010) Multicenter phase II study of KW-0761, a defucosylated anti-CCR4 antibody, in relapsed patients with adult T-cell leukemia-lymphoma (ATL). Blood 116:285 (ASH Annual Meeting Abstracts)
75. Vose J, Armitage J, Weisenburger D (2008) International peripheral T-cell and natural killer/T-cell lymphoma study: pathology findings and clinical outcomes. J Clin Oncol 26:4124–4130

76. Jantunen E, Relander T, Lauritzsen GF et al (2010) Intensive induction chemotherapy followed by autologous stem cell transplantation (ASCT) in patients with enteropathy-associated T-cell lymphoma: a prospective study by the nordic lymphoma group (NLG-T-01). Blood 116:3565 (ASH Annual Meeting Abstracts)
77. Go RS, Wester SM (2004) Immunophenotypic and molecular features, clinical outcomes, treatments, and prognostic factors associated with subcutaneous panniculitis-like T-cell lymphoma: a systematic analysis of 156 patients reported in the literature. Cancer 101:1404–1413
78. Salhany KE, Macon WR, Choi JK et al (1998) Subcutaneous panniculitis-like T-cell lymphoma: clinicopathologic, immunophenotypic, and genotypic analysis of alpha/beta and gamma/delta subtypes. Am J Surg Pathol 22:881–893
79. Kong YY, Dai B, Kong JC et al (2008) Subcutaneous panniculitis-like T-cell lymphoma: a clinicopathologic, immunophenotypic, and molecular study of 22 Asian cases according to WHO-EORTC classification. Am J Surg Pathol 32:1495–1502
80. Willemze R, Jansen PM, Cerroni L et al (2008) Subcutaneous panniculitis-like T-cell lymphoma: definition, classification, and prognostic factors: an EORTC Cutaneous Lymphoma Group Study of 83 cases. Blood 111:838–845
81. Alpdogan O, Ornstein D, Subtil T, Seropian S, Cooper DL, Foss F (2008) Outcomes in subcutaneous panniculitis-like T-cell Lymphoma (STCL). Blood 112:3750 (ASH Annual Meeting Abstracts)
82. Rojnuckarin P, Nakorn TN, Assanasen T, Wannakrairot P, Intragumtornchai T (2007) Cyclosporin in subcutaneous panniculitis-like T-cell lymphoma. Leuk Lymphoma 48:560–563
83. Chim CS, Loong F, Ng WK, Kwong YL (2008) Use of fludarabine-containing chemotherapeutic regimen results in durable complete remission of subcutaneous panniculitis-like T-cell lymphoma. Am J Clin Dermatol 9:396–398
84. d'Amore F, Relander T, Lauritzen G et al (2006) Dose-dense induction followed by autologous stem cell transplant (ASCT) as 1st line treatment in peripheral T-cell lymphomas (PTCL) - A phase II study of the Nordic Lymphoma Group (NLG) [ASH abstract 401]. Blood 108(11):123a
85. Jantunen E, Wiklund T, Juvonen E et al (2004) Autologous stem cell transplantation in adult patients with peripheral T-cell lymphoma: a nation-wide survey. Bone Marrow Trans 33(4):405–410
86. Smith SD, Bolwell BJ, Rybicki LA et al (2007) Autologous hematopoietic stem cell transplantation in peripheral T-cell lymphoma using a uniform high-dose regimen. Bone Marrow Trans 40(3):239–243
87. Chen AI, McMillan A, Negrin RS, Horning SJ, Laport GG (2007) Long term results of autologous hematopoietic cell transplantation (AHCT) for peripheral T cell lymphoma: The Stanford experience [ASH abstract 1906]. Blood 110(11):566a
88. Reimer P, Rudiger T, Geissinger E et al (2009) Autologous stem-cell transplantation as first-line therapy in peripheral T-cell lymphomas: results of a prospective multicenter study. J Clin Oncol 27(1):106–113

Overview of Stem Cell Transplantation for Lymphoma

Karen Ballen

Abstract Although the cure rate for many types of lymphoma has increased with the use of chemotherapy and monoclonal antibody treatment, approximately 50% of lymphoma patients will relapse and be candidates for either autologous or allogeneic transplantation. In this section, we examine the results of clinical transplantation in low-grade, intermediate, and high-grade lymphoma. We also review the results of older patients with lymphoma. Finally, we discuss the emerging and exciting results with the use of umbilical cord blood for patients without matched related or unrelated donors.

Low-Grade Lymphoma

Follicular lymphoma is a slowly growing lymphoma, but patients treated with conventional chemotherapy eventually succumb to the disease, with a median survival of 10 years. Therefore, Phase II studies of transplant compared to conventional controls are challenging. Rohatiner et al. performed a retrospective review of 121 adults with follicular lymphoma treated with high-dose chemotherapy and autologous bone marrow rescue [1]. With a median follow-up of 13.5 years, 48% of patients are alive and disease free with an apparent plateau on the survival curve. Patients in second remission treated with transplant were compared with age-matched controls treated with conventional therapy and the transplanted patients experienced improved remission duration and prolonged survival. The German Low Grade Lymphoma group randomized 307 patients in first remission to autologous stem cell transplantation or interferon maintenance, after all patients received conventional

K. Ballen, M.D. (✉)
Division of Hematology/Oncology, Massachusetts General Hospital, Zero Emerson, Suite 118, Boston, MA 02214, USA
e-mail: kballen@partners.org

P.J. Quesenberry and J.J. Castillo (eds.), *Non-Hodgkin Lymphoma: Prognostic Factors and Targets*, Cancer Drug Discovery and Development,
DOI 10.1007/978-1-4614-5851-7_13,

chemotherapy [2]. The 5-year progression-free survival (PFS) was 65% for the transplanted patients and 33% for the interferon patients.

The encouraging results with autologous transplant have encouraged investigators to study allogeneic transplant, in an attempt to improve disease control by utilizing the graft versus lymphoma effect. Thirty-seven patients with high-risk disease (median of three prior chemotherapy regimens) underwent myeloablative allogeneic transplant from a matched sibling or matched unrelated donor with a conditioning regimen of cyclophosphamide and total body radiation or busulfan and cyclophosphamide [3]. Median overall survival was 79% and disease-free survival 75% at 5 years post transplantation. Reduced intensity regimens may be particularly beneficial for patients with low-grade lymphoma, with an attempt to decrease toxicity and exploit the graft versus lymphoma immunologic benefit. The MD Anderson group treated 47 patients with a reduced intensity regimen of fludarabine, cyclophosphamide, and rituximab followed by matched sibling or unrelated donor allogeneic stem cell transplant [4]. With a median follow-up of 107 months, the 11-year overall and PFS rates were 78% and 72%, respectively, suggesting that nonmyeloablative allogeneic stem cell transplant is curative for relapsed follicular lymphoma.

Large-Cell Lymphoma

The Parma Study established autologous transplantation as the treatment of choice for relapsed, chemotherapy-sensitive large-cell lymphoma [5]. However, approximately 50% of patients will relapse after autologous transplant. Several investigators have added rituximab pre-transplantation to improve outcomes [6]. A randomized study from the Collaborative Trial in Relapsed Aggressive Lymphoma showed no benefit to rituximab maintenance after autologous stem cell transplant [7].

High-risk, younger patients with relapsed large-cell lymphoma may be considered for allogeneic stem cell transplantation. Forty-eight patients with relapsed large-cell lymphoma underwent a reduced intensity allograft after the conditioning regimen of alemtuzumab, fludarabine, and melphalan; cyclosporine was used for GVHD prophylaxis [8]. Four-year PFS was 48%. The non-relapse mortality was 32%, and patients with chemotherapy refractory disease did poorly. Fifty patients with relapsed or refractory lymphoma were treated with allogeneic stem cell transplant and an aggressive multiple drug and total body radiation (TBI) containing regimen [9]. Transplant-related mortality was 30% and at 3 years, the PFS was 55%. There have been no randomized studies comparing autologous and allogeneic transplant in this population. Given the high transplant-related mortality, autologous transplant may be preferred, except in circumstances of bone marrow involvement, or for patients who have relapsed after autologous transplantation.

High-Grade Lymphoma

Lymphoblastic lymphoma is an aggressive lymphoma, akin to acute lymphoblastic leukemia. Many centers treat these patients with acute lymphoblastic leukemia regimens.

The International Bone Marrow Transplant Registry (IBMTR) studied 126 patients who underwent autologous stem cell transplant and 76 patients who underwent HLA-matched sibling allogeneic transplant for lymphoblastic lymphoma [10]. As expected, allogeneic patients had a higher treatment-related mortality, 18% versus 3%, but a lower relapse rate, 34% versus 56%. Disease-free survival at 5 years was similar in both groups at 36% and 39%, respectively, for the allogeneic and autologous groups.

Rossi et al. reported on 18 patients with a chemotherapy-only conditioning regimen of cyclophosphamide, BCNU, and etoposide for patients with non-Hodgkin's lymphoma [11]. Patients had a variety of disease histologies. Two-year disease-free survival was 56%. There is limited data on the use of reduced intensity regimens for allogeneic transplant for patients with lymphoblastic lymphoma.

Mantle Cell Lymphoma

Mantle cell lymphoma, although histologically similar to the low-grade lymphomas, has an aggressive clinical course, with a median survival of only 3–4 years [12]. Thus, these patients are often candidates for transplantation in first or subsequent remission. A prospective randomized study by the European Mantle Cell Lymphoma Network randomized 122 patients in first remission to autologous stem cell transplant or interferon after a CHOP (cyclophosphamide, vincristine, adriamycin, prednisone)-based chemotherapy regimen [13]. The 3-year PFS was significantly higher in the transplant arm, 54% versus 25%, respectively. The Nordic group used a regimen of rituximab, cyclophosphamide, doxorubicin, vincristine, and prednisone alternating with high-dose cytarabine, followed by autologous stem cell transplant using rituximab-based mobilization therapy [14]. The 6-year PFS was 66%, with no relapses after 5 years.

More recent work has focused on allogeneic transplant for mantle cell lymphoma, utilizing the graft versus lymphoma effect from an allograft. Reduced intensity or nonablative allogeneic transplant might be particularly appealing in an older population. A risk adapted strategy has been adopted by the MD Anderson group [15]. The addition of rituximab resulted in an improvement in PFS for patients undergoing autologous stem cell transplant in first remission, but did not affect results for patient transplanted with more advanced disease. Reduced intensity transplant was used in 35 patients with disease advanced beyond first remission. There was no 100-day mortality and the 6-year PFS was 46%.

The timing of transplantation for mantle cell lymphoma is challenging. The optimal approach to transplantation for mantle cell lymphoma has been reviewed by Dr. Vose [16]. Registry data suggests an improved outcome for patients transplanted in first complete remission [17]. Intensive regimens such as HyperCVAD and the addition of rituximab may improve results for patients treated with either chemotherapy or autologous stem cell transplant. Results of allogeneic transplantation were mixed, with poor results in patients with chemotherapy-resistant disease [18]. Allogeneic transplantation might be considered in first complete remission for patients with a good performance status and chemotherapy-sensitive disease, or for patients with elevated Ki-67 levels who do poorly with autologous stem cell transplantation, but many centers are proceeding first to autologous transplant, followed by allogeneic transplant in patients who relapse.

Special Considerations

Elderly Patients

The median age of patients with lymphoma is in the seventh decade, yet few studies have focused specifically on patients in their sixties and seventies. We treated 35 patients over the age of 60 years, including 8 patients over the age of 70 years, with a regimen of high-dose intravenous busulfan and cyclophosphamide followed by autologous stem cell transplant [19]. There was no transplant-related mortality and the PFS at 2 years was 52%. These findings suggest that carefully selected older patients may tolerate myeloablative autologous transplant safely. Absolute age should not necessarily be a contraindication to a potentially curative transplant.

Central Nervous System Lymphoma

Primary central nervous system lymphoma is a difficult and rare clinical problem, accounting for only 1–2% of all lymphomas, and traditionally is associated with low survival rates. High-dose methotrexate with or without radiotherapy has been used, with a high rate of toxicity and low incidence of cure [20]. Several small Phase II studies report survival rates of 40–60% [21]. The appropriate timing of transplant, the optimal conditioning regimen, and the use of concomitant intrathecal treatment are all under investigation.

Alternative Donor Transplant: Umbilical Cord Blood Transplantation

The potential benefit of allogeneic transplant is outlined in the pages above. Unfortunately, only 30% of patients in the United States will have a matched sibling donor. Matched unrelated volunteer donors have been established as an alternative stem cell source, and in some scenarios results approach those seen with matched sibling donors [22]. However, only 50% of patients will be able to find a suitably matched unrelated donor in a timely fashion; the chances of finding a donor are worse for non-Caucasians and for ethnic minorities. Umbilical cord blood has been established as an alternative, with initial promising results in children [23, 24]. Initially, the low cell dose was an impediment to success in adults. To overcome this obstacle, we and others have employed double cord blood transplantation, with the infusion of two partially matched units [25–27].

The Eurocord group studied lymphoma specifically in 104 adult patients [28]. Sixty-four percent of patients received a reduced intensity regimen and 26% received double cord blood transplant. PFS was 40% at 1 year. The use of double cord blood transplantation as opposed to single cord blood transplant was associated with a decreased risk of relapse. A study from the University of Minnesota and Fred Hutchinson Cancer Research Center showed comparable survival in patients receiving either unrelated umbilical cord blood transplant or unrelated donor transplant [29]. Thus, patients who do not have a matched sibling or unrelated donor but are otherwise candidates for transplant may proceed to transplant with umbilical cord blood. A large randomized study comparing outcomes after reduced intensity double umbilical cord and haploidentical (mismatched related donor) is ongoing in the United States.

Future Directions

Lymphoma is now a curable disease for many patients but challenges remain with the toxicity of allogeneic transplant and the incidence of relapse. Therefore, more studies are designed to reduce the risk of relapse and reduce transplant-related mortality. Targeted therapies with radiolabelled antibodies are a new technique to reduce relapse rates. Other ideas in development include anti-angiogenesis agents and immunomodulators [30]. For allogeneic transplant, better HLA typing and donor selection may reduce transplant-related complications.

Conclusions

The last 20 years have been exciting for lymphoma patients and their caregivers. Many patients are cured with conventional chemotherapy alone. For patients who have relapsed or at high risk, there are many options including autologous, allogeneic, or alternative donor transplant. The next 20 years will hopefully bring additional advances.

References

1. Rohatiner AZS, Nadler L, Davies AJ et al (2007) Myeloablative therapy with autologous bone marrow transplantation for follicular lymphoma at the time of second or subsequent remission: long-term follow-up. J Clin Oncol 25:1–6

2. Lenz G, Dreyling M, Schiegnitz E et al (2004) Myeloablative radiochemotherapy followed by autologous stem cell transplantation in first remission prolongs progression-free survival in follicular lymphoma: results of a prospective, randomized trial of the German Low-Grade Lymphoma Study Group. Blood 104:2667–2674
3. Kuruvilla J, Pond G, Tsang R et al (2008) Favorable overall survival with fully myeloablative allogeneic stem cell transplantation for follicular lymphoma. Biol Blood Marrow Transplant 14:775–782
4. Khouri IF, Saliba RM, Erwin WD et al (2012) Nonmyeloablative allogeneic transplantation with or without ^{90}yttrium ibritumomab tiuxetan is potentially curative for relapsed follicular lymphoma: 12 year results. Blood 119:6373–6378
5. Philip T, Guglielmi C, Hagenbeek A et al (1995) Autologous bone marrow transplantation as compared with salvage chemotherapy in relapses of chemotherapy-sensitive non-Hodgkin's lymphoma. N Engl J Med 333:1540–1545
6. Bacher U, Klyuchnikov E, Le-Rademacher J et al (2012) Conditioning regimens for allotransplants for diffuse large B-cell lymphoma: myeloablative or reduced intensity. Blood (epub ahead of print)
7. Gisselbrecht C, Schmitz N, Mounier N et al (2012) Rituximab maintenance therapy after autologous stem cell transplantation in patients with relapsed CD20+ diffuse large B-cell lymphoma: final analysis of the Collaborative Trial in Relapsed Aggressive Lymphoma. J Clin Oncol (epub ahead of print)
8. Thomson KJ, Morris EC, Cook G et al (2008) Favorable long-term survival after reduced-intensity allogeneic transplantation for multiple-relapse aggressive non-Hodgkin's lymphoma. J Clin Oncol 27:426–432
9. O'Meara A, Halter J, Heim D et al (2012) Allogeneic stem cell transplantation for relapsed or refractory lymphoma after conditioning with BEAM/Fludarabine/TBI. Bio Blood Marrow Transplant (e pub ahead of print)
10. Levine JH, Harris RE, Loberiza FR et al (2003) A comparison of allogeneic and autologous bone marrow transplantation for lymphoblastic lymphoma. Blood 101:2476–2482
11. Rossi HA, Becker PS, Emmons RVB et al (2003) High-dose cyclophosphamide, BCNU, and VP-16 (CBV) conditioning before allogeneic stem cell transplantation for patients with non-Hodgkin's lymphoma. Bone Marrow Transplant 31:441–446
12. Velders GA, Kluin-Nelemans JC, De Boer CJ et al (1996) Mantle-cell lymphoma: a population-based clinical study. J Clin Oncol 14:1269–1274
13. Dreyling A, Lenz G, Hoster E et al (2005) Early consolidation by myeloablative radiochemotherapy followed by autologous stem cell transplantation in first remission significantly prolongs progression-free survival in mantle-cell lymphoma: results of a prospective randomized trial of the European MCL Network. Blood 105:2677–2684
14. Geisler CH, Kolstad A, Laurell A et al (2008) Long-term progression free survival of mantle cell lymphoma after intensive front-line immunochemotherapy with in-vivo purged stem cell rescue: a nonrandomized phase 2 multicenter study by the Nordic Lymphoma Group. Blood 112:2687–2693
15. Tam CS, Bassett R, Ledesma C et al (2009) Mature results of the MD Anderson Cancer Center risk-adapted transplantation strategy in mantle cell lymphoma. Blood 113:4144–4152
16. Vose JM (2012) Autotransplantation for mantle cell lymphoma. Cancer J 18:427–431
17. Vandenberghe E, Ruiz de Elvira C, Loberiza FR et al (2003) Outcome of autologous transplantation for mantle cell lymphoma: a study by the European blood and marrow transplant and autologous blood and marrow transplant registries. Br J Haematol 120:793–800
18. Khouri IF, Champlin RE (2012) Nonmyeloablative allogeneic stem cell transplantation for non-Hodgkins lymphoma. Cancer J 18:457–462
19. Yusuf RZ, Dey B, Yeap BY et al (2009) Autologous stem cell transplantation with a dose reduced busulfan and cyclophosphamide regimen in older patients with non-Hodgkin's lymphoma. Bone Marrow Transplant 43:37–42
20. Plotkin SR, Betensky RA, Hochberg FH et al (2004) Treatment of relapsed central nervous system lymphoma with high-dose methotrexate. Clin Cancer Res 10:5643–5645

21. Ferreri AJM, Crocchiolo R, Assanelli A et al (2008) High-dose chemotherapy supported by autologous stem cell transplantation in patients with primary central nervous system lymphoma: facts and opinions. Leuk Lymphoma 49:2042–2047
22. Ballen KK, King RJ, Chitphakdithai P et al (2008) The National Marrow Donor Program experience: the first 20 years of unrelated donor stem cell transplantation. Biol Blood Marrow Transplant 14:2–7
23. Kurtzberg J, Laughlin M, Graham ML et al (1996) Placental blood as a source of hematopoietic stem cells for transplantation into unrelated recipients. N Engl J Med 335:157–166
24. Zhang MJ, Davies SM, Camitta BM et al (2012) Comparison of outcomes after HLA-matched sibling and unrelated donor transplantation for children with high-risk acute lymphoblastic leukemia. Biol Blood Marrow Transplant 18:1204–1210
25. Cutler C, Stevenson K, Kim HT et al (2011) Double umbilical cord blood transplantation with reduced intensity conditioning and sirolimus based GVHD prophylaxis. Bone Marrow Transplant 46:273–277
26. Brunstein CG, Fuchs EJ, Carter SL et al (2011) Alternative donor transplantation after reduced intensity conditioning: results of parallel phase 2 trials using partially HLA-mismatched related bone marrow or unrelated donor umbilical cord blood grafts. Blood 118:282–288
27. Chen YB, Aldridge J, Kim HT et al (2012) Reduced intensity conditioning stem cell transplantation: comparison of double umbilical cord blood and unrelated donor grafts. Biol Blood Marrow Transplant 18:805–812
28. Rodrigues CA, Sanz G, Brunstein CG et al (2008) Analysis of risk factors for outcomes after unrelated cord blood transplantation in adults with lymphoid malignancies: a study by the Eurocord-Netcord and Lymphoma Working Party of the European Group for Blood and Marrow Transplantation. J Clin Oncol 27:256–263
29. Brunstein CG, Gutman JA, Weisdorf DJ et al (2010) Allogeneic hematopoietic cell transplantation for hematologic malignancy: relative risks and benefits of double umbilical cord blood. Blood 116:4693–4699
30. Fernandez HF, Escalon MP, Pereira D et al (2007) Autotransplant conditioning regimens for aggressive lymphoma: are we on the right road? Bone Marrow Transplant 40:505–513

Autologous Hematopoietic Stem Cell Transplantation in Non-Hodgkin Lymphomas

Natthapol Songdej and Eric S. Winer

Abstract Non-Hodgkin Lymphoma is a heterogeneous group of lymphoid malignancies that involves mature B-cells, mature T-cells, and their progenitors. Although novel chemotherapy and immunotherapy regimens have improved rates of complete response and overall survival, autologous stem cell transplant (ASCT) is used in both the front-line and relapsed setting to further improve these markers and potentially cure. Even in indolent lymphomas, ASCT shows a definite improvement in progression-free survival, although no improvement in overall survival. The most promising results for front-line ASCT are in mantle cell lymphoma (MCL), where there is evidence of long-term progression-free and overall survival with evidence of a cured fraction. In the relapsed setting, ASCT is the standard of care in diffuse large B-cell lymphoma, though results of ASCT in the relapsed setting for MCL and Burkitt lymphoma are disappointing. The role and timing of ASCT in peripheral T-cell lymphomas are yet to be defined, but front-line ASCT in enteropathy-associated T-cell lymphoma and advanced-stage cutaneous T-cell lymphoma shows promise for improving long-term outcomes. Additional studies on front-line and relapsed ASCT with novel chemotherapy and immunotherapy regimens may demonstrate further improved responses and survival, especially for high-risk patients.

N. Songdej, M.D./M.P.H.
Department of Medicine, Rhode Island Hospital,
The Warren Alpert Medical School of Brown University, Providence, RI, USA

E.S. Winer, M.D. (✉)
Division of Hematology and Oncology, Rhode Island Hospital,
The Warren Alpert Medical School of Brown University, Providence, RI, USA

Comprehensive Cancer Center, University Medicine,
593 Eddy St, Providence, RI 02903, USA
e-mail: ewiner@lifespan.org

P.J. Quesenberry and J.J. Castillo (eds.), *Non-Hodgkin Lymphoma: Prognostic Factors and Targets*, Cancer Drug Discovery and Development,
DOI 10.1007/978-1-4614-5851-7_14, © Springer Science+Business Media New York 2013

Introduction

Non-Hodgkin's Lymphoma (NHL) is a heterogeneous group of lymphoid malignancies that involves mature B-cells, mature T-cells, and their progenitors. The World Health Organization recently published a new classification system to differentiate between this diverse group of diseases [1]. Although multiple novel agents such as the monoclonal antibodies or novel chemotherapies have improved complete response and overall survival, there are still patients who succumb to the disease. Autologous Stem Cell Transplant (ASCT) has been used in attempts to prolong overall survival and other measures such as progression-free survival and event-free survival in the front line and relapsed setting. In 2008, over 3,000 patients with NHL received an ASCT. [2] This chapter will summarize the data of ASCT for NHL.

Follicular Lymphoma

Follicular Lymphoma (FL) is the second most common NHL, accounting for 15–30% of newly diagnosed lymphomas. The majority of patients have a clinical course characterized by a series of remissions and relapses with minimal patients being cured [3]. While new prognostic systems such as the Follicular Lymphoma International Prognostic Index (FLIPI) [4] have been helpful in stratifying patients in terms of survival, it is not clear if more aggressive treatment in the high-risk patients is beneficial. Many patients also have the potential to transform to a Diffuse Large B-cell Lymphoma, which usually conveys a poor prognosis. One treatment that has been attempted to prolong remissions and attempt cure is high-dose chemotherapy with ASCT.

The initial studies of ASCT in FL were a series of phase II trials performed in the relapsed/refractory setting. The study by Freedman et al. [5] evaluated patients who had ≤2 cm residual disease and <20% bone marrow involvement, and conditioned them with a standard cyclophosphamide/TBI regimen and gave purged marrow. The disease-free survival was found to be 42% at 8 years, with an overall survival at 66% in 8 years; the 12-year survival for the 153 patients in the study was 69%. A similar study was published by Apostolidis et al. [6] which treated 99 patients in second or subsequent remission also conditioned with cyclophosphamide/TBI and given purged marrow. The freedom from recurrence at 5-years was 63% and OS was 69%. In this study, seven of ten late deaths were due to secondary myelodysplastic syndrome (s-MDS) or acute myelogenous leukemia (AML), with 12 of the 99 patients developing s-MDS. In both studies, laboratory correlates were performed evaluating PCR for Bcl-2/IgH rearrangements, with absence of the rearrangement associated with a lower risk of recurrence.

Brice et al. evaluate front-line treatment of 566 patients with FL, and 372 with relapsed disease [7]. Eighty-two of the relapsed patients received physicians choice salvage therapy followed by ASCT. Patients undergoing conditioning with either TBI (71%) or BEAM (29%) followed by ASCT had a prolonged 5-year freedom from second failure (42% vs. 16%; $p=0.0001$) and 5-year survival (58% vs. 38%; $p=0.0005$). The authors noted that the two groups were not similar because median age in ASCT arm was 45 compared to standard treatment are of 58, with remaining parameters showing no statistical differences. The authors tried to negate bias of age, and compared only patients <65 years, and benefit of ASCT showed 5-year OS at 60% vs. 40% ($p=0.001$). A further study by Grigg et al. evaluated ASCT with maintenance interferon, which did not show an extended survival but did have minority of patients with durable remissions [8].

Two further groups retrospectively evaluated ASCT in a phase II relapsed setting. Bierman et al. reviewed data on 100 follicular lymphoma patients who underwent ASCT. Failure-free survival was found to be 44% at 4-years while the OS was 65% [9]. Cao et al. reported on 92 patients with relapsed or refractory follicular lymphoma. The 4-year overall survival in this group was 60% with a disease-free survival at 44%; total body irradiation and treatment with three or fewer regimens was associated with an increased overall survival [10].

The European Group for Blood and Marrow Transplantation (EBMT) Lymphoma Working Party conducted the "CUP" trial to assess the utility of ASCT in a randomized trial [11]. Patients were treated with three cycles of CHOP, and if a CR or PR was obtained, they were randomized to either three further cycles of chemotherapy (C), ASCT with unpurged cells (U) or ASCT with immunomagnetically purged cells (P). Eighty-nine patients were randomized; 69% of patients had only one prior therapy. Progression-free survival at 2 years demonstrated 26% in the chemotherapy alone arm, with 58% and 55% in the unpurged and purged groups, respectively. Similarly, the overall survival at 4 years for the C, U, and P arms were 36%, 71%, and 77% respectively. No benefit was seen between the purged and unpurged group.

Furthermore, the EBMT performed a registry study that evaluated 693 patients that had ASCT for follicular lymphoma [12]. Thirty percent had received only one line of treatment, 62% had received two lines, and 8% had received three or more treatments. The median overall survival was 12 years, with the multivariate analysis demonstrating shorter overall survival in patients with age >45, and chemoresistant disease, Bone marrow as stem cell source, and TBI conditioning regimens. Sixty four patients (9%) developed second malignancies.

There have been numerous phase II studies evaluating the use of ASCT in first remission for FL. These studies all show excellent results. The study from Freedman et al. demonstrated a 3-year disease-free survival and overall survival of 63% and 89% respectively in patients treated with CHOP and were transplanted even though they were positive for t(14;18) by PCR at the time of harvest [13]. Horning et al. evaluated 37 patients in first CR who received TBI, etoposide and cyclophosphamide followed by purged autologous bone marrow. In this group, the estimated 10-year survival was 86%, with a 10-year disease-specific survival of 97% [14]. A third study by Ladetto et al. examined 92 patients under age 60 with advanced FL who had a first line ASCT. The disease-free survival and overall survival at 4 years was 67 and 84% [15].

In order to better examine the question of benefit of ASCT in first remission of FL, four randomized trials were performed (Table 1). The German trial by Lenz

Table 1 Randomized trials for autologous stem cell transplant in first remission follicular lymphoma

Study	Patients(n)	Chemotherapy	Transplant/maintenance	PFS	OS	Secondary malignancy
GLSG[4]	$N=307$	CHOP/MCP×6	IFN Maintenance	33.3%	N/A	N/A
	Advanced fl	CHOP/MCP×4–6	Dexa -Beam	64.7%	N/A	3.87 at 5 years
				$p<0.001$		
GOELAMS [3]	$N=172$	CHVP×6	CHVP+IFN	39%—years	80%—9 years	$N=1$
	FLIPI Scores	VCAP +1MVP-16	CY/TPI	64%	76%	$N=12$
		I6<PR-DHAP		$p=0.004$	$p=0.05$	$p=0.02$
GELA [17]	$N=401$	CHVP×12	IFN	29%—7 years	71%	$N=4$ (21%)
	Advanced FL	CHOP×4	CY/VP16/TBI	38%	76%	
				$p=11$	$p=0.05$	
GITMO IIL [16]	$N=136$	CHOP	Rituxan×4	38%	80%	6.6%
	Advanced FL	APO±DHAP	Cytoxan+Rituxan	61%	81%	
				$p<0.061$	$p=0.96$	

CHOP/MCP cyclophosphamide, doxorubicin, vincristine, prednisone, mitoxantrone, chlorambucil, and prednisone, *CHVP* cuclophosphamide, low-dose doxorubicin, teniposide, and prednisone, *CY/VP/TBI* cyclosphamide, VP-16 and TBI, *DexaBEAM*, dexamethasone, BCNU, etoposide, cytarabine, and melphalan, *APO* (doxorubicin, vincristine, prednisone) DHAP, dexamethasone, high-dose cytarabine, and cisplatin, *IFM* interferon, *IMVP-16*, ifosfamide, methotrexate, and VP-16, *NA* not available, *PFS* progression-free survival, *TBI/CY* total body irradiation and cyclosphamide, *VCAP*, cyclophosphamide, high-dose doxorubicin, prednisone, and vincristine et al. randomized 307 patients with untreated advanced (stage III or IV) follicular lymphoma. Patients received two cycles CHOP (75%) or mitoxantrone, chlorambucil and prednisone (MCP-35% of patients) then were randomized to ASCT or interferon-α maintenance. The patients in the autologous arm received an additional two to four cycles of CHOP and then ASCT with Dexa-BEAM conditioning, while the others received a total of six cycles of CHOP followed by IFN-α maintenance. Crossover was permitted. Progression-free survival was 64.7% in Autologous transplant arm and 33.3% in the IFN- α arm ($p<0.0001$). Data for overall survival was not mature for reporting initially. Further analysis of this study demonstrated a significant risk for secondary malignancy with 5 of 195 developing secondary malignancies and an estimated 5-year risk of 3.8% [4].

The GOELAMS group randomized 172 newly diagnosed follicular lymphoma patients to chemotherapy (cyclophosphamide, doxorubicin, teniposide, prednisone and interferon) or high-dose therapy followed by purged ASCT [16]. The response rate was higher in the high-dose therapy arm (81% vs. 69%; $p=0.045$) and a longer event-free survival (not reached at time of publication vs. 45 months); when the data was stratified by FLIPI score a 5-year event-free survival was noted for patients with poor risk FLIPI (>2) of 67% v. 20% ($p=0.018$), but still no difference in overall survival. Patients with good risk FLIPI had similar event-free survival in the two groups. In this study, overall survival was affected by older age, elevated initial LDH, and poor risk FLIPI. No benefit was noted in overall survival due to increase in secondary malignancies, with 10 of the 172 patients developing secondary malignancies (three leukemias, three s-MDS, two breast cancers, one renal cancer, and one prostate cancer) with an actuarial risk of 18.6% at 5 years. Further analysis of this study was published which still did not demonstrate a difference in overall survival (76% in HDT v. 80% in the chemotherapy alone group). The 9-year progression-free survival and event-free survival were higher in the ASCT group compared to the chemotherapy group (64% vs. 39%; $p=0.004$ and 56% vs. 39%; $p=0.03$, respectively) [3]. No effect on event-free survival was noted with FLIPI, but patients with low FLIPI scores had a longer progression-free survival when treated by ASCT, with a plateau noted at 7 years. This plateau suggests that a subgroup might be cured by ASCT, but the risk of secondary malignancy (12 total, 6.9%) persisted.

GELA study GELF-94 evaluated 401 patients with untreated advanced follicular randomized to either Cyclophosphamide, doxorubicin, teniposide, and prednisone for a total of 12 doses with Interferon-α or four cycles of standard CHOP with responders having ASCT with cyclophosphamide/etoposide/TBI [17]. Event-free survival at 7 years was not significant between the two arms (28 vs. 38%, $p=0.11$), nor was 7-year overall survival (71 vs. 76%, $p=0.53$). When stratified by FLIPI, there was a trend towards longer event-free survival in the ASCT arm compared to the chemotherapy arm in patients with a FLIPI >2. In the ASCT arm, four secondary hematologic malignancies were noted (2.1%).

A final study called the GITMO-IIL trial randomized 136 stage III or IV FL patients to six cycles of CHOP followed by four rituximab infusion compared with four doses of doxorubicin, vincristine and prednisone (APO) with two cycles of

DHAP if not in a complete response followed by etoposide mobilization, rituximab treatment, and cyclophosphamide/rituximab conditioning [15]. The 4-year event-free survival was 38% for the chemotherapy alone arm v. 61% for the ASCT arm ($p<0.001$); there was no significant difference in 4-year OS (80% chemotherapy vs. 81% ASCT; $p=0.96$). There was a significant difference in molecular remission evaluated by PCR for Bcl-2/IgH of 44% vs. 80% ($p<0.001$). It was also noted that even though the ASCT arm had improved molecular outcomes, the chemotherapy only patients had good outcomes after salvage ASCT, recommending the use of transplant in the relapsed or refractory setting. The risk of sMDS/AML was 6.6% in the ASCT arm.

Patients who transform from follicular lymphoma to diffuse large B-cell lymphoma (DLBCL) have a poor prognosis. The Ohio State University group retrospectively evaluated 24 patients with histologically confirmed DLBCL [18]. These patients received salvage chemotherapy and ASCT. The 3-year progression-free and overall survival was 40% and 52%, respectively. More studies are needed in this patient population.

The use of rituximab has revolutionized the way lymphomas are treated. Frontline trials using the regimen CVP showed that the addition of rituximab improved time to progression from 15 to 32 months and overall survival at 4 years of 84% vs. 77% [19]. In further analysis of the GELA study, Sebban et al. investigated two cohorts of patients of patients in two randomized studies, the GELF-86 and GELF 94 studies and evaluated the role of rituximab and ASCT in relapsed FL after first relapse. ASCT was found to be associated with an increase of event-free survival, but rituximab was associated with a greater benefit than ASCT for event-free survival and overall survival after relapse [20]. Witzens-Harig et al. also reviewed the studies of ASCT with rituximab and concluded that although ASCT did not show an overall survival benefit, there may be a role for combination ASCT in addition to rituximab in the relapsed setting [21].

Overall, the data show that ASCT demonstrates an improvement in disease-free survival and event-free survival, but has not shown a benefit over conventional chemotherapy in overall survival. Some studies show that there may be a benefit of ASCT in patients with a high FLIPI score or in transformed lymphoma. There is also a notable plateau in overall survival which may indicate that a small population has potential for cure with ASCT, although the characteristics of these patients are still to be determined.

Diffuse Large B-Cell Lymphoma

Diffuse large B-cell lymphoma (DLCBL) is the most common type of NHL, comprising approximately 30% of newly diagnosed cases. DLBCL is a heterogeneous, intermediate-grade lymphoma; prognostic scores such as the International Prognostic Index or Revised Prognostic Index score can be used to stratify patients in terms of survival. In the rituximab era, 4-year overall survival rates range from

94% for very good Revised IPI (0 IPI factors) score to 55% for poor Revised IPI score (3–5 IPI factors) [22].

Newly diagnosed patients with DLBCL usually undergo treatment with immunotherapy and chemotherapy-based regimen. Currently, up-front ASCT is not recommended for any IPI group. The lack of efficacy for up-front ASCT has been best demonstrated by two meta-analyses published in 2003 and 2007. In the most recent meta-analysis done in 2007, Greb et al. [23] reviewed 15 randomized controlled trials between 1990 and 2005 that pooled together 2,728 patients between the ages of 27 and 48 years. The trials were heterogeneous in terms of types of conventional chemotherapy and induction regimens used. Eight trials employed abbreviated conventional chemotherapy prior to ASCT, five used standard therapy, and two used sequential high-dose chemotherapy. Most trials employed BEAM (carmustine, etoposide, cytarabine and melphalan) or a similar regimen for the ASCT conditioning regimen. When compared with conventional therapy, there were no differences in overall and event-free survival. There was conflicting data regarding high-risk patients, mostly owing to study heterogeneity, with some studies demonstrating improved overall and event-free survival [23]. However, as high-risk patients have poorer 5-year survival rates, the use of ASCT as up-front therapy in these patients is an active area of investigation.

The recent inclusion of rituximab into up-front regimens has yielded promising results. In a 2009 study, Vitolo et al. [24] employed dose dense chemotherapy followed by an intensification phase and ASCT in 94 patients between the ages of 18–60 with stage III-IV DLBCL with intermediate/high or high-risk age-adjusted-IPI. The induction regimen consisted of R-MegaCEOP14 (rituximab, cyclophosphamide, epirubicin, vincristine and prednisone) for two cycles. This was followed by two cycles of R-MAD (rituximab, mitoxantrone, cytarabine and dexamethasone). Autologous stem cell transplant was then performed after myeloablation from a BEAM regimen. Compared with a historical control group of 41 patients who had received a regimen of weekly MACOP-B (methotrexate, doxorubicin, cyclophosphamide, vincristine, prednisone, and bleomycin) for 8 weeks followed by two cycles of MAD and then BEAM with ASCT, there was evidence of improved overall and failure-free survival. At 4 years, overall and failure-free survival for the rituximab plus up-front ASCT group was 80% and 73%, respectively, compared with 54% and 44% in the historical control group.

More recently, Glass et al. [25] also demonstrated improved overall and event-free survival in patients between the age of 18–60 years with high-risk DLBCL who received a rituximab-containing regimen with up-front ASCT. In this study, 64 patients were given four cycles of dose escalated CHOP with the addition of etoposide (MegaCHOEP). Six total infusions of rituximab were given—the first prior to chemotherapy, the second through fifth 12 days after the start of each chemotherapy cycle, and the final 33 days after the final cycle. ASCT was performed after cycles 2–4. This regimen was compared to a historical control group that included 29 patients who had received MegaCHOEP and ASCT without rituximab. Overall and event-free survival in the R-MegaCHOEP plus ASCT group were 78.7% and 72.7% at 3 years, respectively, compared with 55% and 47.2% in the historical control group, though there was a higher frequency of grade 3/4 infections in the R-MegaCHOEP plus ASCT group (18.5% versus 6.0%).

Lastly, a recent phase III randomized SWOG study evaluated the benefit of ASCT in first remission for patients with bulky stage II, III, or IV intermediate-high or high IPI DLBCL. Three hundred ninety-seven patients were enrolled and received either R-CHOP or CHOP alone and then were randomized to ASCT. Preliminary data shows an improved PFS in the transplant arm, especially for the high IPI patients [26].

For patients with relapsed DLBCL, ASCT is currently the standard of care for patients <60 years of age with chemosensitive disease. In the landmark study by the PARMA group, [27] Two-hundred fifteen relapsed patients (188 their first relapse and 27 patients in their second relapse) between the ages of 18 and 60 were given two courses of DHAP (dexamethasone, cisplatin, and cytarabine) chemotherapy. All had intermediate grade (163 patients) or high grade (52 patients) disease. The responders, which included 109 patients, were then randomized to receive either an additional four courses of DHAP chemotherapy every 3–4 weeks plus radiation (54 patients) or intensive chemotherapy followed by ASCT (55 patients). Patients assigned to the ASCT group were given prior treatment with BEAC (carmustine, etoposide, cytarabine, cyclophosphamide, and MESNA) and radiation, if indicated. At 5 years, overall survival, event-free survival, and response rate were 53%, 46%, and 84%, respectively, in the ASCT group compared with 32%, 12%, and 44%, respectively, in the chemotherapy group.

The use of ASCT for patients >60 years of age has not been traditionally routinely recommended and remains a matter of investigation. However, ASCT in patients >60 years of age is of great interest as diagnosis of DLBCL is often made beyond the age of 60 and carries a poorer prognosis beyond that age. Recent studies have suggested that ASCT may be of benefit for older patients. Baudi et al. [28] retrospectively reviewed data from the Mayo clinic Rochester BMT database for 93 patients aged 60 and over (median age 66 years) who underwent ASCT for intermediate grade non-Hodgkin's lymphoma (57 patients with DLBCL) compared with a younger cohort of 178 patients (median age 50 years). There was no difference in treatment-related mortality or event-free survival at 4 years (42% for the younger group and 38% for the older group), although the estimated median survival was 25 months in the older cohort and 56 months in the younger cohort.

In another retrospective review using the European Blood and Marrow Transplant registry, Jantunen et al. [29] compared outcomes in 463 patients aged 60 and over at the time of ASCT with 2,149 younger patients. Of the 463 patients in the 60 and over cohort, the majority were between 60 and 64 years old, with only 12 patients between the ages of 70–74. The median age of the younger cohort was 47 years. At 3 years, the overall and progression-free survival for the elderly group was 60% and 51% compared with 70% and 62%, respectively, for the younger group, with non-relapse mortality higher in the elderly group (10.8% versus 6.5%). Despite poorer outcome of ASCT in patients aged 60 and over when compared to a younger cohort, these studies are nonetheless encouraging when taken in light of the poor prognosis of relapsed DLBCL, especially in elderly individuals.

In summary, ASCT in DLBCL should not be used as part of up-front therapy as thus far there have been no difference in overall survival demonstrated; however, recent data may show that there is a potential benefit in high-risk patients. ASCT is part of the standard of care in relapsed and refractory disease. Further, there is evidence that ASCT is effective and can feasibly be performed in an older age cohort in the relapsed and refractory setting.

Mantle Cell Lymphoma

Mantle cell lymphoma (MCL) is a relatively rare B-cell NHL that has traditionally been an incurable malignancy with poor response to treatment with a median survival between 3 and 5 years. Previous initial treatments consisted of chemotherapy with a CHOP-like regimen. However, the majority of patients treated with such a regimen did not achieve complete remission; those that did relapsed after a median of 1–2 years [30]. Due to the lack of efficacy of initial chemotherapy, there has long been interest in the use of up-front ASCT in patients with mantle cell lymphoma. Disappointingly, chemotherapy in the pre-rituximab era with up-front ASCT only produced median remission duration of approximately 3–4 years with evidence of ongoing relapses [30]. More recently, however, the use of rituximab and cytarabine-containing regimens with up-front ASCT has resulted in significant prolongation of event-free survival and overall survival.

In a landmark study, Geisler et al. [31] gave 160 previously untreated newly diagnosed stage II–IV mantle cell lymphoma patients between the ages of 32 and 65 years (median age 56 years) with alternating cycles of dose-intensified CHOP-21 (maxi-CHOP-21) and high-dose cytarabine-21 for a total of six cycles. Rituximab was given during both the induction phase (first day of cycle 4 and 5) and during stem cell mobilization for in vivo purging (first and ninth day of cycle 6), with a total of four doses of rituximab given. Patients who had evidence of response were then given either high-dose BEAM or BEAC followed by ASCT. Results demonstrated 6-year overall, progression, and event-free survival of 70%, 66%, and 56%, respectively, with a plateau apparent at 5 years, suggesting that some patients may be cured.

Similar promising results were obtained by Dreger et al. [32], who treated 34 newly diagnosed mantle cell lymphoma patients between the ages of 30 and 67 with CHOP induction, followed by stem cell mobilization with either Dexa-BEAM or DHAP, with two doses of rituximab added to myeloablative therapy with cyclophosphamide and total body irradiation. Event-free survival at 4 years was 83% for the rituximab group versus 47% for the non-rituximab group, with a plateau apparent at 4 years. Some studies have suggested that similar good results can be obtained from intensive chemotherapy alone, for example, with a regimen of rituximab-hyperCVAD alternating with rituximab plus high-dose methotrexate and cytarabine [33]. Thus far, there have been no trials that have directly compared a rituximab-containing regimen and up-front ASCT with initial intensive chemoimmunotherapy.

The use of ASCT in individuals >65 years of age appears to yield similar outcomes as ASCT done in a younger cohort. Jantunen et al. [34] retrospectively reviewed data from the European Group for Blood and Marrow Transplantation registry for 79 patients with mantle cell lymphoma who received ASCT beyond the age of 65 (range of 65–73 years with a median age of 67 years). When compared with the younger cohort of 655 patients (range of 29–64 years with a median age of 56 years), at 5 years there were no differences in non-relapse mortality (5.0 vs. 5.6%), rate of relapse (66% vs. 55%), progression-free survival (40% vs. 29%), or overall survival at 5 years (67 vs. 61%).

For relapsed or refractory mantle cell lymphoma, the use of ASCT is not nearly as effective as when employed in up-front treatment. In a series of 36 patients (median age 59, range 42–76) who underwent variable conditioning regimens prior to ASCT (median of two prior chemotherapy regimens) for relapsed or refractory disease, Tam et al. documented a median overall survival of approximately 2 years, with evidence of ongoing relapses [30]. These unfavorable results remained unchanged in the rituximab era, as there was no difference in outcome between the 19 patients who underwent ASCT with rituximab as compared to the 17 patients who underwent ASCT without rituximab. Therefore, patients with relapsed or refractory mantle cell lymphoma are generally offered salvage chemotherapy regimens or allogeneic HSCT if they are suitable candidates.

In summary, up-front ASCT for MCL in the era of rituximab results in long-term overall and progression-free survival with evidence of a cured fraction, although it is unclear if there is a difference in outcome when compared with intensive chemotherapy alone. The outcome of ASCT in the relapsed and refractory setting remains disappointing, and patients with relapsed and refractory MCL should proceed to other salvage therapies.

Burkitt Lymphoma

Burkitt lymphoma (BL) is a rare and aggressive B-cell neoplasm. There are three defined clinical variants, which include the sporadic, endemic, and immunodeficiency types. In the USA, the sporadic type is the most common, and comprises 1–2% of NHLs. Standard up-front therapy for BL consists of intensive chemotherapy and therapy for potential CNS disease (e.g., high-dose methotrexate and cytarabine), with some regimens also including immunotherapy. With intensive regimens in adults, complete remission ranges from 75 to 97% with 5-year overall survival between 70 and 92% [35].

The role for up-front ASCT in BL is limited, owing to the mentioned good response rates from intensive chemotherapy and the lack in improvement or worse outcomes from up-front ASCT. For example, Jost et al. [36] gave 17 patients with BL 12 weeks of chemotherapy with MACOP-B or VACOP-B chemotherapy, followed by high-dose therapy and ASCT in responding patients. At 3 years, overall and event-free survivals were 48% and 31%, respectively.

Better results were reported by Sweetenham et al. [37] in a retrospective analysis of patients from the European Group for Blood and Marrow Transplantation registry who had undergone ASCT. A total of 70 patients (median age 31 years, range 16–57) with BL or Burkitt-like lymphoma (BLL) underwent ASCT in their first complete remission. Induction regimens varied, and included ALL-type regimens, CHOP-like regimens, as well as regimens such as MACOP-B and PACEBOM. The most common high-dose regimens used were BEAM and cyclophosphamide with total body irradiation. At 3 years, the overall and progression-free survival was 72% and 73%, respectively.

Song et al. [38] have provided more recent data regarding outcome of up-front ASCT in BL. The investigators reviewed 43 cases of BL (BLL patients were excluded) in British Columbia from 1987 to 2003 that had intention to proceed to up-front transplant. Of the 43 patients, 27 (age range 16–62, median age 36) proceeded to HSCT (21 autologous, 6 allogenic). Prior to transplant, patients received either a regimen of cyclophosphamide and methotrexate with leucovorin rescue (79% of patients), a CHOP-like regimen (19%), or CODOX-M (cyclophosphamide, doxorubicin, vincristine, and methotrexate with leucovorin rescue; 2%), with all patients receiving intrathecal methotrexate and/or cytarabine. Patients received conditioning with cyclophosphamide with or without etoposide and total body irradiation. The 3-year overall and event-free survival for all 43 patients were 45% and 42%, respectively. Patients who underwent transplant had a 3-year event-free survival of 51%, improving to 57% in the 24 patients with controlled disease at the time of transplant. No differences were noted in outcome between patients undergoing autologous versus allogeneic transplant, though overall number of patients in both groups were small.

Additional data from van Imhoff et al. [39] documented better outcomes. In this series, 27 BL and BLL patients (age range 15–64, median age 36) were given two successive intensive courses of chemotherapy, which included cyclophosphamide, doxorubicin, prednisone, etoposide, and mitoxantrone without high-dose methotrexate or cytarabine. Patients who responded (81% were complete responders, 11% were partial responders) were then given BEAM with ASCT. At 5 years, overall and event-free survivals were 81% and 73%, respectively. Despite these relatively good results, as previously stated, similar and in most cases better outcomes can be achieved with intensive chemotherapy alone.

In relapsed or refractory BL, there may be a role for ASCT; however, the overall response rate in this setting is significantly lower than with up-front HSCT, especially for patients who have chemoresistant disease. In the retrospective analysis by Sweetenham et al. [37] described above, 37 patients with relapsed or refractory disease underwent ASCT. The 3-year overall survival in patients with chemosensitive relapse and chemoresistant relapse was 37% and 7%, respectively.

In summary, the role of ASCT in BL is limited. ASCT does not improve outcome in the up-front setting but may have a role for patients with chemosensitive disease in the relapsed or refractory setting.

Peripheral T-Cell Lymphoma

The peripheral T-cell lymphomas are a heterogeneous group of malignancies that account for approximately 10% of NHL [40]. The subtypes of peripheral T cell lymphomas include peripheral T cell lymphoma-not otherwise specified (PLCL-NOS), anaplastic large cell lymphoma (ALCL)—either anaplastic lymphoma kinase (ALK) protein positive or negative, angioimmunoblastic T-cell lymphoma (AITL), extranodal NK/T-cell lymphoma-nasal type, enteropathy-associated T-cell lymphoma, hepatosplenic T-cell lymphoma, primary cutaneous T-cell lymphoma (e.g., mycosis fungoides/Sezary syndrome), and subcutaneous panniculitis-like T-cell lymphoma. Compared with patients with B-cell lymphomas, patients with peripheral T-cell lymphomas present with more-aggressive disease and advanced-stage disease. Further, patients with peripheral T-cell lymphomas have shorter overall survival and time to relapse [41], with long-term overall survival of 20–40% [42]. ALK+ALCL and primary cutaneous T-cell lymphomas are the exception to this, and generally confer a favorable prognosis [40, 43]. Most conventional chemotherapy regimens consists of CHOP or CHOP-like therapy, as it is not clear that more intensive regimens achieve better results[40]. In an effort the improve outcome, many studies have investigated the role of ASCT in the treatment of peripheral T-cell lymphomas. Unfortunately, no study has directly compared conventional chemotherapy to up-front ASCT. Further studies on ASCT are difficult to interpret and apply, as they have been heterogeneous in terms of the subtypes of peripheral T-cell lymphomas included (including ALK+ALCL), induction and conditioning regimens used, and setting employed (up-front versus salvage). The following section will be a discussion of ASCT in peripheral T-cell lymphomas, though there are separate sections dedicated to enteropathy-associated T-cell lymphoma (EATL) and cutaneous T-cell lymphomas.

Table 2 lists selected studies that employed up-front ASCT while Table 3 lists selected studies for ASCT in the salvage setting of peripheral T-cell lymphomas.

Although the studies are heterogeneous, both prospective and retrospective studies suggest that long-term outcome may be improved with up-front ASCT, even when ALK positive status is excluded. For example, Reimer et al. [44] and Mercadal et al. [45] showed overall survival of 48% (at 3 years) and 39% (at 4 years), respectively. It must be noted, however that in prospective studies only 41–74% of eligible patients completed transplant [44–46].

ASCT also appears to have a role in the salvage setting, as outcomes of transplanted patients improve and approach that of ASCT in relapsed B-cell lymphomas (Table 2). An important prognostic marker for both the up-front and salvage settings is chemosensitive disease. For example, Feyler et al. [47] showed improved outcome with patients who had undergone transplant with chemosensitive disease versus patients with chemoresistant disease, with documented progression-free survival of 53% and 38% and overall survival of 58% and 36%, respectively.

In summary, up-front ASCT for peripheral T-cell lymphomas may improve outcome, though there are no randomized controlled trials directly comparing treatment with ASCT with conventional treatment. The use of ASCT in the relapsed setting likely approaches that of its use in relapsed B-cell lymphomas.

Table 2 Selected studies of up-front ASCT in peripheral T-cell lymphomas (excluding enteropathy-associated T-cell lymphoma)

Year	Study (*N*)	Study type	Subtypes	% Transplant	Regimen	Median follow-up	PFS or EFS/OS
2009	Reimer et al. (83)	P	All (exc ALK+)	66%	CHOP-Cy/TBI	33 months	36%/48% (3 years)
2008	Mercadal et al. (41)	P	All (exc mycosis fungoides, ALK+)	41%	CHOP/ESHAP-BEAM/BEAC	3.2 years	30%/39% (4 years)
2008	Kyriakou et al. (122)	R	Angioimmunoblastic		Variable	31 months	56%/69% (for complete remission) (4 years)
2007	Rodríguez et al. (74)	R	All (unk ALK status)		Variable	67 months	63%/68% (5 years)
2007	Feyler et al. (31)	R	All (inc ALK+, T-cell leukemia, lymphoma)		Variable	37 months	61%/64% (2 years)
2007	Rodríguez et al. (26)	P	u-PTCL, ALCL (ALK-), AIL	73%	MegaCHOP-BEAM	35 months	56%/73% (3 years)
2007	Rodríguez et al. (15)	R	Angioimmunoblastic		Variable	25 months	59%/67% (3 years)
2006	Corradini et al. (62)	P	All (inc ALK+, exc CTCL, lymphoblastic lymphoma)	74%	Mito/Mel or BEAM	76 months	34% OS (21% OS for ALK-) (12 years)
2004	Jantunen et al. (18)	R	All (unk ALK status)		Anthracycline-based BEAM/BEAC	24 months	64%/63% (5 years)
2003	Rodríguez et al. (37)	R	All (unk ALK status)		Variable	37 months	79%/80% OS (5 years)
2003	Schetelig et al. (14)	R	Angioimmunoblastic		Variable	5 years	37%/60%

Table 3 Selected studies of salvage ASCT in peripheral T-cell lymphomas (excluding enteropathy-associated T-cell lymphoma)

Year	Study (*N*)	Type	Subtypes	Regimen	Median follow-up	EFS or PFS/OS
2008	Kyriakou et al. (24)	R	Angioimmunoblastic	Variable	31 months	23%/25% (chemorefractory disease) (4 years)
2007	Smith et al. (26)	R	u-PTCL, ALCL (inc ALK+)	Cisplatin-based busulfan, etoposide, cyclophosphamide	30 months	18%/34% (5 years)
2007	Feyler et al. (13)	R	All (inc ALK+, T-cell leukemia, lymphoma)	Variable	37 months	37%/34% (3 years)
2007	Feyler et al. (20)	R	All (inc ALK+, T-cell leukemia, lymphoma)	Variable	37 months	49%/49% (2 years)
2007	Rodríguez et al. (4)	R	Angioimmunoblastic	Variable	25 months	50%/50% (2 years)
2006	Kewalramani (24)	R	All (exc ALK+)	Unknown	6 years	24%/33% (5 years)
2004	Jagasia et al. (21)	R	All (inc ALK+, CTCL)	CyVpTBI/CBV	3.07 years	62% OS (91% OS for ALCL) (3 years)
2004	Jantunen et al. (19)	R	All (unk ALK status)	anthracycline-based BEAM/BEAC	24 months	28%/45%
2004	Zamkoff et al. (16)	R	ALCL (ALK-)	anthracycline-based		12 weeks/72 weeks
2003	Rodríguez et al. (35)	R	All (no data re: ALK status)	Variable	37.5 months	36%/37%
2003	Rodríguez et al. (78)	R	All (unk ALK status)	Variable	37 months	45% OS (no difference OS for ALCL) (5 years)
2003	Song et al. (36)	R	All (unk ALK status)	Cisplatin-based/mini BEAM	42 months	48% OS (78% OS for ALCL) (3 years)
2003	Schetelig et al. (15)	R	Angioimmunoblastic	Variable	5 years	39%/44%

Enteropathy-Associated T-Cell Lymphoma

Enteropathy-associated T-cell lymphoma (EATL) is a rare form of peripheral T-cell lymphoma (yearly incidence of 0.14/100,000) that occurs primarily in the gut (most commonly jejunum) [48]. It results from type II refractory celiac disease, a clinical phenotype characterized by therapy resistance (i.e., lack of improvement on a gluten-free diet) and intraepithelial clonal expansion of lymphocytes of an aberrant phenotype. The prognosis of EATL has traditionally been poor, with 5-year overall survival of 8% [49]. Therefore, the use of ASCT in treatment has been a continuing area of exploration.

Early documentation of ASCT performed in two patients was reported by Gale et al. [50] within a series of 31 patients with EATL. One patient was a 54-year-old man who had achieved initial complete remission for 20 months with CHOP. After relapse, he underwent treatment with six cycles of PEACE-BOM, then BEAM; he remained in clinical remission 64 months after original diagnosis. The other patient was a 56-year-old woman who had achieved complete remission for 60 months with CHOP. After relapse, she underwent treatment with four cycles of PEACE-BOM, then BEAM; she died of treatment-related sepsis.

Another early study of ASCT in EATL was done by Jantunen et al. [51] in 2003. The investigators enrolled five patients (age range 39–60). One patient had stage I disease, two patients had stage IE disease, one patient had stage IIE disease, and one patient had stage IV disease. Four patients had undergone surgery; all had received chemotherapy. Median time from diagnosis of EATL to transplant was 17 months. Three patients relapsed prior to undergoing transplant. Patients underwent conditioning with either BEAM or BEAC. Of the five patients transplanted, two died from transplant-related complications, while the other three patients had early relapse or progress (range 0–14 months after transplant). Median overall survival after transplant was 2 months.

In 2006, Rongey et al. [52] reported successful treatment with ASCT in a 46-year-old woman with stage IVA EATL. The patient was initially treated with four cycles of CDE (cyclophosphamide, doxorubicin, and etoposide), then three cycles of CHOP. After conditioning with BEAM, she underwent ASCT with continued remission 18 months post-transplant.

More recently in 2007, Al-Toma et al. [53] reported outcomes on a series of four patients (mean age 65 years, range 60–69) with EATL undergoing ASCT. Three patients were undergoing up-front HSCT and one patient was undergoing ASCT for relapsed disease. Three patients had stage IIIA disease and one patient had stage IIIB disease. The patients had received heterogeneous induction and conditioning regimens. Only one patient had long-term complete remission (32 months post transplant). The other three patients died from relapse 3–9 months after transplant.

However, also in 2007, Bishton et al. [54] reported encouraging outcomes on a series of six patients (median age 56, range 40–59) with EATL undergoing up-front ASCT. Five patients had stage IE disease and one patient had stage II disease. All patients received treatment with two cycles of IVE (ifosfamide, etoposide, epirubicin), then two cycles of high-dose methotrexate (with folinic acid rescue) followed by conditioning with BEAM. Two patients relapsed and died (0.21, 1.71 years post transplant). However, four patients were alive and remained in complete remission 1.83–4.32 years post transplant.

It appears that the use of this novel chemotherapy regimen combined with ASCT results in markedly improved outcomes for eligible patients that are able to complete transplant. In 2010, Sieniawski et al. [48] conducted a review of patients diagnosed with EATL in Scotland and the Northern region of England from 1994 onward. Of the 54 patients reviewed (median age 57 years, range 28–82) from 1994 to 1998, the median overall and progression-free survival were 7.1 months and 3.4 months, respectively. Treatment prior to 1998 consisted of anthracycline-based chemotherapy and surgery. Since 1998, IVE/MTX-ASCT has been utilized for 26 patients (median age 56 years, range 36–69). Of the 26 patients evaluated, 14 (54%) underwent transplant with a conditioning regimen of either high-dose melphalan/TBI or BEAM. For patients who underwent transplant, the median overall and progression-free survival was 60% and 52%, respectively. Of note, there were no significant differences in the percentage of patients with extensive disease (70% for earlier cohort vs. 66% for later cohort as defined by Lugano stage IIE, II1E, II2E, IV or Manchester stage IIb, IIc, III, IV) or who discontinued treatment with IVE/MTX-ASCT versus a CHOP-like regimen.

In summary, although traditionally associated with an extremely poor prognosis with previous treatments of conventional therapy and ASCT, the IVE/MTX-ASCT regimen shows promise for improving long-term outcomes in eligible patients that can complete ASCT.

Primary Cutaneous T-Cell Lymphomas

Primary cutaneous T-cell lymphomas (CTCLs) are rare malignancies, comprising 1–2% of NHLs with the most common subtypes being mycosis fungoides and Sezary syndrome. Although CTCLs are often indolent, advanced-stage disease carries a poor prognosis, with median survival between 1 and 4 years. Treatment for CTCLs consists of both topical and systemic therapy [43]. To improve outcome in advanced-stage disease, the use of ASCT has been explored, though the number of documented studies have been limited.

The initial study on the use of ASCT in cutaneous T-cell lymphoma was performed by Biger et al. [55] Six patients were included in the study. There were three patients with stage IIB disease, one patient with IVA disease, and two patients with IVB disease. All patients had undergone conventional treatment, including with local radiotherapy, psoralens with ultraviolet A (PUVA), interferon-α, total skin electron beam therapy, topical chemotherapy, and systemic chemotherapy. At the time of study entry, disease was progressing in all six patients. Conditioning regimen varied, but total skin electron beam radiotherapy for disease control was used prior to transplant in four patients. Of six patients, five achieved complete remission; however all patients achieving complete remission relapsed (range 64 days–1 year), with three relapses occurring within 100 days. Four patients died after relapse (range 286–1,687 days).

In 2001, Olavarria et al. [56] reported the results of a series of nine patients (median age 47 years) (range 27–67 years) and median duration of disease 61 months (range 2–340 months) with tumor-stage mycosis fungoides who had undergone T-cell depletion and ASCT. There were five patients with stage IIB disease and four patients with IVA disease per the Bunn-Lamberg staging system. Four patients had histological lymph node involvement. All patients had undergone numerous and varied treatments (median number 3) (range 3–5), including local superficial radiotherapy, PUVA, interferon-α, total skin electron beam therapy, and high-voltage radiotherapy. At the time of study entry, disease was progressing in all nine patients and five patients had evidence of large cell transformation (three were CD30-positive). Immunomagnetic methods were used to deplete T-cells. Seven patients were conditioned with BEM and two patients were conditioned with TBI and etoposide or melphalan. One patient died of sepsis; the other eight patients engrafted went into complete remission. Of the eight patients, three patients died from progressive disease, four patients relapsed, and one remained in complete remission at 10 months. Median survival post-transplant was 11 months and median relapse-free survival was 7 months. However, in four of the patients that relapsed, disease form was of a less-aggressive stage that responded to conventional therapy (e.g., PUVA, nitrogen mustard, local radiotherapy). Estimated overall survival at 3 years was 53%.

In summary, most patients with advanced-stage CTCL respond to ASCT, although remissions are generally short-lived. However, there is evidence that relapsed patients may do so with less-aggressive disease that is responsive to conventional therapy.

Conclusion

NHL is a very heterogeneous group of diseases that have varied responses to multiple chemoimmunotherapy regimens. Autologous stem cell transplant definitely has a role in the aggressive, in both the relapsed and in some cases front line setting. Even in indolent lymphomas, autologous stem cell transplant shows a definite improvement in progression-free survival, although no improvement in overall survival. Further studies with novel agents such as the monoclonal antibodies and radioimmunoisotopes when used in combination with autologous stem cell transplant may show improved responses and survival.

References

1. Swerdlow AJ (2008) World Health Organization classification of tumours of haematopoietic and lymphoid tissues. IARC, Lyon, France
2. http://www.cibmtr.org/ReferenceCenter/SlidesReports/SummarySlides/pages/index.asp

3. Gyan E, Foussard C, Bertrand P et al (2009) High-dose therapy followed by autologous purged stem cell transplantation and doxorubicin-based chemotherapy in patients with advanced follicular lymphoma: a randomized multicenter study by the GOELAMS with final results after a median follow-up of 9 years. Blood 113(5):995–1001
4. Lenz G, Dreyling M, Schiegnitz E et al (2004) Myeloablative radiochemotherapy followed by autologous stem cell transplantation in first remission prolongs progression-free survival in follicular lymphoma: results of a prospective, randomized trial of the German Low-Grade Lymphoma Study Group. Blood 104(9):2667–2674
5. Freeman BJ, Roberts MS, Vogler CA et al (1999) Behavior and therapeutic efficacy of beta-glucuronidase-positive mononuclear phagocytes in a murine model of mucopolysaccharidosis type VII. Blood 94(6):2142–2150
6. Apostolidis J, Gupta RK, Grenzelias D et al (2000) High-dose therapy with autologous bone marrow support as consolidation of remission in follicular lymphoma: long-term clinical and molecular follow-up. J Clin Oncol 18(3):527–536
7. Brice P, Simon D, Bouabdallah R et al (2000) High-dose therapy with autologous stem-cell transplantation (ASCT) after first progression prolonged survival of follicular lymphoma patients included in the prospective GELF 86 protocol. Ann Oncol 11(12):1585–1590
8. Grigg AP, Stone J, Milner AD et al (2010) Phase II study of autologous stem cell transplant using busulfan-melphalan chemotherapy-only conditioning followed by interferon for relapsed poor prognosis follicular non-Hodgkin lymphoma. Leuk Lymphoma 51(4):641–649
9. Bierman PJ, Vose JM, Anderson JR et al (1997) High-dose therapy with autologous hematopoietic rescue for follicular low-grade non-Hodgkin's lymphoma. J Clin Oncol 15(2):445–450
10. Cao TM, Horning S, Negrin RS et al (2001) High-dose therapy and autologous hematopoietic-cell transplantation for follicular lymphoma beyond first remission: the Stanford University experience. Biol Blood Marrow Transplant 7(5):294–301
11. Schouten HC, Qian W, Kvaloy S et al (2003) High-dose therapy improves progression-free survival and survival in relapsed follicular non-Hodgkin's lymphoma: results from the randomized European CUP trial. J Clin Oncol 21(21):3918–3927
12. Montoto S, Canals C, Rohatiner AZ et al (2007) Long-term follow-up of high-dose treatment with autologous haematopoietic progenitor cell support in 693 patients with follicular lymphoma: an EBMT registry study. Leukemia 21(11):2324–2331
13. Freedman AS, Gribben JG, Neuberg D et al (1996) High-dose therapy and autologous bone marrow transplantation in patients with follicular lymphoma during first remission. Blood 88(7):2780–2786
14. Horning SJ, Negrin RS, Hoppe RT et al (2001) High-dose therapy and autologous bone marrow transplantation for follicular lymphoma in first complete or partial remission: results of a phase II clinical trial. Blood 97(2):404–409
15. Ladetto M, Corradini P, Vallet S et al (2002) High rate of clinical and molecular remissions in follicular lymphoma patients receiving high-dose sequential chemotherapy and autografting at diagnosis: a multicenter, prospective study by the Gruppo Italiano Trapianto Midollo Osseo (GITMO). Blood 100(5):1559–1565
16. Deconinck E, Foussard C, Milpied N et al (2005) High-dose therapy followed by autologous purged stem-cell transplantation and doxorubicin-based chemotherapy in patients with advanced follicular lymphoma: a randomized multicenter study by GOELAMS. Blood 105(10):3817–3823
17. Sebban C, Mounier N, Brousse N et al (2006) Standard chemotherapy with interferon compared with CHOP followed by high-dose therapy with autologous stem cell transplantation in untreated patients with advanced follicular lymphoma: the GELF-94 randomized study from the Groupe d'Etude des Lymphomes de l'Adulte (GELA). Blood 108(8):2540–2544
18. Hamadani M, Benson DM Jr, Lin TS et al (2008) High-dose therapy and autologous stem cell transplantation for follicular lymphoma undergoing transformation to diffuse large B-cell lymphoma. Eur J Haematol 81(6):425–431
19. Marcus R, Imrie K, Belch A et al (2005) CVP chemotherapy plus rituximab compared with CVP as first-line treatment for advanced follicular lymphoma. Blood 105(4):1417–1423

20. Sebban C, Brice P, Delarue R et al (2008) Impact of rituximab and/or high-dose therapy with autotransplant at time of relapse in patients with follicular lymphoma: a GELA study. J Clin Oncol 26(21):3614–3620
21. Witzens-Harig M, Dreger P (2010) Autologous transplant of follicular lymphoma in the era of rituximab. Leuk Lymphoma 51(6):967–974
22. Sehn LH, Donaldson J, Filewich A et al (2007) Rapid infusion rituximab in combination with corticosteroid-containing chemotherapy or as maintenance therapy is well tolerated and can safely be delivered in the community setting. Blood 109(10):4171–4173
23. Greb A, Bohlius J, Trelle S et al (2007) High-dose chemotherapy with autologous stem cell support in first-line treatment of aggressive non-Hodgkin lymphoma—results of a comprehensive meta-analysis. Cancer Treat Rev 33(4):338–346
24. Vitolo U, Chiappella A, Angelucci E et al (2009) Dose-dense and high-dose chemotherapy plus rituximab with autologous stem cell transplantation for primary treatment of diffuse large B-cell lymphoma with a poor prognosis: a phase II multicenter study. Haematologica 94(9):1250–1258
25. Glass B, Ziepert M, Reiser M et al (2010) High-dose therapy followed by autologous stem-cell transplantation with and without rituximab for primary treatment of high-risk diffuse large B-cell lymphoma. Ann Oncol 21(11):2255–2261
26. Stiff PJ, Unger JM, Cook J, Constine LS, Couban S, Shea TC, Winter JN, Miller TP, Tubbs RR, Marcellus DC, Friedberg JW, Barton K, Mills GM, LeBlanc ML, Rimsa L, Forman SJ, Fisher RI (2011) Randomized phase III U.S./Canadian intergroup trial (SWOG S9704) comparing CHOP +/− R for eight cycles to CHOP +/− R for six cycles followed by autotransplant for patients with high-intermediate (H-Int) or high IPI grade diffuse aggressive non-Hodgkin lymphoma (NHL). J Clin Oncol 29:8001, Meeting Abstract
27. Philip T, Guglielmi C, Hagenbeek A et al (1995) Autologous bone marrow transplantation as compared with salvage chemotherapy in relapses of chemotherapy-sensitive non-Hodgkin's lymphoma. N Engl J Med 333(23):1540–1545
28. Buadi FK, Micallef IN, Ansell SM et al (2006) Autologous hematopoietic stem cell transplantation for older patients with relapsed non-Hodgkin's lymphoma. Bone Marrow Transplant 37(11):1017–1022
29. Jantunen E, Canals C, Rambaldi A et al (2008) Autologous stem cell transplantation in elderly patients (> or =60 years) with diffuse large B-cell lymphoma: an analysis based on data in the European Blood and Marrow Transplantation registry. Haematologica 93(12):1837–1842
30. Tam CS, Bassett R, Ledesma C et al (2009) Mature results of the M.D. Anderson Cancer Center risk-adapted transplantation strategy in mantle cell lymphoma. Blood 113(18):4144–4152
31. Geisler CH, Kolstad A, Laurell A et al (2008) Long-term progression-free survival of mantle cell lymphoma after intensive front-line immunochemotherapy with in vivo-purged stem cell rescue: a nonrandomized phase 2 multicenter study by the Nordic Lymphoma Group. Blood 112(7):2687–2693
32. Dreger P, Rieger M, Seyfarth B et al (2007) Rituximab-augmented myeloablation for first-line autologous stem cell transplantation for mantle cell lymphoma: effects on molecular response and clinical outcome. Haematologica 92(1):42–49
33. Romaguera JE, Fayad L, Rodriguez MA et al (2005) High rate of durable remissions after treatment of newly diagnosed aggressive mantle-cell lymphoma with rituximab plus hyper-CVAD alternating with rituximab plus high-dose methotrexate and cytarabine. J Clin Oncol 23(28):7013–7023
34. Jantunen E, Canals C, Attal M et al (2011) Autologous stem-cell transplantation in patients with mantle cell lymphoma beyond 65 years of age: a study from the European Group for Blood and Marrow Transplantation (EBMT). Ann Oncol 23:166–171
35. Sweetenham JW. Highly aggressive lymphomas in adults. *Hematology/oncology clinics of North America* 2008; 22(5): 965–78, ix.
36. Jost LM, Jacky E, Dommann-Scherrer C et al (1995) Short-term weekly chemotherapy followed by high-dose therapy with autologous bone marrow transplantation for lymphoblastic and Burkitt's lymphomas in adult patients. Ann Oncol 6(5):445–451

37. Sweetenham JW, Pearce R, Taghipour G et al (1996) Adult Burkitt's and Burkitt-like non-Hodgkin's lymphoma–outcome for patients treated with high-dose therapy and autologous stem-cell transplantation in first remission or at relapse: results from the European Group for Blood and Marrow Transplantation. J Clin Oncol 14(9):2465–2472
38. Song KW, Barnett MJ, Gascoyne RD et al (2006) Haematopoietic stem cell transplantation as primary therapy of sporadic adult Burkitt lymphoma. Br J Haematol 133(6):634–637
39. van Imhoff GW, van der Holt B, MacKenzie MA et al (2005) Short intensive sequential therapy followed by autologous stem cell transplantation in adult Burkitt, Burkitt-like and lymphoblastic lymphoma. Leukemia 19(6):945–952
40. Hosing C, Champlin RE (2011) Stem-cell transplantation in T-cell non-Hodgkin's lymphomas. Ann Oncol 22:1471–1477
41. Coiffier B, Brousse N, Peuchmaur M et al (1990) Peripheral T-cell lymphomas have a worse prognosis than B-cell lymphomas: a prospective study of 361 immunophenotyped patients treated with the LNH-84 regimen. The GELA (Groupe d'Etude des Lymphomes Agressives). Ann Oncol 1(1):45–50
42. Rodriguez J, Conde E, Gutierrez A et al (2007) The results of consolidation with autologous stem-cell transplantation in patients with peripheral T-cell lymphoma (PTCL) in first complete remission: the Spanish Lymphoma and Autologous Transplantation Group experience. Ann Oncol 18(4):652–657
43. Duarte RF, Schmitz N, Servitje O et al (2008) Haematopoietic stem cell transplantation for patients with primary cutaneous T-cell lymphoma. Bone Marrow Transplant 41(7):597–604
44. Reimer P, Rudiger T, Geissinger E et al (2009) Autologous stem-cell transplantation as first-line therapy in peripheral T-cell lymphomas: results of a prospective multicenter study. J Clin Oncol 27(1):106–113
45. Mercadal S, Briones J, Xicoy B et al (2008) Intensive chemotherapy (high-dose CHOP/ESHAP regimen) followed by autologous stem-cell transplantation in previously untreated patients with peripheral T-cell lymphoma. Ann Oncol 19(5):958–963
46. Rodriguez J, Conde E, Gutierrez A et al (2007) Prolonged survival of patients with angioimmunoblastic T-cell lymphoma after high-dose chemotherapy and autologous stem cell transplantation: the GELTAMO experience. Eur J Haematol 78(4):290–296
47. Feyler S, Prince HM, Pearce R et al (2007) The role of high-dose therapy and stem cell rescue in the management of T-cell malignant lymphomas: a BSBMT and ABMTRR study. Bone Marrow Transplant 40(5):443–450
48. Sieniawski M, Angamuthu N, Boyd K et al (2010) Evaluation of enteropathy-associated T-cell lymphoma comparing standard therapies with a novel regimen including autologous stem cell transplantation. Blood 115(18):3664–3670
49. Al-Toma A, Verbeek WH, Hadithi M et al (2007) Survival in refractory coeliac disease and enteropathy-associated T-cell lymphoma: retrospective evaluation of single-centre experience. Gut 56(10):1373–1378
50. Gale J, Simmonds PD, Mead GM et al (2000) Enteropathy-type intestinal T-cell lymphoma: clinical features and treatment of 31 patients in a single center. J Clin Oncol 18(4):795–803
51. Jantunen E, Juvonen E, Wiklund T et al (2003) High-dose therapy supported by autologous stem cell transplantation in patients with enteropathy-associated T-cell lymphoma. Leuk Lymphoma 44(12):2163–2164
52. Rongey C, Micallef I, Smyrk T et al (2006) Successful treatment of enteropathy-associated T cell lymphoma with autologous stem cell transplant. Dig Dis Sci 51(6):1082–1086
53. Al-toma A, Verbeek WH, Mulder CJ (2007) The management of complicated celiac disease. Dig Dis 25(3):230–236
54. Bishton MJ, Haynes AP (2007) Combination chemotherapy followed by autologous stem cell transplant for enteropathy-associated T cell lymphoma. Br J Haematol 136(1):111–113
55. Bigler RD, Crilley P, Micaily B et al (1991) Autologous bone marrow transplantation for advanced stage mycosis fungoides. Bone Marrow Transplant 7(2):133–137
56. Olavarria E, Child F, Woolford A et al (2001) T-cell depletion and autologous stem cell transplantation in the management of tumour stage mycosis fungoides with peripheral blood involvement. Br J Haematol 114(3):624–631

The Role of Hematopoietic Stem Cell Transplantation for HIV-Associated Lymphomas

Pascual Balsalobre, David Serrano, Jorge Gayoso, Juan Berenguer, and José L. Díez-Martín

Abstract The effective long-term suppression of HIV replication following HAART, and the subsequent beneficial effects on immune and performance status, has been followed by a growing trend to treat HIV-associated hematological malignancies in a similar way than that used for the HIV-negative counterparts. Regarding HIV patients with lymphoma, autologous hematopoietic stem cell transplantation (HSCT), a cellular therapy procedure aimed to restore a previously impaired lympho-hematopoietic system by a healthy one able to establish a long-term normal hematopoiesis, has shown outcomes comparable to those seen in the similar non-HIV lymphoma population.

Although the use of allogeneic HSCT in HIV-infected patients has been still limited, the potential usefulness of this therapeutic approach to treat both hematological malignancy and the HIV infection itself is a field to keep under research.

Introduction

The incidence of cancer is higher in patients with AIDS than in the general population [1]. In 1985 the Centers for Disease Control and Prevention (CDC) included aggressive B-cell non-Hodgkin´s lymphomas (NHL) as AIDS-defining entities [2].

P. Balsalobre (✉)
Department of Hematology, Pabellón de Oncología, 1ª pta.
Hospital General Universitario Gregorio Marañón,
C/Dr Esquerdo, 46, Madrid 28007, Spain
e-mail: pbalsalobre.hgugm@salud.madrid.org

D. Serrano • J. Gayoso • J.L. Díez-Martín
Department of Hematology, Hospital General Universitario
Gregorio Marañón, Madrid, Spain

J. Berenguer
Unit of Infectious Diseases, Hospital General Universitario
Gregorio Marañón, Madrid, Spain

P.J. Quesenberry and J.J. Castillo (eds.), *Non-Hodgkin Lymphoma: Prognostic Factors and Targets*, Cancer Drug Discovery and Development,
DOI 10.1007/978-1-4614-5851-7_15,

Nevertheless, other lymphoproliferative disorders with increased incidence in HIV-infected patients, such as Hodgkin's lymphoma (HL), have not been established as AIDS-defining malignancies [3].

HIV patients with lymphoma usually present with high-risk features, including advanced stage with frequent extranodal involvement of bone marrow, liver, CNS, gastrointestinal tract, etc. Apparently, the underlying immunosuppression (usually CD4+ T cell counts below 200/μL) and the frequent coinfection with EBV and HHV-8 seem to play a key role in the particular features of HIV-associated lymphomas [4].

Before the broad introduction of Highly Active Antiretroviral Therapy (HAART) in 1996, the outcome of HIV-associated lymphoma patients was markedly poorer than that observed in the non-HIV infected population, usually showing a more aggressive clinical course and worse response to chemotherapy. Furthermore, treatment with standard-dose chemotherapy yielded a high incidence of infections and a subsequently higher treatment-related mortality in this population. Attempts to decrease treatment toxicity reducing the chemotherapy doses resulted in higher rates of disease relapse. At that time, complete remission (CR) rates were around 50%, with a median survival between 5 and 8 months [5, 6].

The effective long-term suppression of HIV replication following the introduction of HAART was followed by a decreased incidence of AIDS-defining entities, including AIDS-related lymphomas. This decline was initially related to the incidence of primary CNS lymphomas, while the decline in the incidence of systemic lymphomas has been observed more recently [7–9]. Furthermore, despite the changes seen in the incidence of hematological malignancies in this population, high-risk features at presentation in terms of stage, bone marrow involvement, performance status, B symptoms, etc., remain similar to those observed in the pre-HAART era. Nevertheless, patients seem to be older and to show a better immunological status at diagnosis of lymphoma. In this regard, the introduction of HAART seems to have led to changes in the population at risk rather than in the biology of the lymphomas [10].

Regarding chemotherapy for HIV-positive patients, the better hematologic reserves related to HAART allowed the use of full-dose standard chemotherapy regimens. This resulted in significantly better clinical outcomes in terms of CR and overall survival (OS) rates. Within this context, prognosis of HIV-related lymphomas has been mainly related to the International Prognostic Index (IPI) and response to HAART [11, 12]. Nonetheless, the better tolerance to standard chemotherapy did not yield outcomes as favourable as those observed in the non-HIV lymphoma population, particularly in those relapsing or progressing after front-line standard chemotherapy [13, 14].

Within this scenario, the addition of rituximab (Rituxan®, Genentech Inc., South San Francisco, CA, USA) to chemotherapy schemes, broadly used in the HIV-negative lymphoma population, was explored in the HIV-related lymphoma setting showing promising response rates. However, unexpectedly high rates of associated infectious complications were reported, mainly in severely immunosuppressed patients (CD4+ T cell counts below $50/mm^3$) [15, 16]

Hematopoietic Stem Cell Transplantation

Hematopoietic stem cell transplantation (HSCT) is a cellular therapy procedure aimed to restore a previously impaired lympho-hematopoietic system, usually related to a malignant condition, by a new healthy one able to establish a long-term normal lympho-hematopoiesis. Progenitor cells derive from bone marrow, (mobilized) peripheral blood, or umbilical cord blood, and may be obtained from the patient itself—autologous (Auto) HSCT—or from a related or a nonrelated closely HLA-matched donor (allogeneic (Allo) HSCT). The therapeutic rationale of HSCT is based on the chemotherapy dose intensification by using high-dose chemotherapy and/or radiotherapy (Auto-HSCT), in addition to the graft versus tumor effect related to the immune-mediated allo-reactivity of donor cells [17].

In general, this therapeutic approach, requires a pre-transplant period of tumor debulking with standard chemotherapy and/or radiotherapy, collection of hematopoietic progenitors, usually after a leukapheresis procedure following a mobilizing treatment based on the use of stem cell growth factors (sometimes in combination with chemotherapy), and the eventual cryopreservation of progenitors until transplantation. Once the reduction of the tumor burden is considered optimal, a conditioning regimen including high-dose chemotherapy/radiotherapy is administered followed by the intravenous infusion of the harvested progenitors. The pancytopenia induced by the conditioning regimen is reversed about 10–20 days after transplant, once the infused progenitors engraft in the host bone marrow and begin to produce new blood cells. The general scheme of HSCT, including all the procedures related, is shown in Fig. 1.

Autologous-HSCT in HIV Patients with Lymphoma

High-dose chemotherapy/radiotherapy followed by autologous HSCT is the therapy of choice in relapsed or partially responding HIV-negative lymphoma patients. Moreover this treatment is used in first-remission patients showing poor-risk features at diagnosis [18, 19]. Since the beneficial effect of HAART on the response to chemotherapy in HIV-related lymphomas has been clearly established, it was reasonable to think that the treatment of HIV patients with neoplasms should not be different from that applied in the general population [12]. This included the use of high-dose chemotherapy followed by autologous progenitor cells rescue in order to offer a number of HIV patients with lymphoma (either in first complete remission showing high-risk features, in partial response or after relapse) a better chance for long-term remission. In this regard, since the pioneered experience of Gabarre J et al. [20], a number of European and American transplant groups have published several series of HIV lymphoma patients undergoing Auto-HSCT.

Dr. Gabarre's group, from France [21], reported in 2000 on their initial experience in HIV-associated relapsed or refractory NHL and HL patients undergoing salvage treatment with second-line chemotherapy and high-dose chemotherapy or TBI

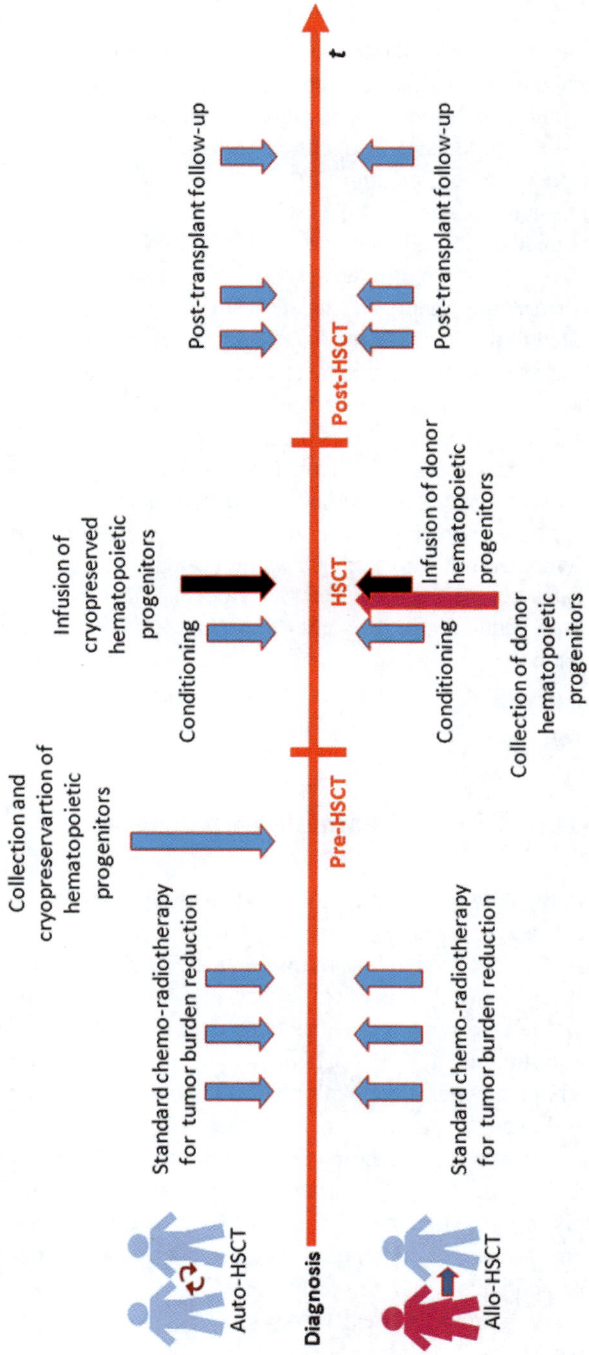

Fig. 1 General scheme of autologus and allogeneic hematopoietic stem cell transplantation

followed by Auto-HSCT. This initial series included eight patients and was updated in 2004, including 14 patients between Sep 98 and Jan 01. At the time of transplantation around 60% of the patients were beyond first CR, 20% in partial remission (PR)/chemotherapy-sensitive (chemo-S) relapse and the remaining 20% showed a refractory disease or a chemotherapy-resistant (chemo-R) relapse. The projected OS at 3 years post-ASCT was around 30%, with a disease-free survival (DFS) lower than 20%. No transplant-related deaths were reported.

In 2001, Dr. Krishnan and colleagues published the experience of the City of Hope Comprehensive Cancer Center, in California. The initial series of nine patients was updated in 2005 [22], becoming the largest series to date published from a single centre. Twenty HIV-associated lymphoma patients, failing to achieve CR after standard front-line chemotherapy, with chemo-S relapse or in first CR but showing high-risk IPI at diagnosis were included between 1998 and 2003. The event-free and overall survival for the whole series at a median follow-up of 32 months were 85%, slightly falling to 81% for those patients not in first CR at transplantation. A non-relapse mortality (NRM) rate of 5% was reported.

The multicentric Italian experience, initially published in 2003 by Dr. Re and colleagues, was updated in 2009 [23]. In an intention to treat trial, 50 unselected HIV-associated lymphoma patients failing to achieve CR after standard-dose first-line chemotherapy or experiencing first or subsequent relapses were eligible for debulking treatment, stem cell mobilization and Auto-HSCT. Since 23 patients did not receive the transplant due to early toxic death (2), chemotherapy-resistant disease (10), mobilization failure (6), disease progression after collection (4) and patient refusal (1), only 54% of patients finally underwent high-dose chemotherapy and Auto-HSCT. After a median follow-up of 44 months 21 patients remained alive and disease-free (OS 74.6%, DFS 75.9%), with no cases of non-relapse mortality reported. In multivariate analyses both lymphoma stage and low CD4-count at protocol entry negatively influenced the probability to reach transplantation.

Finally, in 2010 the Spanish cooperative experience, previously published in 2005, was updated by Dr. Serrano and colleagues [24, 25]. Since April 2000, 33 relapsed, partially responding or high-risk first CR HIV-associated lymphoma patients were auto-transplanted. Histologies were large-B cell NHL (13), HL (10), T cell NHL (4), and other (6). Conditioning regimen used was BEAM/BEAC (30) or TBI-based (3). All patients showed chemo-S disease at transplantation (CR in 24, 14 of them in first CR). HAART was aimed to be maintained throughout the transplant procedure although it was temporarily withdrawn in 13 patients, mainly due to gastrointestinal mucositis. With a median follow-up of 5 years, OS and DFS at 61 months after transplant were reported as 61% and 53%, respectively, with a cumulative incidence (CI) of NRM of 6%, 16% and 24% at 3 months, 1 year and 5 years, respectively. NRM was related to multiorgan failure (1), early (2) or late infection (2) and secondary acute leukemia (2).

The largest multi-institutional series reporting on auto-HSCT in HIV patients with lymphoma was published by the Lymphoma Working Party of the European Group for Blood and Marrow Transplantation (EBMT-LWP) [26]. This study included 68 patients, almost 75% of them with NHL (mainly Large B-Cell lymphomas), and over 20% of them in first CR at time of transplantation. This analysis yielded a CI of relapse at

2 years after transplant of 30%, and a CI of 1-year NRM of 7.5%. With a median follow-up of 32 (2–81) months, the PFS and OS were 56% and 61% at 3 years, respectively.

In the multivariate analysis, TRM was increased in patients over the age of 50 years (relative risk (RR) 4.5; $P=0.04$). Relapse was increased in patients receiving more than two lines of treatment prior to transplantation (RR 3; $P=0.03$), in NHL with histological pattern other than diffuse large B cell lymphoma (RR 3.4; $P=0.03$), and in those patients not in CR at transplantation (RR 3.6; $P=0.01$). Finally, OS was found to be worse in patients not achieving CR prior to transplantation as well as in those showing chemo-R disease at HSCT (RR 3; $P=0.01$; and RR 6.5; $P=0.004$, respectively).

After reporting the feasibility, security, and usefulness of Auto-HSCT in HIV+patients with lymphoma, the EBMT-LWP also launched a comparative analysis to test whether the reported outcomes were comparable to those seeing in the HIV-negative lymphoma setting [27]. This analysis included two cohorts (HIV-positive versus HIV-negative), with 53 lymphoma patients per arm (66% NHL, of which 80% were large B cell lymphomas, being the 22% of all included cases in first CR at transplant). Both cohorts were well balanced according to the main prognostic factors, including at least histology, stage, and IPI at diagnosis and disease status at transplantation. At a median follow-up of 30 months, outcomes (HIV-positive vs. HIV-negative) were comparable in terms of survival (OS 61.5% vs. 70%; and PFS 61% vs. 56%, $P=\text{NS}$); and relapse rates (29% vs. 42%; $P=\text{NS}$), regardless histological subtype (NHL/HL) and lymphoma status at transplantation (first CR vs. any other chemo-S status). Nevertheless, a trend towards a higher CI of 1-year NRM was observed within the HIV pos cohort (8% vs. 2%; $P=0.2$), mainly related to early bacterial infections.

According to these results, the authors stated that, within the HAART era, HIV infection should not preclude lymphoma patients from undergoing Auto-HSCT based on the same eligibility criteria adopted for HIV-negative lymphoma patients. Nevertheless, HIV candidates to Auto-HSCT should show an effective suppression of HIV replication and HAART should be maintained throughout the pre- and posttransplant procedures. Furthermore, particular attention should be paid to drug interactions [28] and, in the event of toxic events requiring HAART withdrawal, it should be reintroduced as soon as the toxic event is resolved. Given the significant occurrence of infectious-related deaths reported after Auto-HSCT, optimal infection prophylaxis and cautious immune recovery surveillance should take place early after ASCT.

Allogeneic-HSCT in HIV Patients with Lymphoma

Although pre-HAART experiences showed poor outcomes, allo-HSCT is a potential curative option for a number of hematological malignancies also in the HIV setting [29]. Since 2000, four case reports of HIV patients with lymphoma treated with allo-HSCT have been published from single institutions [30–32]. Interestingly, graft-versus-tumor effect in this population has been reported [32]. In this context, it would be of interest to comment on the case from our institution of a 44-year-old, stage C3 HIV-positive man, on HAART for 4 years prior to a diagnosis of an Ann-Arbor stage IV-A (skin and bone marrow involvement) diffuse large B-cell lymphoma, showing a low-intermediate IPI at time of diagnosis. After six courses of CHOP in combination with rituximab (R) and five courses of R-ESHAP, the patient underwent high-dose chemotherapy (BEAM scheme) and auto-HSCT rescue in chemo-sensitive first relapse, reaching a second CR. Seven months after auto-HSCT, skin and marrow relapse was documented. The patient showed partial response after rescue chemotherapy (MINE-R × 3 courses and GEMOX-R × 1 course) and received a non-myeloablative allo-HSCT from an HLA-identical sibling donor following conditioning with fludarabine, melphalan, rituximab and yttrium-90-ibritumomab tiuxetan. GvHD prophylaxis with cyclosporin A and methotrexate and infectious antifungal, viral, and *Pneumocystis* prophylaxis according to the center protocol were set up. At the time of transplant, CD4+ T cell count was 72/mm^3 and HIV viral load was lower than 50 copies/mL. Full donor chimerism was observed on day +32. Grade II acute GvHD and a subsequent CR were documented. A new skin relapse was found 1 year later completely resolved after immunosuppressive treatment withdrawal, four weekly doses of rituximab and the infusion of 5×10^7/kg donor T-lymphocytes. In the absence of GvHD, a second donor lymphocyte infusion with the same cell dose was performed 8 weeks later. Late-onset extensive chronic GvHD was well controlled with steroid therapy. Thirty nine months after transplant and 29 months after first DLI, the patient died due to a *Streptococcus viridans* septic shock. At the time of death, the patient was free of immunosuppressive drugs and showed no evidence of GvHD or lymphoma relapse. HIV viral load was lower than 50 copies/mL and CD4+ T cell count was 290 cells/mm^3.

Promising experiences of Allo-HSCT using donors with homozygous genotype for the CCR5 Δ32 deletion, which confers resistance against HIV-1 infection [33], or eventual gene therapy procedures which may provide donor hematological cells with a natural protection against HIV, are potential uses of Allo-HSCT to treat both HIV infection and hematological malignancies in these individuals.

As stated before for Auto-HSCT, potential drug interactions between antiretroviral therapy and the constellation of drugs related to Allo-HSCT (chemotherapy, antimicrobial drugs, immunesuppresive agents, etc.) should be cautiously evaluated and optimized.

HSCT in HIV-Associated Lymphoma Patients: Practical Issues

Mobilization and Collection of Hematopoeitic Progenitors

Although marrow stem cells are not subject to be infected by HIV, hematopoiesis in HIV-infected population has shown to be impaired by indirect mechanisms [34, 35]. In this context, mobilization of CD34+ progenitor cells into peripheral blood has been considered an issue in HIV patients who are candidates to Auto-HSCT.

An efficient mobilizing effect of G-CSF administered at standard doses has been reported in HIV patients showing more than 500 CD4+ cells/mm^3, while the same dose of filgrastim usually fails to mobilize CD34+ cells in patients with advanced HIV disease (less than 500 CD4+ cells/mm^3) [36]. Furthermore, a significant proportion (22%) of HIV lymphoma patients undergoing mobilization of hematopoietic progenitor cells failed to mobilize at least 2×10^6 CD34+ cells/kg, even after more than one mobilizing attempt. The use of high-dose cyclophosphamide (more than 3 g/m^2) in combination with G-CSF was found to be a predictor for effective collection while low doses of cyclophosphamide and refractory lymphoma were reported as negative predictors [37].

Since the use of HAART has shown favorable effects on the hematologic reserves by means of increasing white blood cell and platelet counts as viral loads decline, its administration should be maintained throughout the mobilizing procedure, although avoiding marrow toxic agents as zidovudine or cotrimoxazol [38, 39]. Finally, in order to prevent viral cross contamination, cryopreserved progenitor cells from HIV patients should be stored in a specifically designated container.

Conditioning

Although an eventual increased toxicity related to the combination of HAART, high-dose chemotherapy, and concomitant drugs in the setting of HIV patients undergoing HSCT emerged as an issue of concern, experiences from different groups have essentially reported gastrointestinal and mild liver toxicity. These toxic events are usually resolved after a limited time of HAART discontinuation and supportive treatment. Since the observed drug-related toxicity has been generally considered comparable to that seen in the HIV-negative counterparts, to keep patients on HAART throughout the transplant, if possible, is generally highly recommended [21–23, 32].

Posttransplant Engraftment and Immune Reconstitution

Myeloid engraftment of stem cells in HIV-infected patients undergoing Auto-HSCT is not different from that observed in the non-HIV-infected setting, with a median of 10–12 days to achieve more than 0.5×10^9/L neutrophils and 11–20 days to achieve more than 20×10^9/L platelets [32]. Administration of G-CSF until neutrophil recovery is a generalized practice in this population.

Given the impaired immune system of HIV lymphoma patients, damaged by the HIV infection itself, chemotherapy or tumor-related factors, post-HSCT immune reconstitution in this population has also been specifically approached by researchers.

In HIV-negative patients treated with Auto-HSCT a fast and profound decrease of CD4+ lymphocyte counts is expected during the first 3-months after transplant, with a rapid expansion of CD56+ NK and CD8+ cell populations during the first month or shortly after. Low counts of CD19+ B cells during the first 3–6 months (or even longer if previous treatment with rituximab) and a decreased age-related thymic function (monitored by TRECs) lasting 6–12 months have also been described in these patients.

Simonelli et al. recently analyzed immune recovery after Auto-HSCT in 24 HIV lymphoma patients compared with nine non-HIV infected controls [40]. These authors reported that no significant differences could be detected in pre-HSCT CD4+ cell subsets and TRECs, although HIV patients showed an inverted CD4+/CD8+ ratio due to higher CD8+ T cell counts. Furthermore, CD4+ cells showed similar kinetic of recovery post-HSCT, with a temporary setback in HIV-infected population 3 months after transplant, as well as similar TRECs dynamics and no significant changes in HIV viremia with levels 24-months after HSCT lower than those reported at baseline.

Conclusions

The markedly better control of HIV infection related to the advent of HAART, becoming a chronic condition, has been followed by a growing trend to treat HIV conditions in a similar way than that offered to the HIV-negative counterparts. In the field of HIV-related hematological malignancies, a number of studies have shown that similar approaches have yielded comparable outcomes in both HIV-infected and noninfected patients. Furthermore, HSCT has been widely reported to show a feasibility, efficacy, and safety similar to that of the general population, particularly in the field of auto-HSCT for the treatment of HIV patients with poor-prognosis lymphomas. According to these studies, provided an adequate infection prophylaxis and surveillance, HIV infection should not preclude lymphoma patients from undergoing Auto-HSCT according to the same eligibility criteria adopted for HIV-negative lymphoma patients.

Although the use of allo-HSCT in hematological HIV-infected patients has been limited to date, the potential of this therapeutic approach to treat not only eligible hematological malignancies but also the HIV infection itself remains an interesting field to be explored.

References

1. International Agency for Research on Cancer (1996) IARC monographs on the evaluation of carcinogenic risks to humans, volume 67: human immunodeficiency viruses and human T-cell lymphotropic viruses. International Agency for Research on Cancer, Lyon, France
2. CDC (1985) Current trends revision of the case definition of acquired immunodeficiency syndrome for national reporting—United States. MMWR 34:373–375
3. Frisch M, Biggar RJ, Engels EA et al (2001) Association of cancer with AIDS-related immune suppression in adults. JAMA 285:1736–1745
4. Sparano JA (2001) Clinical aspects and management of AIDS-related lymphoma. Eur J Cancer 37(10):1296–1305

5. Kaplan LD, Straus DJ, Testa MA et al (1997) Low-dose compared with standard-dose m-BACOD chemotherapy for non-Hodgkin's lymphoma associated with human immunodeficiency virus infection: National Institute of Allergy and Infectious Diseases AIDS Clinical Trials Group. N Engl J Med 336:1641–1648
6. Levine AM (2000) Acquired immunodeficiency syndrome-related lymphoma: clinical aspects. Semin Oncol 27:442–453
7. Kirk O, Pedersen C, Cozzi-Lepri A et al (2001) Non-Hodgkin lymphoma in HIV-infected patients in the era of highly active antiretroviral therapy. Blood 98:3406–3412
8. Besson C, Goubar A, Gabarre J et al (2001) Changes in AIDS-related lymphoma since the era of highly active antiretroviral therapy. Blood 98(8):2339–2344
9. Herida M, Mary-Krause M, Kaphan R et al (2003) Incidence of non-AIDS-defining cancers before and during the highly active antiretroviral therapy era in a cohort of human immunodeficiency virus-infected patients. J Clin Oncol 21:3447–3453
10. Matthews GV, Bower M, Mandalia S et al (2000) Changes in acquired immunodeficiency syndrome-related lymphoma since the introduction of highly active antiretroviral therapy. Blood 96:2730–2734
11. Bower M, Gazzard B, Mandalia S et al (2005) Prognostic index for systemic AIDS-related non-Hodgkin lymphoma treated in the era of highly active antiretroviral therapy. Ann Intern Med 143(4):265–273
12. Miralles P, Berenguer J, Ribera JM et al (2007) Prognosis of AIDS-related systemic non-Hodgkin lymphoma treated with chemotherapy and highly active antiretroviral therapy depends exclusively on tumor-related factors. J Acquir Immune Defic Syndr 44:167–173
13. Spina M, Vaccher E, Juzbasic S et al (2001) Human immunodeficiency virus-related non-Hodgkin's lymphoma: Activity of infusional cyclophosphamide, doxorubicin, and etoposide as second-line chemotherapy in 40 patients. Cancer 92:200–206
14. Bi J, Espina BM, Tulpule A et al (2001) High-dose cytosinearabinoside and cisplatin regimens as salvage therapy for refractory or relapsed AIDS-related non-Hodgkin lymphoma. J Acquir Immune Defic Syndr 28:416–421
15. Kaplan LD, Lee JY, Ambinder RF et al (2005) Rituximab does not improve clinical outcome in a randomized phase 3 trial of CHOP with or without rituximab in patients with HIV-associated non-Hodgkin lymphoma: AIDS-Malignancies Consortium Trial 010. Blood 5:1538–1543
16. Spina M, Jaeger U, Sparano JA et al (2005) Rituximab plus infusional cyclophosphamide, doxorubicin, and etoposide in HIV-associated non-Hodgkin lymphoma: pooled results from 3 phase 2 trials. Blood 10:1891–1897
17. Blume KG, Forman SJ, Appelbaum FR (eds) (2004) Thomas' hematopoietic cell transplantation (3ª edición). Blackwell Publishing, Malden
18. Nademanee A, Molina A, O'Donnell MR et al (1997) Results of high-dose therapy and autologous bone marrow/stem cell transplantation during remission in poor-risk intermediate- and high-grade lymphoma: international index high and high-intermediate risk group. Blood 90:3844–3852
19. Milpied N, Deconinck E, Gaillard F et al (2004) Initial treatment of aggressive lymphoma with high-dose chemotherapy and autologous stem-cell support. N Engl J Med 350:1287–1295
20. Gabarre J, Azar N, Autran B et al (2000) High-dose therapy and autologous haematopoietic stem-cell transplantation for HIV-1-associated lymphoma. Lancet 355:1071–1072
21. Gabarre J, Marcelin AG, Azar N et al (2004) High-dose therapy plus autologous hematopoietic stem cell transplantation for human immunodeficiency virus (HIV)-related lymphoma: results and impact on HIV disease. Haematologica 89(9):1100–1108
22. Krishnan A, Molina A, Zaia J et al (2005) Durable remissions with autologous stem cell transplantation for high-risk HIV-associated lymphomas. Blood 105(2):874–878
23. Re A, Michieli M, Casari S et al (2009) High-dose therapy and autologous peripheral blood stem cell transplantation as salvage treatment for AIDS-related lymphoma: long-term results of the Italian Cooperative Group on AIDS and Tumors (GICAT) study with analysis of prognostic factors. Blood 114:1306–1313
24. Serrano D, Carrion R, Balsalobre P et al (2005) HIV-associated lymphoma successfully treated with peripheral blood stem cell transplantation. Exp Hematol 33(4):487–494

25. Serrano D, Miralles P, Carrion R et al (2010) Long term follow-up of autologous stem cell transplant in AIDS related lymphoma patients. Results of Spanish cooperative registry GELTAMO/GESIDA [abstract 822]. In: 36th annual meeting of the European group for blood and marrow transplantation, Vienna, Austria
26. Balsalobre P, Diez-Martin JL, Re A et al (2009) Autologous stem-cell transplantation in patients with HIV-related lymphoma. J Clin Oncol 27:2192–2198
27. Diez-Martin JL, Balsalobre P, Re A et al (2009) Comparable survival between HIV+and HIV−non-Hodgkin and Hodgkin lymphoma patients undergoing autologous peripheral blood stem cell transplantation. Blood 113:6011–6014
28. Department of Health and Human Services. Panel on antiretroviral guidelines for adults and adolescents. Guidelines for the use of antiretroviral agents in HIV-1-infected adults and adolescents, 10 Jan 2011, p 1–174. Available at http://www.aidsinfo.nih.gov/ContentFiles/AdultandAdolescentGL.pdf. Accessed 10 Jun 2011
29. Gupta V, Tomblyn M, Pedersen TL et al (2009) Allogeneic hematopoietic cell transplantation in human immunodeficiency virus-positive patients with hematologic disorders: a report from the center for international blood and marrow transplant research. Biol Blood Marrow Transplant 15:864–871
30. Kang EM, de Witte M, Malech H et al (2002) Nonmyeloablative conditioning followed by transplantation of genetically modified HLA-matched peripheral blood progenitor cells for hematologic malignancies in patients with acquired immunodeficiency syndrome. Blood 99:698–701
31. Bryant A, Milliken S (2008) Successful reduced-intensity conditioning allogeneic HSCT for HIV-related primary effusion lymphoma. Biol Blood Marrow Transplant 14:601–602
32. Serrano D, Miralles P, Balsalobre P et al (2010) Hematopoietic stem cell transplantation in patients infected with HIV. Curr HIV/AIDS Rep 7(3):175–184
33. Hutter G, Nowak D, Mossner M et al (2009) Long-term control of HIV by CCR5 Delta32/Delta32 stem-cell transplantation. N Engl J Med 360:692–698
34. Weichold FF, Zella D, Barabitskaja O et al (1998) Neither human immunodeficiency virus-1 (HIV-1) nor HIV-2 infects most primitive human hematopoietic stem cells as assessed in long term bone marrow cultures. Blood 91:907–915
35. Koka PS, Jamieson BD, Brooks DG, Zack JA (1999) Human immunodeficiency virus type 1-induced hematopoietic inhibition is independent of productive infection of progenitor cells in vivo. J Virol 73:9089–9097
36. Schooley RT, Mladenovic J, Sevin A et al (2000) Reduced mobilization of CD34+ stem cells in advanced human immunodeficiency virus type 1 disease. J Infect Dis 181:148–157
37. Re A, Balsalobre P, Michieli M, Ribera JM et al (2010) Peripheral blood stem cell mobilization in HIV positive patients with lymphoma candidates to autologous transplantation: predictive factors analysis for failure or suboptimal stem cell collection [abstract 2250]. In: 2010 ASH Annual Meeting, Orlando, USA
38. Huang SS, Barobour JD, Deeks SG et al (2000) Reversal of human immunodeficiency virus type 1 associated hematosuppression by effective antiretroviral therapy. Clin Infect Dis 30:504–510
39. Krishnan A, Zaia J, Forman SJ (2003) Should HIV-positive patients with lymphoma be offered stem cell transplants? Bone Marrow Transplant 32:741–748
40. Simonelli C, Zanussi S, Pratesi C et al (2010) Immune recovery after autologous stem cell transplantation is not different for HIV-infected versus HIV-uninfected patients with relapsed or refractory lymphoma. Clin Infect Dis 50(12):1672–1679

The Role of Hematopoietic Stem Cell Transplantation in Peripheral T-Cell Lymphomas

Jenna D. Goldberg, Carla Casulo, and Steven M. Horwitz

Abstract Peripheral T-cell lymphomas (PTCL) include a group of heterogeneous and rare lymphomas. The T-cell phenotype is an independent poor prognostic feature and these lymphomas have a lower cure rate with chemotherapy than with their B-cell counterparts. Retrospective studies suggest that high-dose therapy and autologous stem cell transplant (HDT-ASCT) may be feasible and effective for some patients in the salvage setting. However, many of these studies are biased by the inclusion of patients with ALK+anaplastic large cell lymphoma, an entity known to have a relatively positive prognosis with chemotherapy. Because PTCL have a generally poor prognosis, HDT-ASCT has been studied in first complete or partial remission for these patients as consolidation with favorable outcomes noted. However, there are currently no randomized trials that establish upfront HDT-ASCT as standard of care for patients with PTCL. Allogeneic transplantation is becoming more frequently used for these patients, as there is growing evidence for a graft-versus-lymphoma effect in these diseases and a growing acceptance for reduced intensity conditioning regimens. But, there continues to be limited data describing allogeneic transplantation for these diseases and, thus, the application of this modality of therapy for PTCL is still unclear.

J.D. Goldberg
Adult Bone Marrow Transplantation Service, Memorial Sloan-Kettering Cancer Center, New York, NY, USA

C. Casulo • S.M. Horwitz (✉)
Division of Hematology and Oncology, Memorial Sloan-Kettering Cancer Center, 1275 York Avenue, New York, NY 10021, USA
e-mail: horwitzs@mskcc.org

P.J. Quesenberry and J.J. Castillo (eds.), *Non-Hodgkin Lymphoma: Prognostic Factors and Targets*, Cancer Drug Discovery and Development, DOI 10.1007/978-1-4614-5851-7_16,

Introduction

T-cell lymphomas represent a very heterogenous array of aggressive Non-Hodgkin lymphomas (T-NHL) and typically account for less than 20% of aggressive lymphomas and 10% of all newly diagnosed cases of NHL in the United States (US) [1, 2]. However, in Asia 70–80% of NHL may be of the T-cell phenotype [3]. According to the World Health Organization (WHO) classification schema, T-cell lymphomas are divided into either precursor T/(natural killer) NK-cell neoplasms or peripheral T/NK-cell neoplasms. The most common subtypes of peripheral T/NK neoplasms are peripheral T-cell lymphoma NOS (PTCL-nos) and anaplastic large cell lymphoma (ALCL) accounting for 50% and 25% of T-NHL respectively.

In general T- and NK-cell lymphomas are associated with a poorer prognosis following chemotherapy than their B-cell counterparts, with the exception of anaplastic lymphoma kinase (ALK)-positive ALCL. In a large prospective study, 1,883 NHL patients including 288 T-NHL patients were treated with different anthracycline-containing regimens [4]. The T-NHL group had significantly lower complete remission, OS and EFS relative to the B-cell lymphomas. The international prognostic factor index has been validated in T-NHL [5] and a median survival of 6 months in high-risk patients and 15 months in high-intermediate patients was reported. In addition, other groups have proposed prognostic models specific for T-NHL including the prognostic index for peripheral T cell lymphoma (PIT) [6]. Finally, molecular profiling may prove to be prognostic [7].

Currently, there is no universally accepted treatment approach for T-NHL. The heterogeneous nature of this group further complicates the issue. Chemotherapeutic regimens alone have generally not been curative for the majority. High-dose therapy and autologous stem cell transplant have been studied in both the upfront and relapsed setting. However, due to the lack of randomized studies, its best use remains ill defined. The role of allogeneic hematopoietic stem cell transplant (allo-HSCT) remains undefined.

Chemotherapy for PTCL

While there is no prospective data to support its use in PTCL, CHOP (cyclophosphamide, doxorubicin, vincristine, prednisone) and CHOP-like regimens are frequently used first line extrapolating from large B-cell lymphoma data. Survival following these regimens is poor [8–10]. Thus, many attempts have been made to administer more intensive chemotherapeutic regimens.

Escalon et al. at M.D. Anderson Cancer Center (MDACC) performed a retrospective study comparing CHOP with other more intensive regimens including HyperCVAD, ASHOP, MBACOS, MINE and HCVID-Doxil in 135 with T-NHL [11]. The treatment plan was at the discretion of the treating physician. They found no significant difference in overall survival (OS) between patients treated with CHOP or other more intensive therapies (56% versus 62%, respectively). This lack of advantage with more intense treatment regiments was maintained even when patients with ALK-positive ALCL were excluded.

The Groupe d'Etude des Lymphomes de l'Adulte (GELA) LNH-84 study evaluated the effects of intensification of chemotherapy in 737 patients with advanced-stage NHL. They later performed subset analyses on patients whose immunophenotype was known. Thirty percent of these patients had T-NHL. All patients received induction with three to four cycles of ACVB (Adriamycin, cyclophosphamide, vindesine, bleomycin, and methylprednisolone) with intrathecal methotrexate, followed by consolidation chemotherapy with high-dose methotrexate, ifosfamide plus etoposide, cytarabine, and L-asparaginase. They were then randomized to either intensification with two more cycles of consolidation chemotherapy or nothing. While the patients with B-cell NHL had a similar complete response (CR) rate as patients with T-NHL (71% vs. 72%), relapse rates were higher for patients with T-NHL compared to B-cell NHL (43% vs. 23%, at 30 months though NS). The authors found that late intensification offered no survival or relapse advantage [12].

Modeled on the success of rituximab (Rituximab®) with diffuse large B-cell lymphoma (DLBCL), the monoclonal antibody, alemtuzumab (Campath®) has recently been added to CHOP for PTCL. Alemtuzumab is an anti-CD52 monoclonal antibody that has shown activity in PTCL. However, unlike rituximab, alemtuzumab is broadly immunosuppressive and is associated with grade 3–4 infections. The GITIL (Gruppo Italiano Terapie Innovative nei Linfomi), is a prospective multicenter trial, combining alemtuzumab with CHOP for newly diagnosed PTCL in 24 patients [13]. After preliminary safety was demonstrated in the first four patients, the next 20 patients received eight cycles of CHOP with alemtuzumab at 30 mg on day −1 of each course. Complete responses were seen in 17/24 (71%) patients. At a median follow-up of 16 months 13/24 (54%) were disease-free with an estimated 2 year OS and failure-free survival (FFS) of 53% and 48%, respectively. However, secondary to immunosuppression from the combination of alemtuzumab with cytotoxic therapy, major infections included JC virus reactivation, aspergillosis, staphylococcal sepsis, and pneumonia as well as CMV reactivation were observed in this trial.

Recently, new agents have been approved for the treatment of PTCL. Pralatrexate (Folotyn®) is approved for relapsed or refractory PTCL based on the PROPEL trial, a 111 patient phase II study [14]. Of 109 evaluable patients, the overall response rate was 29% (32 of 109). The most common grade 3/4 adverse events were thrombocytopenia (32%), mucositis (22%), neutropenia (22%), and anemia (18%). Pralatrexate was the first drug approved specifically for the treatment of PTCL. Romidepsin was approved subsequently for the treatment of relapsed or refractory PTCL based on a Phase II, NCI-sponsored study in 47 subjects with PTCL or other T-cell lymphomas. Of these 47 subjects, 27 had PTCL-nos and 20 had other T-cell lymphomas, including AITL, primary cutaneous large T-cell, gamma-delta T-cell, and ALCL [15]. Among all 47 subjects, the overall response rate (ORR, CR+PR) was 38% (17/45). The CR and PR rates were 17% (8/45) and 20% (9/45), respectively. The overall median duration of response was 8.9 months. Among the 18 patients who had undergone prior high dose therapy with autologous stem cell transplant (HDT-ASCT), six experienced a response to therapy, including three CR and three PR.

Autologous Transplant for PTCL

Clinicians have evaluated HDT-ASCT in various settings for the treatment of PTCL. Based on favorable results utilizing HDT-ASCT in relapsed and refractory high-grade B cell lymphomas, clinicians have evaluated the role of intensifying treatment with HDT-ASCT for relapsed and refractory PTCL. Because the T cell phenotype has been demonstrated to be an independent poor prognostic factor and chemotherapy alone is rarely curative, upfront HDT-ASCT as consolidation has been studied.

Autologous Transplant for PTCL in the Salvage Setting

There are no prospective studies evaluating HDT-ASCT for the treatment of PTCL in the salvage setting. However, there are multiple retrospective studies evaluating autologous transplant for relapsed or refractory patients. They demonstrate overall survival rates following stem cell transplantation in this setting that are similar to those for B cell lymphomas. However, the results of many studies are impacted by their inclusions of patients with the more favorable ALK+ALCL.

Rodriguez et al. from MDACC performed a retrospective analysis on 36 patients with relapsed or refractory PTCL who received either an autologous ($n=29$, 80%) or an ablative allo-HSCT ($n=7$, 19%) between 1989 and 1998 [16]. Patients were heavily pretreated; with a median of three prior therapies. Seven patients (19%) had a diagnosis of ALK-positive ALCL. Eleven out of 29 patients (38%) entered HDT-ASCT in CR. Patients who received HDT-ASCT had a higher 3 year OS compared with those who received allo-HSCT (39% vs. 29%), respectively. Median PFS for HDT-ASCT was 32%, versus 14% for allo-HSCT. This study demonstrated that even in heavily pretreated patients with PTCL, HDT-ASCT is a feasible option with a fraction of long-term survivors.

Another small study published by Kahl et al. reported on 15 relapsed or refractory patients with PTCL who received either HDT-ASCT ($n=10$) or an allo-HSCT ($n=5$) [17]. Patients were heavily pretreated with a mean of 4.6 prior chemotherapeutic regimens. This patient group included three patients with ALCL without mention of ALK status. Prior to HDT-ASCT, only two out of ten patients had CR. However, OS at 12 months for HDT-ASCT was still improved compared to allo-HSCT (58% vs. 40%). Although this study is small with a short follow-up of only 12 months, it demonstrates that patients with relapsed or refractory PTCL may benefit from HDT-ASCT even in the heavily pretreated setting.

Song et al. performed a study comparing outcomes with HDT-ASCT between patients with T NHL and B cell malignancies. They evaluated 36 patients with relapsed or refractory PTCL who underwent HDT-ASCT, and matched them to similar patients with aggressive B cell lymphoma treated at the same institution [18]. Patients were similar with respect to age, stage at relapse, presence of extranodal disease, and chemosensitivity to salvage treatment. The preparative regimen consisted of high-dose melphalan and etoposide with or without total body irradiation.

Seven patients (19%) with ALCL (ALK status unknown) were included. For the PTCL cohort the 3 year OS was 48% and the event-free survival (EFS) was 37%. The 3 year EFS of patients with the PTCL-nos subtype was significantly inferior to that of DLBCL (23% vs. 42%, $p=0.02$). However, there was no statistical difference for OS ($p=0.11$). In addition, patients with PTCL-nos had a lower EFS when compared with ALCL (3 year EFS 23% vs. 67%), possibly as a result of improved outcomes with ALK+ALCL.

Kewalramani et al. also compared outcomes following HDT-ASCT between patients with PTCL or B-cell NHL [19]. They compared 24 patients with relapsed or refractory PTCL who responded to first or second line chemotherapy with 86 consecutive patients with chemosensitive relapsed or primary refractory DLBCL. In this study, patients with ALK-positive ALCL or ALK status unknown ALCL were excluded. No significant difference in 5 year PFS was demonstrated between PTCL and DLBCL (24% vs. 34%, $p=0.14$). No significant differences were found between the two groups with respect to time to disease progression or survival after progression. Therefore, this study also suggests the outcomes following HDT-ASCT for patients with chemosensitive relapsed or primary refractory PTCL is similar to those for patients with DLBCL.

In summary, these data demonstrate that HDT-ASCT is a viable option for patients with relapsed or refractory PTCL with a proportion of patients salvaged. Because some of these studies included ALK+ALCL, the data can be difficult to interpret. Moreover, as transplanted patients only were included in these analyses, the likelihood of benefit with this strategy from the time of relapse is not known. Chemosensitivity likely predicts for improved outcome.

Autologous Transplant for PTCL in the Upfront Setting

Retrospective Studies—HDT-ASCT in the Upfront Setting Compared to the Salvage Setting

Retrospective studies have also been performed that compare HDT-ASCT performed in first complete remission (CR1) or first partial remission (PR1) with HDT-ASCT in the salvage setting. The Gel-Tamo group studied 115 patients with PTCL who received HDT-ASCT [20]. Seven percent of patients had ALCL (ALK status unknown). Conditioning regimens were varied. Two-thirds of patients had two or three risk factors according to the International Prognostic Index (IPI), and 32% of patients were transplanted in first CR. For all patients, the 5 year OS was 56% and disease-free survival (DFS) was 60%. In addition, this study reported a survival benefit for patients receiving HDT-ASCT as consolidation in CR1 compared with a later time. At 5 years, the patients who received HDT-ASCT had an OS was 80% with a DFS 79%, compared to those in second or more remission who had a 5 year OS of 50% ($p=0.007$) and DFS of 42% ($p=0.002$). However, inequalities between the two groups may have biased the outcome. For example, the median age for patients in CR1 was 31 years. It is important to note that both the OS and DFS for refractory patients at transplant were 0%, supporting a lack of benefit for HDT-ASCT in chemotherapy-refractory patients.

Jantunen et al. also compared upfront HDT-ASCT to transplant in more advanced settings. This study assessed 37 patients with different histologies of PTCL who received HDT-ASCT over a 11 year period of time at multiple centers [21]. The conditioning regimen was either BEAM or BEAC. Disease status at time of ASCT was CR1 or PR1 in 18 patients (48%), and CR2 or PR2 in 14 patients (37.8%). This study again suggested a benefit to receiving HDT-ASCT in CR1. For example, the 5 year OS for patients transplanted in CR1 was 63% compared to 45% for patients transplanted later (p=ns) and the PFS for patients in CR1 was 64% vs. 28% (p=ns). The projected 5 year OS for the entire group was 54%, with significantly better outcomes in patients with ALCL compared to other subtypes (85% vs. 35%, $p=0.007$), again likely related to the inclusion of ALK-positive patients.

Feyler et al. published a study of 82 patients with PTCL identified through national transplant registries in the United Kingdom and Australia. This study included both HDT-ASCT ($n=64$, 78%) and allo-HSCT ($n=18$, 22%) [22] A significant number of patients had ALCL (31%), with many patients having an unconfirmed ALK status. Thirty-one patients (48%) receiving HDT-ASCT were transplanted in CR1. For the entire group, 3 year OS and PFS was 53% and 50%, respectively. However, patients who received HDT-ASCT in CR1 experienced a 2 year OS and PFS of 64 and 61%. The authors found that chemosensitivity was an important prognostic marker with responders having an improved 3 year OS at 58% compared to 38%. In fact, chemosensitivity emerged as the only factor to significantly impact outcome in multivariate analysis. Similarly, for patients receiving HDT-ASCT in CR1, OS was 64%, similar to the data reported by Jantunen et al. [21]

The Stanford experience with HDT-ASCT for PTCL also suggests that outcomes in the relapsed or refractory setting are inferior to those when transplant is used in the upfront setting to consolidate a first remission [23]. Fifty-three patients with ALCL ($n=18$), PTCL-nos ($n=17$), angioimmunoblastic lymphoma (AITL; $n=9$), nasal type extranodal NK/T ($n=7$), hepatosplenic ($n=2$) and adult T cell leukemia/lymphoma ($n=1$) were included. Fifteen patients were transplanted in CR1 or first partial remission (PR1), 32 in second or beyond CR or PR and 11 with primary refractory disease. With a median follow-up of 5 years, the 5-year progression-free survival (PFS) for the entire group was 25% and OS was 48%. Disease status at time of transplant was significantly associated with PFS and OS. The 5-year PFS for patients transplanted in CR1 or PR1 was 51%, for patients transplanted in second or greater CR or PR was 12% and for refractory patients was 0% ($p<0.01$). The 5 year OS for patients transplanted in CR1 or PR1 was 76%, for patients transplanted in second or greater CR or PR was 40% and for refractory patients was 30%.

Yang et al. presented data on 64 patients who received HDT-ASCT for PTCL at 14 different institutions in Korea [24]. Most patients received CHOP-based chemotherapy with different mobilization strategies. Twenty eight patients underwent HDT-ASCT either in CR1 or PR1. The 3 year OS and PFS rates for the entire group were 53% and 44.3%, respectively. Upfront transplantation had predicted for improved OS, as demonstrated by other studies. The 3 year OS rates for patients receiving HDT-ASCT in CR1/PR1 was 60% compared to 37.7% in the salvage setting. High-dose therapy-ASCT showed no benefit in patients with high a-IPI or PIT.

These retrospective studies suggest the possibility that HDT-ASCT in the frontline setting may offer improved outcomes compared with transplantation in the salvage setting. However, given the inherent limitations of retrospective studies such as patient selection, other bias and treatment heterogeneity, definitive conclusions cannot be made without well designed prospective studies. A common thread in most studies, however, was the less significant role played by HDT-ASCT for patients with adverse prognostic factors and chemoresistant disease. Age adjusted-IPI and PIT also emerged as important prognostic indices in several studies.

Retrospective Studies—HDT-ASCT in the Upfront Setting Alone

One retrospective study evaluated HDT-ASCT in the upfront setting only. In this study, Rodriguez et al. evaluated 74 patients with advanced-stage PTCL who received HDT-ASCT in first CR [25]. A significant proportion of patients, 31%, had a diagnosis of ALCL (ALK status unknown). Patients received mostly CHOP or other anthracycline-based regimens, followed by BEAM or BEAC (91%). With a median follow-up of 67 months, 5 year OS was 68% and PFS was 63%. When analyzing patients with ALCL, 5 year OS was significantly better, 84% versus 61% compared to other histologies ($p=0.05$). In both univariate and multivariate analyses, patients with two factors or less according to the PIT system had a 74% 5 year OS compared to 31% of patients with more than two factors, implying that patients with a high PIT score should be considered for allo-HSCT or other therapies on a clinical protocol.

Prospective Studies for HDT-ASCT as Consolidation in CR1 or PR1

Only five prospective studies evaluating HDT-ASCT for PTCL in the upfront setting have been published. The largest such trial to date has only thus far appeared in abstract form. The Nordic group evaluated the impact of a dose-intensified chemotherapy schedule consisting of CHOEP-14×6, followed by consolidation with HDT-ASCT for patients in CR1 or PR1 (d'Amore F, et al., EHA abstract 2009). The preparative regimen consisted of BEAM for all patients. A total of 166 patients were enrolled, excluding ALK+ALCL, most of whom (81%) had advanced-stage disease. Out of 155 evaluable patients, 85% were in CR/Cru ($n=132$) or in PR ($n=51$). Seventy-five percent of patients received HDT-ASCT. The reasons patients did not reach HDT-ASCT included disease progression, toxicity, or failure to mobilize. After a median follow-up of 3 years and 9 months, OS at 3 years and 5 years for the entire cohort was 57% and 50%, respectively, while PFS at 3 years and 5 years was 48% and 43%, respectively.

The second-largest prospective study evaluating upfront therapy for PTCL and the largest study presented thus far in manuscript form was conducted by Reimer et al. [26].

Eighty three patients with PTCL (excluding ALK+ALCL) received four cycles of CHOP chemotherapy, and those achieving CR moved on to receive mobilization therapy with BEAM or etoposide, methylprednisolone, cytarabine and cisplatin. The predominant histologies included PTCL-nos ($n=32$) and AITL ($n=27$). The cohort included a high-risk patient population. Three quarters of patients had stage III or IV disease and 51% had a high or high-intermediate risk a-IPI. Although the median age was only 46.5 years. Patients achieving less than CR after CHOP received two more cycles, and after a total of six, at least a PR was required for mobilization. The preparative regimen was uniformly radiochemotherapy with high-dose cyclophosphamide and TBI. The overall response rate to CHOP was 79 and 39% of patients received a CR. Eighteen patients had progressive disease and were treated off study. Sixty-five patients (78%) started stem-cell mobilizing therapy (39 in CR). Only 55 patients (66%) received transplantation. The most common reason for not receiving HDT-ASCT was progression of disease. Seventy-three percent of patients were in CR pre-transplantation. A trend was seen for superior OS with a CR documented before transplantation. For patients in CR, 3 year OS, DFS and PFS rates were 48% and 53% and 36% respectively. The estimated 3 year OS was 71% for patients undergoing ASCT, vs. 11% for those that did not. This study also demonstrated the prognostic value of PIT and simplified PIT on OS

A smaller study by Rodriguez et al. evaluated 26 patients with high-risk PTCL (excluding ALK+ALCL) [27]. Patients received three cycles of MegaCHOP (cyclophosphamide 2 g/m^2, doxorubicin 90 mg/m^2, vincristine 1.4 mg, prednisone 60 mg/m^2), and those that were gallium scan negative received another cycle of MegaCHOP followed by HDT-ASCT. Patients remaining gallium scan positive received two courses of IFE (ifosfamide and etoposide). Patients were required to achieve at least a PR to proceed to HDT-ASCT. Twenty six percent of patients did not reach HDT-ASCT secondary to progression of disease or lethal toxicity. After a median follow-up of 35 months, OS and PFS at 3 years was 73% and 53%, respectively. For patients who received a transplant, the OS and PFS at 2 years were 84 and 56%. No difference was seen between patients with positive and negative gallium scans after three cycles of MegaCHOP though there was a trend towards improved OS and EFS for patients who had negative scans. However, patients in CR or PR after MegaCHOP had superior OS at 3 year (83%) vs. those with refractory disease (43%, $p=0.035$).

Corradini et al. performed two prospective phase II trials to answer this question [28]. Sixty two patients with PTCL (including ALK-positive ALCL) were enrolled. Patients received either high-dose sequential chemotherapy ($n=32$), or MACOP-B/MAD (methotrexate, doxorubicin, cyclophosphamide, vincristine, bleomycin)/(mitoxantrone, cytarabine) chemotherapy ($n=30$), followed by HDT-ASCT. High-dose therapy consisted of two courses of APO (doxorubicin, vincristine, prednisone), followed by DHAP (cisplatin, cytarabine, dexamethasone), and high-dose cyclophosphamide and cisplatin followed by etoposide. In both trials, if patients were noted to have bulky or residual disease 1 month post-HDT-ASCT they were given radiation therapy. Out of the 62 treated patients, 56% were in CR prior to ASCT, 10 (16%) were in PR and 15 (24%) had POD. Only 46 patients (74%)

ultimately underwent HDT-ASCT. The most common reason to not reach transplant was progression of disease. With a median follow-up of 76 months, the estimated 12-year OS, DFS and EFS rates were 34%, 55% and 30%, respectively. On subgroup analysis, ALK+patients had an OS of 62% at 10 years versus 21% for non ALK+. The OS at 12 years for the entire group was 34%. The disease status on admission to HDT-ASCT was also prognostic, with patients in CR having significantly improved outcomes compared to those not in CR. The 10 year EFS of patients in CR before ASCT was 47%, while it was 11% otherwise, strongly suggesting that patient outcomes are improved if they enter HDT-ASCT in a complete remission.

Mercadal et al. performed a study on 41 patients with PTCL who received intensive chemotherapy with high-dose CHOP (cyclophosphamide 2 g, doxorubicin 90 mg/m^2, vincristine 2 mg, prednisone 60 mg/m^2) and three doses of ESHAP (etoposide, cisplatin, cytarabine and prednisone) [29]. In this study the transplantation rate was lower than reported in other studies (41%). This was likely a result of a lower than expected response rate seen with chemotherapy. Only 39% of patients achieved a CR (four had Cru, and four had PR). In addition, a rather high number of patients (41%) experienced disease progression on chemotherapy. Out of 24 patients with CR, Cru or PR who were eligible for HDT-ASCT, only 17 proceeded to HDT-ASCT due to various reasons. The achievement of CR after chemotherapy predicted for an improved OS, though no differences were found among the 24 patients in CR or PR, regardless of whether or not they proceeded to transplant. It is difficult to determine if there was a contribution of HDT-ASCT in this dataset because the number of patients who were eligible for transplantation was smaller than expected.

In summary, HDT-ASCT appears to be a reasonable option in either the salvage or frontline setting. It appears that outcomes following HDT-ASCT in either CR1 or PR1 are improved compared to receiving a transplant in a more advanced setting. Autologous transplantation for refractory diseases appears to offer no advantage. However, many of these studies are confounded by inclusion of ALCL patients without excluding ALK-positive patients. Further, at this time, there are no randomized prospective studies comparing outcomes for patients who receive an upfront transplant as consolidation of CR1/PR1 to those patients who are observed. Until such a trial is performed, it will not be definitively known if a patient's outcome is improved by receiving an autologous transplant upfront. This study should also determine if patients who have either a PR or minimal residual disease at admission fare worse with HDT-ASCT than those patients transplanted in CR.

Allogeneic Transplant for PTCL

Because there are few studies evaluating allo-HSCT for the treatment of PTCL, its role in the treatment of these diseases is currently unclear. With the exception of one 17 patient study, all studies evaluating allo-HSCT for these diseases are retrospective. Potential benefits of allo-HSCT over HDT-ASCT include the infusion of a tumor-free graft and a graft versus lymphoma (GVL) effect. However, any potential anti-tumor benefit of allo-HSCT must be weighed against the increased morbidity and mortality with this modality of therapy. For example, patients who receive an allo-HSCT are at an increased risk of infection and graft-versus-host disease (GVHD) regardless of the intensity of their preparative regimen.

Evidence for a GVL Effect

Small case reports/case series provide evidence for a GVL effect, at least with regard to the more indolent PTCL histologies. Burt et al. [30] describe a single report of a nonmyeloablative (NMAT) allogeneic transplant for mycoses fungoides (MF). The patient relapsed 9 months later, but 1 month after withdrawal of the immune suppressant cyclosporine, remission was again achieved. A series of three patients (age 35–49) was reported by Herbert, et al. [31] which describes disease response both in the context of donor lymphocyte infusions (DLI) and reduction of immunosuppression following reduced intensity (RIC) transplants for cutaneous T-cell lymphomas. The three patients entered transplant with active disease and progressed following transplant. The first patient achieved remissions of his MF post transplant both with withdrawal of immune suppression and administration of DLI. These remissions coincided with GVHD flares, demonstrating the increased immune activity of his graft. The second patient, with a history of Sezary Syndrome, was transplanted with active indolent disease after treatment with high-dose cyclophosphamide. He relapsed at day +43 and a partial remission was obtained with removal of cyclosporine. A further progression was treated with DLI that induced cutaneous and oral GVHD. A complete regression of his MF was noted in this context. However, this patient passed away 11 months post transplant from complications related to chronic GVHD. The third patient underwent a transplant for MF with progressive large cell disease. She entered remission following the allo-HSCT. However, a mild cutaneous relapse was documented 4 months post transplant. She first achieved remission with removal of cyclosporine and development of GVHD. A high-grade relapse was documented 2 months later that responded to chemotherapy.

Retrospective Analyses for PTCL

Myeloablative Conditioning

Prior to the adoption of NMAT or RIC preparative regimens, all patients who received an allo-HSCT received a fully myeloablative regimen either with chemotherapy alone or with the addition of TBI. The problems associated with this strategy are apparent in a study published by Kim, et al. [32]. This paper described a 233 patient case series of NHL treated with myeloablative allo-HSCT. This series featured a large number of patients with varied diseases states with PTCL including 22 with PTCL-nos, 19 with extranodal NK/T cell nasal type, two with AITL and eight patients with other PTCLs. Sixty-seven percent of the T-NHL patients with measurable disease entering into transplant had either a complete or partial response. Eighty-nine percent of these patients with a complete response entering into transplant maintained this response. Treatment-related mortality (TRM) was high at 42% for the entire group. However, it is important to note that this group was not selected for their ability to tolerate a myeloablative regimen. Careful patient selection would likely lower the TRM seen in this trial significantly. Chemoresistance and prior auto-graft both were associated with significantly increased TRM in this series. It is notable that the 5-year OS was highest with the PTCL-nos subset of patients at 70%.

Heterogeneous Conditioning

The largest reported experience with allo-HSCT for PTCL was reported by Le Gouill, et al. [33]. The diagnoses were varied, with the most predominant histologies being PTCL-nos ($n=27$), ALCL ($n=27$), AITL ($n=11$). Fifty seven out of 77 patients received a myeloablative transplant. Thirty-one patients were in CR at admission for allo-HSCT and 26 patients were in PR. For the entire group, the 5-year TRM was 33%, the 5-year OS was 57% and the 5-year EFS was 53%. The strongest predictors for poor OS were chemotherapy-resistant disease (greater than PR) and grade III-IV GVHD. Interestingly, receipt of a myeloablative vs. RIC preparative regimen or prior autologous transplant did not impact on OS, EFS or TRM. It is also interesting to note that two patients received DLI for relapse post allo-HSCT and achieved a CR that was maintained for greater than 2 years.

Kyriakou, et al. presented the EBMT experience with allo-HSCT for AITL [34]. Forty-five patients who had undergone allo-HSCT between 1998 and 2005 were included. The patients were heavily pretreated with 11 patients (24%) receiving a prior autologous transplant. The preparative regimens were varied with 25 patients (56%) undergoing a myeloablative regimen and the remainder receiving a RIC transplant. It is also important to note that 18 patients (40%) had refractory disease entering into transplant. For the entire group, the cumulative incidence of non-relapse mortality (NRM) was acceptable at 25% at 12 months. Poor performance status predicted for increased NRM. Relapse rates were low considering the high-risk patient population at 16% at 2 years and 20% at 3 years. The evidence of an allo effect against AITL is implied because the relapse rate was lower with patients who suffered chronic GVHD. At 3 years the PFS was 53% and OS was 64%.

The Japanese experience with allo-HSCT for the treatment of adult T-cell leukemia/lymphoma has been reported in a large retrospective study [35]. Three hundred eighty-six patients were analyzed. The graft sources were varied, with 154 patients receiving HLA-matched related peripheral blood or bone marrow grafts, 43 patients receiving mismatched related marrow or peripheral blood, 99 patients receiving unrelated marrow and 90 patients receiving single-unit umbilical cord blood grafts. After a median follow-up of 41 months, the 3 year OS was 33% for the entire group. Multivariate analysis revealed that age >50 years, male sex, status other than CR and use of cord blood predicted for inferior OS. However, it is important to note that few centers currently perform single-unit, non-expanded umbilical cord blood transplants as was described in this study. It is not well understood why male sex predicted for poor survival, but it may be related to a virus-specific factor. While the 3-year OS reported in this study is inferior to other studies, it is better than what would be expected without allo-HSCT for this patient population.

Jacobsen, et al. report on a single center's experience performing allo-HSCT for PTCL [36]. Fifty-two patients were analyzed and preparative regimens were, again, varied. With a median follow-up for survivors of 49 months, NRM was 27% and relapse was 43%. When patients were analyzed separately by nodal versus extranodal histology, the PFS was significantly different. For nodal histologies (PTCL, AITL and ALCL), the 3-year PFS was 45%, while for extranodal histologies, the 3-year PFS was 6% ($p=0.016$). The overall survival at 3 years for all patients was 41%

At MSKCC, we analyzed our experience with allo-HSCT for PTCL between the years 1992 and 2009 [37]. Thirty four patients were included in this analysis. Preparative regimens were myeloablative for 21 patients (62%). Sixteen patients (47%) received ex-vivo T-cell depletion as GVHD prophylaxis. With a median follow-up of survivors of 45 months, the 2-year OS was 61% with a plateau at 28 months. Ki-67 expression of ≤25% pre-salvage chemotherapy predicted for improved OS ($p<0.01$) and transplant in complete remission was predictive of a decreased cumulative incidence of events ($p=0.04$). Interestingly, receipt of a T-cell depleted graft or intensity of preparative regimen did not predict response. Four patients received DLI; and three patients demonstrated a response, supporting a graft-versus-lymphoma effect.

Prospective Analysis for PTCL

One single prospective trial has analyzed allo-HSCT as treatment for PTCL [38]. Corradini, et al. performed a RIC allo-HSCT on 17 patients with a diagnosis of relapsed or refractory PTCL. Histologies included PTC-nos ($n=9$), ALK-negative ALCL ($n=4$), and AITL ($n=4$). Eight patients (47%) had a disease relapse following HDT-ASCT. With a median follow-up of 28 months, 14 patients were alive, with 12 patients in CR. The estimated 3-year OS and PFS were 81 and 64%, which were better results than predicted by the retrospective studies. The estimated 2-year NRM was 6%. Two patients were noted to respond to post transplant DLI. While these results are positive and encouraging, they must be interpreted with caution. The sample size is quite small and the histologies studied are quite limited. Also, the median time between diagnosis and transplant was 18.7 months, which is longer than expected raising the possibility these patients were selected. For example, five patients were transplanted at least 60 months post diagnosis. One especially intriguing finding of this paper is the low NRM without apparent increased relapse rate using RIC. This finding would need to be confirmed in a larger, more heterogeneous prospective trial.

Allogeneic transplant offers a promising strategy for the treatment of PTCL. There is mounting evidence for a GVL in these diseases. However, there is still limited data to guide who should receive an allo-HSCT or at what disease stage. It is also unclear if patients should receive a myeloablative or RIC regimen. We may discover that strategies for allogeneic transplantation should be tailored to the specific histology. For example, an upfront allo-HSCT may prove to offer an advantage for some rare, higher risk histologies such as hepatosplenic gamma-delta T-cell lymphoma. Therefore, it is imperative that large, prospective trials analyzing allo-HSCT are performed to address these questions.

References

1. (1997) A clinical evaluation of the International Lymphoma Study Group classification of non-Hodgkin's lymphoma. The Non-Hodgkin's Lymphoma Classification Project. Blood 89(11):3909–18
2. Rudiger T, Weisenburger DD, Anderson JR, Armitage JO, Diebold J, MacLennan KA et al (2002) Peripheral T-cell lymphoma (excluding anaplastic large-cell lymphoma): results from the Non-Hodgkin's Lymphoma Classification Project. Ann Oncol 13(1):140–149
3. Nakamura S, Suchi T, Koshikawa T, Suzuki H, Oyama A, Kojima M et al (1993) Clinicopathologic study of 212 cases of peripheral T-cell lymphoma among the Japanese. Cancer 72(5):1762–1772
4. Gisselbrecht C, Gaulard P, Lepage E, Coiffier B, Briere J, Haioun C et al (1998) Prognostic significance of T-cell phenotype in aggressive non-Hodgkin's lymphomas. Groupe d'Etudes des Lymphomes de l'Adulte (GELA). Blood 92(1):76–82
5. Ansell SM, Habermann TM, Kurtin PJ, Witzig TE, Chen MG, Li CY et al (1997) Predictive capacity of the International Prognostic Factor Index in patients with peripheral T-cell lymphoma. J Clin Oncol 15(6):2296–2301
6. Gallamini A, Stelitano C, Calvi R, Bellei M, Mattei D, Vitolo U et al (2004) Peripheral T-cell lymphoma unspecified (PTCL-U): a new prognostic model from a retrospective multicentric clinical study. Blood 103(7):2474–2479
7. Iqbal J, Weisenburger DD, Greiner TC, Vose JM, McKeithan T, Kucuk C et al (2010) Molecular signatures to improve diagnosis in peripheral T-cell lymphoma and prognostication in angioimmunoblastic T-cell lymphoma. Blood 115(5):1026–1036
8. Horwitz SM (2008) Novel therapies and role of transplant in the treatment of peripheral T-cell lymphomas. Hematology Am Soc Hematol Educ Program 289–96
9. Zaja F, Russo D, Silvestri F, Fanin R, Damiani D, Infanti L et al (1997) Retrospective analysis of 23 cases with peripheral T-cell lymphoma, unspecified: clinical characteristics and outcome. Haematologica 82(2):171–177
10. Armitage JO, Greer JP, Levine AM, Weisenburger DD, Formenti SC, Bast M et al (1989) Peripheral T-cell lymphoma. Cancer 63(1):158–163
11. Escalon MP, Liu NS, Yang Y, Hess M, Walker PL, Smith TL et al (2005) Prognostic factors and treatment of patients with T-cell non-Hodgkin lymphoma: the M.D. Anderson Cancer Center experience. Cancer 103(10):2091–2098
12. Coiffier B, Brousse N, Peuchmaur M, Berger F, Gisselbrecht C, Bryon PA et al (1990) Peripheral T-cell lymphomas have a worse prognosis than B-cell lymphomas: a prospective study of 361 immunophenotyped patients treated with the LNH-84 regimen. The GELA (Groupe d'Etude des Lymphomes Agressives). Ann Oncol 1(1):45–50
13. Gallamini A, Zaja F, Patti C, Billio A, Specchia MR, Tucci A et al (2007) Alemtuzumab (Campath-1H) and CHOP chemotherapy as first-line treatment of peripheral T-cell lymphoma:

results of a GITIL (Gruppo Italiano Terapie Innovative nei Linfomi) prospective multicenter trial. Blood 110(7):2316–2323

14. O'Connor OA, Pro B, Pinter-Brown L, Bartlett N, Popplewell L, Coiffier B et al (2011) Pralatrexate in patients with relapsed or refractory peripheral T-cell lymphoma: results from the pivotal PROPEL study. J Clin Oncol 29(9):1182–1189
15. Piekarz RL, Frye R, Prince HM, Kirschbaum MH, Zain J, Allen SL et al (2011) Phase 2 trial of romidepsin in patients with peripheral T-cell lymphoma. Blood 117(22):5827–5834
16. Rodriguez J, Munsell M, Yazji S, Hagemeister FB, Younes A, Andersson B et al (2001) Impact of high-dose chemotherapy on peripheral T-cell lymphomas. J Clin Oncol 19(17):3766–3770
17. Kahl C, Leithauser M, Wolff D, Steiner B, Hartung G, Casper J et al (2002) Treatment of peripheral T-cell lymphomas (PTCL) with high-dose chemotherapy and autologous or allogeneic hematopoietic transplantation. Ann Hematol 81(11):646–650
18. Song KW, Mollee P, Keating A, Crump M (2003) Autologous stem cell transplant for relapsed and refractory peripheral T-cell lymphoma: variable outcome according to pathological subtype. Br J Haematol 120(6):978–985
19. Kewalramani T, Zelenetz AD, Teruya-Feldstein J, Hamlin P, Yahalom J, Horwitz S et al (2006) Autologous transplantation for relapsed or primary refractory peripheral T-cell lymphoma. Br J Haematol 134(2):202–207
20. Rodriguez J, Caballero MD, Gutierrez A, Marin J, Lahuerta JJ, Sureda A et al (2003) High-dose chemotherapy and autologous stem cell transplantation in peripheral T-cell lymphoma: the GEL-TAMO experience. Ann Oncol 14(12):1768–1775
21. Jantunen E, Wiklund T, Juvonen E, Putkonen M, Lehtinen T, Kuittinen O et al (2004) Autologous stem cell transplantation in adult patients with peripheral T-cell lymphoma: a nation-wide survey. Bone Marrow Transplant 33(4):405–410
22. Feyler S, Prince HM, Pearce R, Towlson K, Nivison-Smith I, Schey S et al (2007) The role of high-dose therapy and stem cell rescue in the management of T-cell malignant lymphomas: a BSBMT and ABMTRR study. Bone Marrow Transplant 40(5):443–450
23. Chen AI, McMillan A, Negrin RS, Horning SJ, Laport GG (2008) Long-term results of autologous hematopoietic cell transplantation for peripheral T cell lymphoma: the Stanford experience. Biol Blood Marrow Transplant 14(7):741–747
24. Yang DH, Kim WS, Kim SJ, Bae SH, Kim SH, Kim IH et al (2009) Prognostic factors and clinical outcomes of high-dose chemotherapy followed by autologous stem cell transplantation in patients with peripheral T cell lymphoma, unspecified: complete remission at transplantation and the prognostic index of peripheral T cell lymphoma are the major factors predictive of outcome. Biol Blood Marrow Transplant 15(1):118–125
25. Rodriguez J, Conde E, Gutierrez A, Arranz R, Leon A, Marin J et al (2007) The results of consolidation with autologous stem-cell transplantation in patients with peripheral T-cell lymphoma (PTCL) in first complete remission: the Spanish Lymphoma and Autologous Transplantation Group experience. Ann Oncol 18(4):652–657
26. Reimer P, Rudiger T, Geissinger E, Weissinger F, Nerl C, Schmitz N et al (2009) Autologous stem-cell transplantation as first-line therapy in peripheral T-cell lymphomas: results of a prospective multicenter study. J Clin Oncol 27(1):106–113
27. Rodriguez J, Conde E, Gutierrez A, Arranz R, Leon A, Marin J et al (2007) Frontline autologous stem cell transplantation in high-risk peripheral T-cell lymphoma: a prospective study from The Gel-Tamo Study Group. Eur J Haematol 79(1):32–38
28. Corradini P, Tarella C, Zallio F, Dodero A, Zanni M, Valagussa P et al (2006) Long-term follow-up of patients with peripheral T-cell lymphomas treated up-front with high-dose chemotherapy followed by autologous stem cell transplantation. Leukemia 20(9):1533–1538
29. Mercadal S, Briones J, Xicoy B, Pedro C, Escoda L, Estany C et al (2008) Intensive chemotherapy (high-dose CHOP/ESHAP regimen) followed by autologous stem-cell transplantation in previously untreated patients with peripheral T-cell lymphoma. Ann Oncol 19(5):958–963
30. Burt RK, Guitart J, Traynor A, Link C, Rosen S, Pandolfino T et al (2000) Allogeneic hematopoietic stem cell transplantation for advanced mycosis fungoides: evidence of a graft-versus-tumor effect. Bone Marrow Transplant 25(1):111–113

31. Herbert KE, Spencer A, Grigg A, Ryan G, McCormack C, Prince HM (2004) Graft-versus-lymphoma effect in refractory cutaneous T-cell lymphoma after reduced-intensity HLA-matched sibling allogeneic stem cell transplantation. Bone Marrow Transplant 34(6):521–525
32. Kim SW, Tanimoto TE, Hirabayashi N, Goto S, Kami M, Yoshioka S et al (2006) Myeloablative allogeneic hematopoietic stem cell transplantation for non-Hodgkin lymphoma: a nationwide survey in Japan. Blood 108(1):382–389
33. Le Gouill S, Milpied N, Buzyn A, De Latour RP, Vernant JP, Mohty M et al (2008) Graft-versus-lymphoma effect for aggressive T-cell lymphomas in adults: a study by the Societe Francaise de Greffe de Moelle et de Therapie Cellulaire. J Clin Oncol 26(14):2264–2271
34. Kyriakou C, Canals C, Goldstone A, Caballero D, Metzner B, Kobbe G et al (2008) High-dose therapy and autologous stem-cell transplantation in angioimmunoblastic lymphoma: complete remission at transplantation is the major determinant of Outcome-Lymphoma Working Party of the European Group for Blood and Marrow Transplantation. J Clin Oncol 26(2):218–224
35. Hishizawa M, Kanda J, Utsunomiya A, Taniguchi S, Eto T, Moriuchi Y et al (2010) Transplantation of allogeneic hematopoietic stem cells for adult T-cell leukemia: a nationwide retrospective study. Blood 116(8):1369–1376
36. Jacobsen ED, Kim HT, Ho VT, Cutler CS, Koreth J, Fisher DC et al (2011) A large single-center experience with allogeneic stem-cell transplantation for peripheral T-cell non-Hodgkin lymphoma and advanced mycosis fungoides/Sezary syndrome. Ann Oncol 22:1608–1613
37. Goldberg JD, Chou JF, Horwitz S, Teruya-Feldstein J, Barker JN, Boulad F et al (2012) Long term survival in patients with peripheral T cell lymphomas after allogeneic hematopoietic stem cell transplantation. Leuk Lymphoma 53(6):1124–9
38. Corradini P, Dodero A, Zallio F, Caracciolo D, Casini M, Bregni M et al (2004) Graft-versus-lymphoma effect in relapsed peripheral T-cell non-Hodgkin's lymphomas after reduced-intensity conditioning followed by allogeneic transplantation of hematopoietic cells. J Clin Oncol 22(11):2172–2176

Index

P.J. Quesenberry and J.J. Castillo (eds.), *Non-Hodgkin Lymphoma: Prognostic Factors and Targets*, Cancer Drug Discovery and Development, DOI 10.1007/978-1-4614-5851-7, © Springer Science+Business Media New York 2013

B

Printed by Printforce, the Netherlands